Antibiotic Resistant Bacteria

Antibiotic Resistant Bacteria

Edited by **Sebastian Driussi**

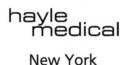

New York

Published by Hayle Medical,
30 West, 37th Street, Suite 612,
New York, NY 10018, USA
www.haylemedical.com

Antibiotic Resistant Bacteria
Edited by Sebastian Driussi

International Standard Book Number: 978-1-63241-046-7 (Hardback)

Contents

Preface

Antibiotic Resistant Bacteria are bacteria that cannot be killed or controlled by antibiotics. Most of the infecting bacteria can become resistant to at least one or two antibiotics. Antibiotic resistance can be a serious disease and is currently, a major medical issue faced by scientists all over the world even though preventive, diagnostic and antibiotherapy techniques have improved significantly. In this book, scientists have presented observations from years of research, to provide an updated account on new strategies and methodologies from interventions against antibiotic resistant bacteria. This book deals with all the novel aspects of anti-biotic resistant organisms, providing insight into all recently developed techniques highlighting antibiotic resistance at a global level, the techniques applied in nursing homes, trends in AR during cold storage of raw milk, and AR staphylococcus species of animal origin. This book is a valuable contribution to the progress of medical research.

This book is a comprehensive compilation of works of different researchers from varied parts of the world. It includes valuable experiences of the researchers with the sole objective of providing the readers (learners) with a proper knowledge of the concerned field. This book will be beneficial in evoking inspiration and enhancing the knowledge of the interested readers.

In the end, I would like to extend my heartiest thanks to the authors who worked with great determination on their chapters. I also appreciate the publisher's support in the course of the book. I would also like to deeply acknowledge my family who stood by me as a source of inspiration during the project.

Editor

Synthesis of New Antibiotics and Probiotics: The Promise of the Next Decade

Current Trends of Emergence and Spread of Vancomycin-Resistant Enterococci

Guido Werner

Robert Koch-Institute, Wernigerode Branch,
Germany

1. Introduction

Enterococci are intestinal colonizers in many mammals including man, birds, reptiles and even invertebrates and are also found in diverse environments such as sewage, soil and water. They have been used for decades for food fermentation and preservation due to their metabolic properties and their capability to produce bacteriocins active against food contaminants like *Listeria*. Within the last two decades enterococcoci became prominent as important hospital-acquired pathogens. Isolates of *Enterococcus faecalis* and *E. faecium* are the third- to fourth-most prevalent nosocomial pathogen worldwide. Among ICU-acquired bloodstream infections enterococci ranked second most prevalent according to data from an European project on Healthcare-Associated Infections.[1] Infections with enterococci hit the very young, the elderly and immuno-compromised patients and are thus mostly restricted to specific hospital wards like haemato-oncological, paediatric, and intensive care units. The growing number of patients at risk of acquiring an enterococcal infection is linked to an aging population, especially in industrialised countries, and an increasing application of invasive medical treatment options.

Non-susceptibility to glycopeptide antibiotics like vancomycin and teicoplanin is the key resistance characteristic in enterococci. Acquired resistance to vancomycin is mediated by various mechanisms (types VanA/B/D/E/G/L; Table 1); the *vanA* and *vanB* resistance genotypes are by far the most prevalent. The reservoir for *vanA*- and *vanB*-type resistance in humans is in *E. faecium* (Christiansen et al., 2004; Willems and van Schaik W. 2009; Johnson et al., 2010; Willems et al., 2011). Consequently, increasing rates of VRE in several European countries are due to an increasing prevalence of vancomycin-resistant *E. faecium* (VREfm). Ampicillin- and/or vancomycin-resistant *E. faecalis* (VREfs) are still rare. Defined clonal groups of *E. faecium* show an enhanced capacity to disseminate in the nosocomial setting and are thus called epidemic or hospital-acquired (Top et al., 2008a; Willems and van Schaik W. 2009; EARSS 2009; Willems et al., 2011). These strains can be assigned to distinct clonal groups or complexes based on various molecular typing schemes and subsequent phylogenetic analyses (Willems and van Schaik W. 2009; Willems et al., 2011). Hospital-acquired *E. faecium* are mostly ampicillin-resistant, partly high-level ciprofloxacin-resistant

---

[1] http://www.ecdc.europa.eu/en/publications/Publications/1011_SUR_Annual_Epidemiological_Report_on_Communicable_Diseases_in_Europe.pdf

and possess additional genomic content (accessory genome), which includes putative virulence traits such as a gene for an enterococcal surface protein, *esp*, genes encoding different cell wall-anchored surface proteins, a putative hyaluronidase gene, *hyl*Efm and a gene encoding a collagen-binding protein, *acm* (Willems et al., 2001; Leavis et al., 2007; Hendrickx et al., 2007; Hendrickx et al., 2008; Heikens et al., 2008; Sillanpaa et al., 2008; Nallapareddy et al., 2008; Hendrickx et al., 2009; van Schaik et al., 2010; Laverde Gomez et al., 2010; van Schaik and Willems 2010).

2. Natural antibiotic resistances in *E. faecium* and *E. faecalis*

Besides their huge arsenal of insusceptibilities to physicochemical and environmental stresses (Murray 1990; Facklam et al., 2002) *E. faecalis* and *E. faecium* possess a broad spectrum of natural antibiotic resistances (Klare et al., 2003; Arias and Murray 2008).

All enterococci are naturally (intrinsically) resistant to the following agents: semisynthetic penicillins (e.g., oxacillin), cephalosporins of all classes, monobactams and polymyxins. Aminoglycosides show insusceptibility at a low level, most probably due to a reduced uptake. At least, isolates of *E. faecalis* and *E. faecium* show clindamycin insusceptibility; in *E. faecalis* this is known to be associated with the expression of an ABC porter designated Lsa (Singh et al., 2002; Singh and Murray 2005). Presence of Lsa also mediates resistance to streptogramin A which in the consequence also leads to resistance to the streptogramin A/B combination (quinupristin/dalfopristin). Insusceptibility to fluoroquinolones, for instance to ciprofloxacin, is most probably associated with expression of chromosomal *qnr* homologues (functionally proven only for *E. faecalis*, (Arsene and Leclercq 2007; Rodriguez-Martinez et al., 2008). Isolates of *E. faecalis* are also resistant to mupirocin, a property that can be used to differentiate them from other enterococcal species. Although not reaching the level of what is defined as resistance, penicillins are generally less active against enterococci than against streptococci and in addition, *E. faecium* is less susceptible than *E. faecalis* (Murray 1990).

3. Acquired antibiotic resistances in *E. faecium* and *E. faecalis*

The already tremendous spectrum of intrinsic insusceptibilities of *E. faecalis* and *E. faecium* is accompanied by the potential to acquire resistance to all antimicrobial drugs available (Tenover and McDonald 2005; Rice 2006). Therapeutically important are resistance properties against penicllin/ampicillin, gentamicin/streptomycin and glycopeptides (vancomycin/teicoplan) as well as resistances against antibiotics of last resort quinupristin/dalfopristin [*E. faecium*], linezolid and tigecycline (maybe also daptomycin).

3.1 Penicillin resistance

Penicillin resistance in *E. faecalis* is rare and if occurring linked to certain clonal lineages expressing beta-lactamases similar or identical to the *S. aureus* penicillinase (Nallapareddy et al., 2005; Ruiz-Garbajosa et al., 2006; McBride et al., 2007). Penicillin resistance in *E. faecium* is mediated via point mutations in the housekeeping *pbp5* gene leading to reduced penicillin binding to the expressed protein (Jureen et al., 2004; Rice et al., 2004; Rice et al., 2009). Mutated *pbp5'* was also found as an integral part of conjugative transposons, like Tn5382, thus encoding transferable ampicillin and VanB-type vancomycin resistance (Carias et al.,

1998; Valdezate et al., 2009). Results of a recent study suggested additional factors independent from pbp5' contributing to acquired ampicillin resistance in hospital strains of *E. faecium* (Galloway-Pena et al., 2011).

3.2 Aminoglycoside resistance

Only the two aminoglycosides gentamicin and streptomycin exemplify a synergistic effect when given in combination with a cell-wall active agent like a penicillin or a glycopeptide (Murray 1990). Certain aminoglycoside-modifying enzymes mediate acquired high-level gentamicin and streptomycin resistance in *E. faecalis* and *E. faecium*. The *aac6'-aph2"* (*aac(6')-Ie-aph(2")-Ia*) gene encodes a bifunctional enzyme encoding high-level resistance to all aminoglycosides except streptomycin (Horodniceanu et al., 1979). It is the most prevalent form of acquired gentamicin resistance in both species and associated with homologues of transposon Tn4001/Tn5281 flanked by two copies of IS256 and most probably originating from staphylococci (Casetta et al., 1998; Hallgren et al., 2003; Saeedi et al., 2004). Gentamicin resistance may also be encoded by other determinants such as *aac(6')-Ii*, *aph(2")-Ie*, and *ant(6)-Ia* (Jackson et al., 2004; Jackson et al., 2005; Zarrilli et al., 2005; Mahbub et al., 2005). High-level streptomycin resistance is encoded by the *aadE* gene which is an integral part of a multi-resistance gene cluster *aadE-sat4-aphA* encoding streptomycin-streptothricin-kanamycin resistance. The *sat4* gene encoding streptothricin (nourseothricin) resistance has first been described in *Campylobacter coli* (Jacob et al., 1994; Bischoff and Jacob 1996). In staphylococci the *aadE-sat4-aphA* gene cluster is flanked by two copies of IS1182 constituting transposon Tn5405 (Derbise et al., 1996; Derbise et al., 1997). The *aadE-sat4-aphA* gene cluster is widespread among many Gram-positive genera and it remains to be speculative where this gene clusters originates from and subsequently spread to other bacteria. Strikingly, in *S. aureus* the *sat4* gene possesses a point mutation within the coding region leading to a pre-mature STOPP codon; whereas it is complete and functional in *C. coli* and enterococci encoding detectable streptothricin (nourseothricin) insusceptibility (Schwarz et al., 2001; Werner et al., 2001a; Teuber et al., 2003; Werner et al., 2003a).

3.3 Fluoroquinolone resistance

The targets of fluoroquinolones are topoisomerases II and IV, and mutational changes among genes encoding mainly subunits A and to a lesser extent also subunits B are associated with increased MICs to ciprofloxacin and other fluoroquinolones (Hooper 2002; Jacoby 2005). Topoisomerase II (DNA gyrase) appears to be the primary target in Gram-negative bacteria and topoisomerase IV is the primary target in Gram-positive bacteria. Corresponding in vitro selection models were also described for enterococci; however, results are somehow conflicting regarding the primary target in *Enterococcus* spp. and the necessity of specific mutations in one or both A subunit genes to confer what is specified as high-level ciprofloxacin resistance (Onodera et al., 2002; Oyamada et al., 2006a; Oyamada et al., 2006b). Molecular studies with high-level ciprofloxacin-resistant clinical isolates revealed mutations in both A subunits associated with different levels of ciprofloxacin resistance, whereas mutations in *gyrB* and *parE* alleles were only infrequently found (Woodford et al., 2003; Leavis et al., 2006; Valdezate et al., 2009; Werner et al., 2010a).

3.4 Resistance to macrolides, lincosamides and streptogramin B (MLS$_B$)

Resistance to MLS$_B$ antibiotics is encoded by the widespread *erm*(B) gene and only occasionally via *erm*(A) or *erm*(C)(Roberts et al., 1999). Erm ("erythromycin resistance methylases") confer resistance by modifying nucleotide A2058 of the bacterial 23S rRNA (methylation) leading to resistance to MLS$_B$ antibiotics. The resistance phenotype is partly overlapping with the spectrum of natural resistances in *Enterococcus* (lincosamides); however, *erm* genes are widespread among other Gram-positive bacteria such as streptococci, staphylococci, lactococci and lactobacilli where the corresponding resistance phenotype has been studied in detail (Shaw and Clewell 1985; Novick and Murphy 1985). Naturally, the expression of *erm* genes is induced with low levels of 14-membered macrolides (i.e. erythromycin) and results in cross-resistance to all 14-, 15- and 16-membered macrolides, lincosamides and streptogramin B antibiotics. Induction results from translational relief of attenuation (Horinouchi and Weisblum 1980). Constitutive expression of *erm*(A) and *erm*(C) in staphylococci results from deletions, duplications, and point mutations in the region of the leader peptide, and is selected for by the use of non-inducing antibiotics (Werckenthin et al., 1999; Werckenthin and Schwarz 2000; Schmitz et al., 2001). In enterococci *erm*(B) is constitutively expressed (Werner et al., 2000; Werner et al., 2002; Martel et al., 2003); however, corresponding modifications in the leader peptide could not be linked unambiguously to cause the corresponding phenotype in wildtype isolates (Rosato et al., 1999; Werner et al., 2002). Recent in vitro studies have linked point mutations rather than deletions and duplications to a corresponding *erm*(B) constitutive phenotype in enterococci (Min et al., 2008). The *erm*(B) determinant is widespread among enterococci, especially *E. faecium* and *E. faecalis* and is part of many multi-resistance plasmids and often linked to Tn*1546*-like *vanA* elements (Aarestrup et al., 2000a; Borgen et al., 2002; Werner et al., 2003a; Werner et al., 2003b; Manson et al., 2003b; Werner et al., 2006; Laverde Gomez et al., 2010). Another mechanism mediating macrolide (and streptogramin B) resistance is conferred by the *msrA-C* genes (Reynolds et al., 2003; Kerr et al., 2005) whereas *msrC* is discussed as a species-specific property in *E. faecium* (Singh et al., 2001; Werner et al., 2001b) shown to encode erythromycin and clarithromycin resistance when expressed in *S. aureus* (Reynolds and Cove 2005). Staphylococcal efflux pumps of the Vgb-type encoding for streptogramin type B resistance remain extremely rare among *E. faecium* (Werner et al., 2002).

3.5 Streptogramin A resistance

Two types of acetyltransferases VatD and VatE mediate resistance to streptogramin A in enterococci, mainly *E. faecium* (Werner et al., 2002). *E. faecalis* is naturally resistant to streptogramin A and thus the synergism of the A and B streptogramin combination is abolished (Werner et al., 2002; Singh et al., 2002). However, a few studies described also *vat* genes to be prevalent among related lactic acid bacteria (Gfeller et al., 2003) and *E. faecalis* isolates (Simjee et al., 2002; Jones and Deshpande 2004). Their relevance for increasing the level of streptogramin resistance in *E. faecalis* is unclear; nevertheless, resistance determinants could further spread to *E. faecium* and other enterococcal species thus rendering their level of streptogramin susceptibility. Staphylococcal efflux pumps of the Vga-type encoding for streptogramin type A resistance remain unknown to *E. faecium* (Werner et al., 2002); except for a single Korean *E. faecium* isolate described recently harbouring streptogramin A resistance genes *vgaD* and *vatG* on a plasmid fragment encoding for a new efflux pump type and a new streptogramin acetyltransferase, respectively (Jung et al., 2010).

3.6 Tetracycline resistance

Resistance to tetracyclines is mediated via different acquired *tet* genes encoding proteins mediating (a) ribosomal protection [*tet*(O)/(M)(S)] or efflux [tet(K)/(L)] [(Roberts 2005). Most wide-spread among enterococci and best studied are elements containing *tet*(M). The *tet*(M) gene mostly resides on conjugative transposons of the Tn916/Tn1545- or Tn5397-types that possess a very wide host range and can exist in several functional copies thus supporting flexibility and recombinational events within a given bacterial genome (Thal et al., 1997; Roberts et al., 2001; Agerso et al., 2006; Rice et al., 2007; Boguslawska et al., 2009; de Vries et al., 2009; Rice et al., 2010; Roberts and Mullany 2011).

3.7 Linezolid resistance

Linezolid is a synthetic oxazolidinone antibiotic of last resort active against multi- and vancomycin-resistant enterococci. It inhibits first steps of ribosome formation [108]. Although being fully synthetic, resistance is selected under therapy and is in relation to the duration of treatment (Prystowsky et al., 2001; Pai et al., 2002; Ruggero et al., 2003; Seedat et al., 2006). However, a few reports documented resistance detection independent from linezolid treatment (Rahim et al., 2003; Bonora et al., 2006). Resistance results from point mutations in 23S rRNA, preferably at position 2576 (G > T)(Sinclair et al., 2003; Werner et al., 2004; Qi et al., 2006; Werner et al., 2007a) and the level of resistance is dependent on the number of mutated alleles per genome (Marshall et al., 2002; Lobritz et al., 2003; Bourgeois-Nicolaos et al., 2007; Boumghar-Bourtchai et al., 2009). Once established, resistance levels quickly arise due to recombinational exchange of mutated 23S rDNA alleles under selective pressure (Willems et al., 2003; Boumghar-Bourtchai et al., 2009). In *Staphylococcus*, a Cfr methylase is able to modify 23S rRNA at position A2503 leading to cross-resistance to a number of antibiotics including oxazolidinones (Toh et al., 2007); however, the corresponding *cfr* gene has not been described in enterococci so far.

3.8 Tigecycline resistance

Tigecycline is a member of a new tetracycline antibiotic class containing a 9-tert-butylglycylamido group named glycylcyclines and acts similar to tetracyclines by inhibiting protein biosynthesis. Tigecycline is active against many Gram-negative and Gram-positive bacteria including isolates of Enterococcus. International surveillance studies revealed in general potent in vitro activity; non-susceptible isolates are very rare. A single resistance mechanism linked to an overexpression of an oxygen- and flavin-dependent monooxygenase, TetX, originating from anaerobic bacteria of the genus Bacteroides was described (Moore et al., 2005). A single tigecycline-non-susceptible *E. faecalis* isolate was reported recently and investigated in greater details; however, the underlying resistance mechanism could not been determined (Werner et al., 2008b).

3.9 Daptomycin resistance

Daptomycin is a cyclic lipopeptide antibiotic disrupting cell membrane composition, function and permeability (Straus and Hancock 2006a; Straus and Hancock 2006b). Daptomycin is active against many Gram-positive bacteria. Its in vivo activity against enterococci is still debatable (Canton et al., 2010). Daptomycin resistance developed under therapy in bacteria other than enterococci and was multifactorial and is still not understood completely (Fischer et al., 2011).

3.10 Vancomycin resistance

Glycopeptide antibiotics consist of a peptide ring to which several sugars are covalently linked. They are produced by actinomycetes and have a quite complex structure. This voluminous structure prevents penetration through the outer membrane of Gram-negative bacteria limiting their therapeutic use only to treat infections with Gram-positive bacteria. Two naturally produced antibiotics have been introduced into antimicrobial treatment, vancomycin and teicoplanin; the latter only outside North-America. Three semisynthetic progenitors designated as lipoglycopeptides or glycolipopeptides (dalbavancin, telavancin, oritavancin) are promising new candidate drugs partially active against multi-resistant and also vancomycin-(intermediate)resistant bacteria (Zhanel et al., 2010a). The primary target of glycopeptides is the C-terminal D-Alanyl-D-Alanine ending of the peptide side chain of the enterococcal peptidoglycan cell wall precursor. Due to steric hindrance the cell wall synthesis enzymes like transglycosylases, transpeptidases and D,D-carboxypeptidases cannot access their target and cell wall synthesis stops. Vancomycin and related glycopeptides act as dimers (Batchelor et al., 2010).

Enterococci were the first pathogens that showed acquired vancomycin resistance and corresponding strains have been isolated from clinical samples from patients in Europe and the USA in the late 1980s (Leclercq et al., 1988; Leclercq et al., 1989; Sahm et al., 1989). The corresponding resistance phenotypes which included inducible resistance to all known glycopeptides or vancomycin only were designated VanA and VanB, respectively. In fact, the structure, localization and functional interplay of the resistance determinants arranged in specific transposable elements in enterococci has been studied with some of the first identified VRE: *E. faecium* BM4147 (*vanA* genotype) from France (Leclercq et al., 1988) and *E. faecalis* V583 (*vanB* genotype) from the USA (Sahm et al., 1989). The latter became prominent as the first *Enterococcus* isolate that has been completely sequenced (Paulsen et al., 2003). To date eight types of acquired vancomycin resistance in enterocooci are known having a related mechanism of resistance and a similar resistance gene cluster composition but show major differences in prevalence (**Table 1** and **Figure 1;** see recent reviews for details: (Courvalin 2005; Courvalin 2006; Werner et al., 2008a; Werner et al., 2008c). Worldwide by far the most prevalent type is *vanA* followed by *vanB*. The *vanA* gene is an integrated part of Tn*1546* or derivatives of this transposon which are usually located on transferable plasmids (Werner et al., 2008a; Werner 2011). *vanB* could be subdivided into three different allele types (*vanB1-3*) with *vanB-2* the most prevalent type worldwide. The *vanB* alleles are part of Tn*1547* or the conjugative transposon Tn*1549/5382* which are mainly chromosomally located and less frequently, on plasmids (Werner et al., 2006; Zheng et al., 2009; Hegstad et al., 2010; Bjorkeng et al., 2011). The main clinical relevant reservoir of *vanA* and *vanB* elements is in *E. faecium*, at least in Europe, Northern and Latin America and Southeast Asia, although they have also been observed occasionally in other enterococcal species (see **Table 1** and below)(Zirakzadeh and Patel 2005; Werner et al., 2008a; Werner 2011).

4. The *van* alphabet in *Enterococcus* spp.

Non-susceptibility to glycopeptide antibiotics like vancomycin and teicoplanin is the key resistance characteristic in enterococci. Acquired resistance to vancomycin is mediated by

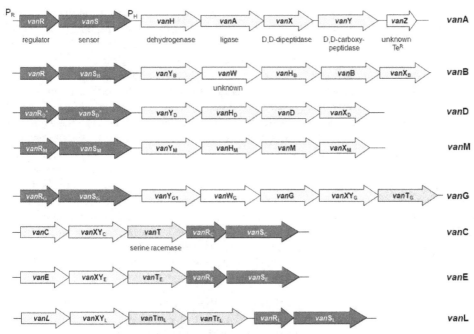

The image of the *vanC* cluster from naturally vancomycin-resistant *E. gallinarum* and *E. casseliflavus* were introduced for reasons of comparability. Arrows indicate genes and arrowheads show the direction of transcription. Colour codes represent functional groups: red, two-component regulatory system; yellow, core genes essential for resistance expression; grey, serine racemase; white, additional or unknown function. Arrow lengths are according to the size of the genes but are not drawn to scale. * denotes point mutations leading to constitutive expression of the VanD-type resistance. For further details see main text or references given there. P$_R$ and P$_H$ are promoters preceding *vanR* and *vanH*, respectively. Te^R, gene associated with decreased teicoplanin susceptibility. For references see legend of Table 1.

Fig. 1. **Structure and composition of the vancomycin resistance clusters *vanA-M*** (see also Table 1). Types *vanA, vanB, vanD* and *vanM* encode D-Ala-D-Lac mediated resistance; types *vanC, vanE, vanL* and *vanG* (also *vanN*, not shown) encode D-Ala-D-Ser mediated resistance (see text and Table for details)

various mechanisms (types VanA/B/D/E/G/L/M/N; **Table 1**); the *vanA* and *vanB* resistance genotypes are by far the most prevalent worldwide. Isolates of *E. gallinarum* and *E. casseliflavus* (= *E. flavescens*) are naturally (intermediate-)resistant to vancomycin at low levels (MIC = 8 mg/L) by a so-called VanC-1/-2 type.

4.1 The VanA resistance type

The original *vanA* gene cluster contains nine genes which are arranged in a transposon structure (Arthur et al., 1993)(Fig. 1). It is flanked by two incomplete inverted repeats and possesses two coding sequences located at the left end (ORFs 1 and 2 not shown in Fig. 1). Their putative proteins show similarity with resolvases and transposases of various transposons or plasmids. The entire element is 10,981 bp and designated Tn*1546*, belonging to transposons of the Tn*3*-family.

Expression of VanA type vancomycin resistance in enterococci is inducible via a complex mechanism. The consequences of a prevented cell wall synthesis are sensed by an as yet still unknown mechanism via a membrane-associated, Tn1546-encoded protein VanS possessing a histidine kinase in its cytoplasmatic C-terminus. The histidine kinase function of the VanS protein is activated by autophosphorylation and the corresponding phosphate moiety is transferred to a cytoplasmic response regulator called VanR also encoded on Tn1546. Phosphorylated VanR functions as a transcriptional activator binding at two promoters P_R and P_H in the vanA resistance gene cluster (Arthur et al., 1997). This leads to the expression of two transcripts of genes that are arranged in an operon structure and that are transcribed unidirectional: the vanRS genes themselves and the gene cluster vanHAXYZ (**Fig. 1**). The proteins VanH, VanA and VanX possess essential functions for the expression of glycopeptide resistance whereas VanY encodes a D,D-carboxypeptidase contributing to elevated resistance levels and a VanZ protein of unknown function but contributing by an unknown mechanism to low-level teicoplanin resistance (**Fig. 2**)(Arthur and Quintiliani, Jr. 2001). VanA type vancomycin resistance is mediated via an alternative pathway synthesizing cell wall precursors ending in D-Alanyl-D-Lactat (D-Ala-D-Lac) showing reduced glycopeptide binding and down-shifting of the regular cell wall synthesis by house-keeping enzymes (**Fig. 1**)(Arthur and Quintiliani, Jr. 2001).

Studies about characterizing the structure of vanA gene clusters in enterococci of different ecological and geographical sources displayed a great variety of point mutations, deletions (in/of non-essential genes), and insertions of additional DNA (mainly IS elements) leading to modified and fragmented Tn1546 structures. This can be demonstrated in a phylogenetic tree of relatedness exemplifying elements typically identified in US hospital VRE, poultry VRE, pig/human commensal VRE, etc. (Willems et al., 1999; Werner et al., 2006). Typing of vanA gene clusters allows elucidating ways of spread of vancomycin resistance either via clonal spread of VRE or via horizontal gene transfer between different enterococci (Park et al., 2007; Sletvold et al., 2010).

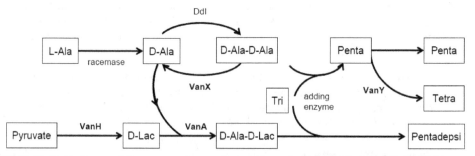

Ddl, D-Ala:D-Ala ligase; adding enzyme is a synthetase; Penta, L-Ala-γ-D-Glu-L-Lys-D-Ala-D-Ala; Pentadepsi, L-Ala-γ-D-Glu-L-Lys-D-Ala-D-Lac; Tetra, L-Ala-γ-D-Glu-L-Lys-D-Ala; Tri, L-Ala-γ-D-Glu-L-Lys. Penta, Tetra, Tri, Pentadepsi represent amino acid side chains linked to the enterococcal peptidoglycan disaccharide precursor N-acetyl-glucosamin-N-acetyl-muramic acid. Resistance enzymes encoded by the vanA cluster are shown in bold. [Figure adapted from (Courvalin 2006)].

Fig. 2. **VanA-type glycopeptide resistance.** Synthesis of an alternative, vancomycin-resistant pentadepsipeptide peptidoglycan precursor in VanA-type resistant strains.

4.2 The VanB resistance type

The typical VanB phenotype is characterized by inducible moderate vancomycin resistance levels (MICs of 8 - 64 mg/L) and teicoplanin susceptibility. *vanB* isolates with high-level vancomycin resistance have also been identified. Differences in the *vanB* gene were found and three different *vanB* ligase alleles were assigned which can be used for subtyping [*vanB*-1/-2/-3; (Dahl et al., 2003; Werner et al., 2006)]. However, the different *vanB* genotypes did not correlate with the level of vancomycin resistance. Despite being slightly different in nucleotide composition, the *vanB* cluster types 1 to 3 all resemble the core structure of the *vanA* gene cluster (**Fig. 1**). Genes of related composition and function are arranged in a similar manner, an equivalent to *vanZ* is lacking and an additional gene *vanW* of unknown function was found. Genes encoding the two-component regulatory system $vanR_BS_B$ are only distantly related to their Tn*1546* counterparts and regulation of gene expression is different, because only vancomycin, but not teicoplanin, is an inducer of the *vanB* cluster. The entire transposon backbone of *vanB* clusters is different to *vanA*; distinct *vanB* cluster types are either flanked by certain IS elements or an integral part of larger mobile and/or conjugative elements that may be composed of several individual elements [Tn*1547*, Tn*1549*, Tn*5382*-like, Tn*vamp*; (Carias et al., 1998; Dahl and Sundsfjord 2003; Werner et al., 2006; Launay et al., 2006; Valdezate et al., 2009; Lopez et al., 2009)]. The conjugative *vanB* transposon Tn*1549* or its backbone is widely prevalent among *vanB* type enterococci and related Gram-positive bacteria such as *Clostridium* spp. (see chapter 5;(Launay et al., 2006; Tsvetkova et al., 2010)). Conjugative transposons have been known for a long time in *Enterococcus* and *Bacteroides* and were lately also identified in Gram-negatives. They have an important function for a wide distribution of (resistance) genes across species and genus barriers and for genomic rearrangements in bacteria in general (Rice et al., 2005; Roberts and Mullany 2009; Rice et al., 2010; Roberts and Mullany 2011).

Whereas teicoplanin does not induce VanB type resistance, constitutively resistant mutants quickly arose in vivo during therapy or in vitro after teicoplanin challenge (Baptista et al., 1999; Kawalec et al., 2001a; Kawalec et al., 2001b; San Millan et al., 2009b). Accordingly, teicoplanin treatment is not recommended for eradicating VanB VRE infections despite a correspondingly suggestive diagnostic result (teicoplanin susceptibility).

Expression via the VanB type two-component regulatory system $VanR_BS_B$ is differently regulated in various Gram-positive hosts. Naturally occurring VanB type *Streptococcus bovis/gallolyticus* isolates retained the VanB phenotype inducible by vancomycin only (Poyart et al., 1997; Mevius et al., 1998). Genetic constructs of *vanB* cluster elements in a *Bacillus subtilis* background did not show an inducible phenotype since $VanS_B$ was active also without vancomycin addition (San Millan et al., 2009a). In addition, it was shown that the phosphorylated regulator $VanR_B$-P was capable of binding to a number of promoter regions and thus controlling expression of genes commonly regulated by response regulators.

4.3 The VanC resistance type

The two motile species *E. gallinarum* and *E. casseliflavus* possess an intrinsic resistance to vancomycin at a low level designated VanC-1 and VanC-2, respectively. The corresponding *vanC*-type ligase gene possessed minor sequence diversity resulting in the two described subtypes *vanC*-1 and *vanC*-2 (Courvalin 2005; Courvalin 2006). The formerly third species *E.*

flavescens described as possessing a supposed *vanC-3* gene was merged recently with the species *E. casseliflavus* (Naser et al., 2006b) thus leading to two subtypes of *E. casseliflavus* with slightly different *vanC-2/-3* subtype variants. Recently, another subtype *vanC-4* was described in another *E. casseliflavus* isolate with 93-95% nucleotide identity with *vanC-2/-3* (Naser et al., 2006a).

Resistance phenotype	VanA	VanB[2]	VanD[2]	VanE	VanG[2]	VanL	VanM	VanN[4]
MIC vancomycin in µg/ml	16 - 1000	4 - 32 (-1000)	16 - 512	8 - 32	16	8	>256	16
MIC teicoplanin in µg/ml	(4-) 16 - 512	0,5 - 1	0,5 - 64	0,5	0,5	S	0.75 / 96[3]	S
expression	inducible	inducible	constitutive	inducible	inducible	inducible	inducible	?
ligase	D-Ala-D-Lac	D-Ala-D-Lac	D-Ala-D-Lac	D-Ala-D-Ser	D-Ala-D-Ser	D-Ala-D-Ser	D-Ala-D-Lac	D-Ala-D-Ser
localization	plasmid/ chrom.	chrom./ plasmid	chrom.	chrom.	chrom.	chrom.?	plasmid	?
transferable by conjugation	+/-	+/-	-	-	+	-	+	?
Distribution among enterococcal species	E. faecium E. faecalis E. durans E. hirae E. gallinarum[1] E. casseliflavus[1] E. raffinosus E. avium E. mundtii	E. faecium E. faecalis E. durans E. gallinarum[1]	E. faecium E. faecalis E. raffinosus E. gallinarum[1]	E. faecalis	E. faecalis	E. faecalis	E. faecium	E. faecium

S, susceptible (no MIC given); [1] Acquisition of *vanA*, *vanB* or *vanD* genes in addition to vanC1/C2 genes – rare event; [2] subtypes exist (*vanB1-3, vanD1-5, vanG1-2*); [3] several strains exist with different teicoplanin MICs; [4] data from a presentation given by R. Leclercq, ESCMID conference on Enterococci, Barcelona/ES, 18.-20.11.2009.

Table 1. **Types of acquired vancomycin resistance in enterococci**

Nucleotide identity varied also along the other elements of the *vanC-4* cluster with genes *vanXY*$_C$, *vanT*$_C$, *vanR*$_C$, and *vanSc* showing 88-93 % identity with corresponding genes of the *vanC-2/-3* cluster (see below and **Fig. 1**). VanC type resistance is mediated via a modified D-Ala-D-Ser moiety similar to VanE/G/L/N types reaching also a similar low level of resistance only (Arias et al., 2000). All these resistance types require activity of a serine racemase converting L-Ser into D-Ser, the first one of these enzymes/genes was described in *E. gallinarum* (Arias et al., 1999). The *vanC-1* gene cluster of *E. gallinarum* contains a ligase gene *vanC-1*, a combined D-Ala-D-Ala dipeptidase/carboxypeptidase *vanXY*$_C$ gene, a *vanT* racemase gene and two genes encoding a sensor kinase/response regular two-component regulatory system *vanR*$_C$ and *vanS*$_C$ (Reynolds et al., 1999; Reynolds and Courvalin 2005). The *vanC-2* cluster in *E. casseliflavus* showed a composition similar to the *vanC-1* cluster in *E. gallinarum* (Dutta and Reynolds 2002). Due to the different VanC resistance mechanism a *vanH* equivalent is functionally not required and missing. Initially it was thought that VanC type resistance was always constitutively expressed as a species-specific property. However,

E. casseliflavus expressed an inducible resistance phenotype which was detected several hours after induction in vitro (Dutta and Reynolds 2002). *E. gallinarum* isolates expressing an inducible and constitutive phenotypes were identified; mutational changes in the amino acid sequences of the corresponding sensor histidine kinases VanS$_C$ in constitutive and inducible strains were demonstrated (Panesso et al., 2005). Acquisition of mobile *vanA*, *vanB* and *vanD* gene clusters additional to the natural *vanC-1/-2* cluster in *E. gallinarum/casseliflavus* may lead to high-level vancomycin resistance in these strains; however, their prevalence remains low (Foglia et al., 2003; Mammina et al., 2005; Haenni et al., 2009; Neves et al., 2009).

4.4 The VanD resistance type

The basic organization of the *vanD* operons, which are located exclusively on the chromosome, is similar to that of the *vanA* and *vanB* clusters (Casadewall and Courvalin 1999; Boyd et al., 2000; Depardieu et al., 2003b; Depardieu et al., 2004; Boyd et al., 2004). Genes equivalent to *vanZ* or *vanW* are absent. The *vanD* resistance clusters appear as a remarkable example of how by certain mutational events regulatory networks adjust and finetune gene expression: VanD-type strains have negligible VanX$_D$ activity, an enzyme that normally shuts down synthesis of vancomycin-susceptible, housekeeping call wall precursors. This otherwise physiological drawback is compensated by an inactivated D-Ala-D-Ala ligase (deletions, point mutations, insertion) host enzyme, preventing synthesis of vancomycin-susceptible precursors ending in D-Ala-D-Ala. However, *vanD* expression and corresponding essential cell wall precursor synthesis would still request induction by glycopeptides (vancomycin dependence). Consequently all investigated VanD type *E. faecalis*, *E. faecium* and *E. avium* strains show a constitutive resistance phenotype resulting from different mutations in the VanS$_D$ sensor or VanR$_D$ regulator. Another unusual feature of VanD-type strains is their only slightly diminished susceptibility to teicoplanin (**Tab. 1**) which cannot be explained on the basis of already known DNA sequence diversities. Due to different strategies in establishing those complex and highly regulated networks independently and via different routes five different *vanD* cluster types had arranged and were characterized so far (Boyd et al., 2000; Depardieu et al., 2004). Up to now, VanD-type resistance still is a rare *van* resistance type among enterococci but has been described in a VanC type *E. gallinarum* N04-0414, too (Boyd et al., 2006b). In this strain the vancomycin resistance phenotype is constitutive but typical VanD strain features are lacking (mutations in *vanS$_D$* linked to constitutive expression; shut-down of housekeeping D-Ala-D-Ala ligase activity, etc.). A *vanD* cluster was also described in *E. raffinosus* (Tanimoto et al., 2006). It showed almost identity to the *vanD4* gene cluster of *E. faecium* 10/96A and expressed all features of typical VanD type resistance such as an inducible resistance phenotype based on VanS$_D$ mutations.

Different VanD-type enterococci present a number of different combinations of mutations (mainly in VanS$_D$) suggesting an independent development and convergent evolution (Depardieu et al., 2009). These various modifications also led to a wide range of resistance phenotypes with low to high-level vancomycin resistant strains (16-512 mg/L) and susceptibility (0,5 mg/L) and low to high-level resistance to teicoplanin (≤ 64 mg/L)(**Tab. 1**). Remarkably, VanD strain *E. faecium* BM4656 had a wildtype Ddl enzyme being the only VanD strain with a functional D-Ala-D-Ala ligase. In this strain, also enzymes VanX$_D$ and VanY$_D$ were active being essentiell for shutting down synthesis of glycopeptide-susceptible cell wall precursors in a background of an active host Ddl enzyme for mediating vancomycin resistance (**Fig. 3**) (Depardieu et al., 2009).

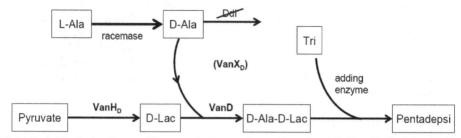

Ddl, D-alanine:D-alanine ligase; adding enzyme is a synthetase; Pentadepsi, L-Ala-γ-D-Glu-L-Lys-D-Ala-D-Lac; Tri, L-Ala-γ-D-Glu-L-Lys. Tri and Pentadepsi represent amino acid side chains linked to the enterococcal peptidoglycan disaccharide precursor N-acetyl-glucosamin-N-acetyl-muramic acid. Resistance enzymes encoded by the *vanD* cluster are shown in bold. [Figure adapted from (Courvalin 2006)].

Fig. 3. **VanD-type glycopeptide resistance.** Synthesis of peptidoglycan precursors in a VanD-type resistant strain. Dependence on the presence of vancomycin in a background of reduced VanX$_D$ activity (VanX$_D$) and a non-functional Ddl is compensated by mutations in VanR$_D$ or VanS$_D$ leading to a constitutive resistance phenotype (not demonstrated in details; see also main text and **Fig. 2**).

4.5 The VanE resistance type

Isolates representing a VanE resistance type were described in a few *E. faecalis* strains from Northern America and Australia (Fines et al., 1999; Abadia Patino et al., 2002; Boyd et al., 2002; Abadia Patino et al., 2004). The *vanE* resistance cluster resembles structures of the *vanC1* cluster naturally occurring in *E. gallinarum* (**Fig. 2**) and shows also highest similarities with the corresponding proteins. Therefore resistance is mediated by producing D-Ala-D-Ser-terminated cell wall precursors (**Tab. 1**). Due to that and as compared to the VanC resistance type, VanE type vancomycin resistance requires a VanT racemase converting L-Ser into D-Ser (Fines et al., 1999; Abadia Patino et al., 2002). VanE strains remain teicoplanin-susceptible and show moderate to low levels of inducible vancomycin resistance. Despite this phenotype, sequence determination suggested a putative non-functional VanS$_E$ protein indicating cross-talk between the VanR$_E$ response regulator and other functional membrane-located kinase activators. All five consecutive genes of the *vanE* gene cluster were cotranscribed from a single promoter (Abadia Patino et al., 2004). Downstream the *vanE* cluster in a single Canadian VanE-type *E. faecalis* an integrase gene is found, which may have been involved in the acquisition of this operon; however, when tested in vitro the *vanE* cluster was in all attempts not transferable (Boyd et al., 2002). Initially a *van* gene cluster designated *vanE* has been described in *Paenibacillus popilliae* showing 74-79 % protein sequence identity with the corresponding essential proteins VanH/A/X in *vanA* clusters (Patel et al., 2000; Patel 2000; Guardabassi et al., 2005; Guardabassi and Agerso 2006). This has later been renamed into *vanF* (see chapter 5).

4.6 The VanG resistance type

E. faecalis possessing a *vanG* cluster were low-level vancomycin-resistant and teicoplanin-susceptible (McKessar et al., 2000; Depardieu et al., 2003a; Boyd et al., 2006a). Resistance is mediated via inducible synthesis of D-Ala-D-Ser-terminated cell wall precursors. Only few isolates have been described and *vanG* gene clusters identified allow differentiation into two subtypes. The chromosomal *vanG* cluster consists of seven genes which according to its order and gene composition appear to be reassembled from different *van* operons (**Fig. 1**). In contrast to all the other *van* operons, the *vanG* cluster encodes three putative gene products with regulatory functions. Besides the common $vanR_G$ and $vanS_G$ determinants a $vanU_G$ gene encoding an additional putative transcriptional activator was identified (Depardieu et al., 2003a; Boyd et al., 2006a). The *vanY* gene is present but a frame-shift mutation resulting in premature termination of the encoded protein accounted for the lack of disaccharide-tetrapeptide prescursors in the cytoplasm (Depardieu et al., 2003a). VanG-type resistance was successfully transferred in vitro and acquisition of the *vanG* cluster was associated with a transfer of a 240 kb chromosomal fragment flanked by imperfect inverted repeats (Depardieu et al., 2003a). Crystallisation and X-ray analysis of the VanG D-Ala-D-Ser ligase in complex with ADP was described recently (Weber et al., 2009).

4.7 The VanL resistance type

A single *E. faecalis* isolate from Canada (N06-0364) expressed low level vancomycin resistance by a new mechanism called VanL (Boyd et al., 2008). The corresponding VanL gene mediates D-Ala-D-Ser ligation. The *vanL* gene cluster was similar in organization to the *vanC* operon, but the VanT serine racemase was encoded by two separate genes, $vanTm_L$ (membrane binding) and $vanTr_L$ (racemase) resembling the two functional domains of the otherwise combined *vanT* type racemase (**Fig. 1**)(Boyd et al., 2008). The putative VanL ligase exhibited 51 and 49% sequence identity to the VanE and VanC ligases, respectively. All attempts to transfer the *vanL* gene cluster in vitro failed. The *E. faecalis* isolate N06-0364 did not demonstrate plasmids assuming that the *vanL* gene cluster was chromosomally encoded.

4.8 The VanM resistance type

The *vanM* genotype was described in seven Chinese VRE isolates originating from a single hospital and revealing three different MLST (ST18, ST78, ST341) and five PFGE types/subtypes (Xu et al., 2010). A single VanM VRE was investigated in greater details. The translated sequence of VanM, the corresponding ligase, showed highest similarity to the VanA, the corresponding VanM gene product mediates ligation of the D-Ala-D-Lac peptide. The *vanM* gene cluster showed a gene arrangement similar to *vanB* and *vanD* with the D,D-carboxypeptidase gene $vanY_M$ preceding the ligase gene (**Fig. 1**). VanM type resistance was transferable by conjugation in vitro and plasmid-located. VanM phenotype showed in vitro resistance against vancomycin and tecioplanin in six of seven isolates investigated (the single ST341 isolate was susceptible to teicoplanin).

4.9 The vancomycin dependence phenotype

Soon after the first appearance of *vanA*- and *vanB*-type VRE, strains with unusual resistance phenotypes were notified including constitutively resistant strains and even vancomycin-dependent isolates of the species *E. faecalis*, *E. faecium* and *E. avium* (Woodford et al., 1994; Rosato et al., 1995; Sifaoui and Gutmann 1997). Features of in vitro selected strains were similar to variants identified from clinical cases mostly associated with long term vancomycin treatment. In vancomycin-dependent VRE the housekeeping D-Ala-D-Ala ligase (*ddl* gene) is not functional due to modifications in the coding sequence (point mutations, deletions, insertions). Consequently depletion of D-Ala-D-Ala dipeptides leads to an impaired cell wall synthesis. The effect could be complemented by providing the missing D-Ala-D-Ala dipeptide (Sng et al., 1998a) or similar di- or depsipeptides. Vancomycin is capable of inducing the VanA or VanB type resistance and thus providing D-Ala-D-Lac as the necessary substrate for a revived cell wall synthesis. These strains remain dependent on the inducing effect of vancomycin for an ongoing cell wall synthesis. Dependence on vancomycin could be circumvented by subsequent mutations targeting the two-component regulatory system of VanR and/or VanS. Mutations in the histidine kinase or the regulator may bypass the inducing property of the antimicrobial compound in leading to a constitutive resistance phenotype not requiring vancomycin anymore. This switch from inducible to constitutive vancomycin resistance phenotype may also appear independently from a previous vancomycin dependence phenotype (Sng et al., 1998b; Baptista et al., 1999). As described recently in a VanB type VRE, a mutation in the transcription terminator of the regulatory genes resulting in transcriptional readthrough of the resistance genes from the P_{RB} promoter in the absence of vancomycin may also circumvent vancomycin dependence and lead to a constitutive phenotype (San Millan et al., 2009b). Expression of vancomycin resistance comes along with a fitness burden under non-selective conditions (in the absence of glycopeptides). Accordingly VRE with a constitutive phenotype are less competitive under non-selective conditions (Foucault et al., 2010).

5. The *van* alphabet in non-enterococcal strains

5.1 The *van* alphabet in intestinal and environmental bacteria and glycopeptide producers

Prevalence studies revealed occurrence of different *van* genes like *vanB*, *vanD* and *vanG* in non-enterococcal, human intestinal colonizers of *Clostridium* spp., *Ruminococcus* spp. and others (Patel 2000; Stinear et al., 2001; Domingo et al., 2005; Ballard et al., 2005b; Domingo et al., 2007). One of these isolates was investigated further and a new, naturally vancomycin-resistant species, *Ruminococcus gauvreauii*, was identified possessing a *vanD* gene cluster (Domingo et al., 2008). In strains of *Clostridium symbiosum* an entire *vanB2* type Tn*1549* cluster was identified which was transferable in vitro and in vivo in the digestive tract of mice highlighting the important role that commensal, intestinal, non-enterococcal hosts may play for acquiring, preserving and distributing (vancomycin) resistance genes to nosocomial pathogens (Launay et al., 2006). The corresponding conjugative transposon Tn*1549* encodes all necessary functions for a successful transfer of the element across species and genus barriers also demonstrating its potential to transfer *vanB* type vancomycin resistance from *Enterococcus* to other important nosocomial pathogens like *Staphylococcus* spp, *C. difficile* and others (Tsvetkova et al., 2010). A large number of the *C. difficile* genome of the multi-drug resistant, clinical strain 630 consisted of mobile, genetic elements (11%) including a *tet*(M)-encoding self-conjugative transposon Tn*5397* (Sebaihia et al., 2006). Conjugative transposons like Tn*5397*/Tn*916* (and also Tn*1549*) are easily exchanged between members of different bacterial species and genera and are identified in a wide range of different, Gram-positive bacterial species capable of self-transfer and mobilisation of other, genetic elements (Roberts et al., 2001; Jasni et al., 2010; Roberts and Mullany 2011). *C. difficile* 630 also contained an element with similarity to a *vanG* type cluster; however, neither this cluster was complete nor was the strain vancomycin-resistant (Sebaihia et al., 2006). *Clostridium innocuum* is naturally intermediate-resistant to vancomycin (MIC = 8 mg/L). The mechanism of resistance was investigated in strain NCIB 10674 and found to be related due to the activity of two chromosomally encoded Ddl ligases and a racemase allowing the synthesis of a peptidoglycan precursor terminating in D-Ser similar to VanC/E/G/L type vancomycin resistance (David et al., 2004).

Certain vancomycin-resistant strains of fecal streptococci belonging to the *Streptococcus bovis* group (e.g., *S. gallolyticus*, *S. lutetiensis*) were found to contain *vanA* and *vanB* genes (Poyart et al., 1997; Mevius et al., 1998); however, these strains were not investigated in greater molecular details. Results of another study revealed that the entire *vanB2* type Tn*5397* conjugative transposon from a *S. lutetiensis* donor was capable to transfer into *E. faecium* and *E. faecalis* recipients in a *recA*-independent manner (Dahl and Sundsfjord 2003).

Strains of *Paenibacillus popilliae* and *Rhodococcus* spp. contain *vanA/B*-like resistance gene clusters originally called *vanE* in *P. popilliae* and later on designated *vanF* (Patel et al., 2000; Guardabassi et al., 2004; Guardabassi et al., 2005; Guardabassi and Agerso 2006). *P. popilliae* ATCC 14706 is high-level vancomycin-resistant and contained a gene cluster with $vanY_F$ and $vanZ_F$ preceding the *vanHFX* co-transcribed gene cluster. Two genes encoding a two-component regulatory system of the VanRS type were identified ca. 3kb upstream $vanY_F$ associated with an inducible VanF phenotype (Fraimow et al., 2005).

A number of *Lactobacillus*, *Pediococcus*, *Leuconostoc* and *Lactococcus* species are naturally resistant to vancomycin. This is an intrinsic property of certain species and, as known so far, mainly linked to a modified cell wall synthesis mediated via alternative precursors, functionally similar but not linked to an acquisition of any *van* gene cluster (Goffin et al., 2005). For instance , in *Leuconostoc mesenteroides* a Ddl enzyme with a residual D-Ala-D-Lac activity was identified allowing the production of vancomycin-resistant cell wall precursors (Kuzin et al., 2000). In *Lactobacillus plantarum* vancomycin resistance is also mediated via a species-specific Ddl ligase capable of synthesising D-Ala-D-Lac depsipeptides and, in addition, an intrinsic VanX-like D-Ala-D-Ala dipeptidase destroying vancomycin-susceptible cell wall precursors (Deghorain et al., 2007).

Certain soil bacteria produce glycopeptide antibiotics including vancomycin (*Amycolatopsis orientalis*) and teicoplanin (*Actinoplanes teichomyceticus*) as secondary metabolites. They prevent themselves from sensitivity against their own products by intrinsic resistance mechanisms similar but not identical to acquired resistance types in *Enterococcus* spp. (Marshall et al., 1997; Marshall et al., 1998; Patel 2000). It was speculated that enterococcal resistance genes originated from corresponding glycopeptide producers (Marshall et al., 1998; Patel 2000); however, comparably weak amino acid and nucleotide similarities among key genes and proteins involved in the resistance mechanism and the comparably high % GC of the VanRS regulatory system in the glycopeptide producers *Streptomyces toyocaensis* and *A. orientalis* suggested that a possible exchange between glycopeptide producers and nosocomial pathogens having acquired resistance properties did not happen recently (Courvalin 2005).

The anaerobic, Gram-positive, dehalogenating bacterium *Desulfitobacterium hafniense* Y51 was vancomycin-resistant by an inducible resistance phenotype (Patel et al., 2000). The strain contained a resistance Ddl enzyme with a preferred D-Ala-D-Lac ligase activity and a vancomycin resistance gene cluster showing a slightly different gene arrangement as compared with *vanA/B* clusters. The essential *vanH* homologue was missing in this cluster element; however, genome analysis of *D. hafniense* Y51 revealed at least four D-isomer-specific 2-hydroxyacid dehydrogenase genes capable in situ to perform the relevant vanH-type reaction. Nevertheless, the physiological role, the overall prevalence of this gene cluster and the phylogenetic relation to acquired resistance gene clusters in *Enterococcus* spp. remain unclear so far (Patel 2000).

It is known that intestinal colonisation could precede subsequent infections with VRE (Donskey 2004). Screening patients at risk for a colonisation with VRE is an important indicator in preventing and controlling VRE infections and outbreaks (Zirakzadeh and Patel 2006). Molecular assays provide certain advantages over microbiological tests in terms of time, sensitivity and accuracy. Prevalence of *van* genes, especially *vanB* in intestinal, non-enterococcal species impairs performance of rapid, molecular screening assays targeting the corresponding resistance genes only (Stamper et al., 2007; Mak et al., 2009; Usacheva et al., 2010). Results of a number of studies performed with various commercially available diagnostic assays in Northern America, Australia, Asia and different countries in Europe also revealed that *vanB* is generally prevalent among human intestinal colonizers and that this is not a specific property of human intestinal colonisers in certain parts of the world (Ballard et al., 2005a; Stamper et al., 2007; Mak et al., 2009; Usacheva et al., 2010; Lee et al., 2010; Marner et al., 2011; Werner et al., 2011c).

5.2 The *vanA* gene cluster in *Staphylococcus aureus*

Vancomycin is the antibiotic of choice for treating MRSA infected patients. Insusceptibility to vancomycin associated with treatment failure is insofar a matter of serious concern. Various microbiological changes could lead to reduced susceptibility against vancomycin including increased cell wall thickness, activated cell wall synthesis and reduced autolysis. The former changes are based on a modified host gene expression of determinants involved in cell wall synthesis leading to a so-called "trapping effect" where more unlinked cell wall precursors are present being able to bind (more) vancomycin ("to trap" the drug)(Cui et al., 2005; Werner et al., 2008c; Nannini et al., 2010). The Vancomycin intermediate-resistant phenotype (VISA) could be expressed homogeneously or only in a subset of investigated strains (1 of 10^5 cells = heterogeneous VISA - hVISA), the latter requires a sophisticated diagnostics via a population-based-analysis profiling (PAP)(Howden et al., 2010). VISA or hVISA phenotypes are not associated with (*van*) gene acquisition.

Early in vitro studies demonstrated the capability of a transfer of the enterococcal VanA type resistance into *S. aureus*/MRSA rendering descendents as vancomycin- and oxacillin-resistant (Noble et al., 1992). The first clinical *van*A-mediated high-level vancomycin-resistant MRSA (VRSA) was isolated from a dialysis patient in Michigan, USA (Weigel et al., 2003; Chang et al., 2003). Since then, less than a dozen additional cases have been described, nine in the United States (Michigan [n= 7], New York and Pennsylvania) and each one in India and in Iran (the latter two were not confirmed elsewhere) (Sievert et al., 2008; Finks et al., 2009; Nannini et al., 2010).

The US VRSA isolates showed high-level vancomycin resistance of >32 mg/L. All US patients affected by VRSA infections had a history of several underlying conditions and accordingly, all of them were treated extensively with antibiotics including vancomycin and most of them were co-colonized with VRE, respectively. The US VRSA isolates exhibited the *Sma*I macrorestriction patterns USA100, SCC*mec*II and USA800, SCC*mec*IV and all isolates could be assigned to sequence type 5 by multilocus sequence typing (MLST). Typing of corresponding strains, their resistance plasmids and corresponding Tn*1546*-like *vanA* clusters revealed that the isolates were unique and had evolved separately (see next paragraph).

From the first case patient a MRSA strain, a *vanA*-type *E. faecalis* and a *vanA*-type MRSA were isolated which allowed constructing a scenario where the MRSA received the *vanA* type resistance from the resistant co-colonising *E. faecalis*. This has been confirmed by molecular analysis of the corresponding *vanA*-type plasmids from related VRSA and MRSA isolates (Weigel et al., 2003; Clark et al., 2005; Zhu et al., 2008). The VRSA isolate contained a 58 kb conjugative plasmid pLW1043, the MRSA a ca. 47 kb pAM829 plasmid and the VRE two plasmids of 45 and 95 kb. Restriction digestion revealed similar patterns for the pLW1043 and pAM829 plasmids but not for the *E. faecalis* plasmids (Weigel et al., 2003). pLW1043 was fully sequenced and revealed a Tn*1546*-like *vanA* cluster integrated between the *blaZ* (beta-lactamase) and the *aacA-aphD* (gentamicin resistance) regions. It showed a mosaic-like structure, but the backbone was similar to staphylococcal type pSK41 plasmids and different from typical enterococcal plasmids suggesting acquisition of the *vanA* cluster by a resident staphylococcal-type plasmid (Kwong et al., 2008; Weaver et al., 2009). Interestingly, majority of other VRSA and co-colonising VRE isolates contained inc18-type *vanA* plasmids investigated in a follow up study (Zhu et al., 2008). The inc18-type plasmids represent broad-host range plasmids widely prevalent among Gram-positive bacteria of different enterococcal, staphylococcal and streptococcal species (Weaver et al., 2009). Plasmids from three VRSA cases were sequenced [plasmids pWZ7140 (47,277 bp), pWZ909 (42,602 bp), and pWZ1668 (48,365 bp)]. They were almost identical among each other and to a corresponding *vanA* plasmid from co-colonising *E. faecalis* strains revealing a possible direct transfer from an *E. faecalis* donor into MRSA (Zhu et al., 2008). Molecular studies with isogenic MRSA and VRSA isolates revealed that acquired VanA-type resistance was highly costly to the host, when induced (Foucault et al., 2009). In the absence of induction, the determined biological cost was minimal suggesting a serious potential for the dissemination of VRSA clinical isolates.

An comparison of US VRSA isolates (Michigan VRSA, Pennsylvania VRSA) to the *vanA*-type *E. faecalis* from the index patient, the possible donor of the resistance gene cluster for the Michigan VRSA, revealed interesting details on the resistance gene regulation and expression in different hosts (Perichon and Courvalin 2004). The Michigan VRSA was highly resistant to both glycopeptides, whereas the Pennsylvania VRSA displayed low-level resistance to vancomycin and reduced susceptibility to teicoplanin. Resistance genes were expressed at similarly high levels in the two VRSA and the *vanA*-type *E. faecalis*; however, resistance expression was notably delayed in the Pennsylvania strain. Resistance was lost at non-selective condition from the Pennsylvania VRSA. In contrast, it was stable in the Michigan VRSA and the VRE (Perichon and Courvalin 2004). Two Michigan VRSA isolates, designated VRSA-7 and VRSA-9 showed a vancomycin dependence phenotype. Molecular studies revealed a similar mechanism as known from enterococci with the corresponding resistance phenotype. VRSA-7 and VRSA-9 contained different mutations in the housekeeping D-Ala-D-Ala ligase leading to a decreased activity and dependence on the *vanA*-type D-Ala-D-Lac ligase for an ongoing cell wall synthesis (Moubareck et al., 2009; Meziane-Cherif et al., 2010). Strikingly, peptidoglycan precursors ending in D-Ala-D-Lac are not processed by PBP2a, the oxacillin-resistant penicillin binding protein encoded by *mecA* and consequently the VRSA-7 and VRSA-9 were fully susceptible to oxacillin, despite the production of a wild-type PBP2a (Moubareck et al., 2009). This also means that the combination of a beta-lactam and a glycopeptide antibiotic shows a synergistic effect for VRSA in general (Perichon and Courvalin 2006). Comparison of the two vancomycin-dependent VRSA isolates (VRSA-7/-9) indicated that the levels of vancomycin dependence and susceptibility to β-lactams correlate with the degree of D-Ala-D-Ala ligase impairment (Meziane-Cherif et al., 2010).

6. Prevalence of VRE among the hospital setting

Modern molecular typing techniques (AFLP, MLVA, MLST)[2] allow differentiating between commensal and hospital-associated/outbreak *E. faecium* isolates including vancomycin-resistant and vancomycin-susceptible variants (Willems and Bonten 2007; Willems and van Schaik W. 2009). Genomic diversity is higher in commensal *E. faecium* isolates (animal/human) as compared to hospital strains types that especially show a predominance of a number of specific MLST or MLVA types (Werner et al., 2007b; Werner et al., 2011a). Results of a comparative genome-based study revealed a distinct composition of the accessory genome in hospital-associated *E. faecium* strains (Leavis et al., 2007). Results have been confirmed by recent comparative analyses of completely sequenced *E. faecium* genomes (van Schaik et al., 2010; Palmer et al., 2010). The current model predicts that spread of ampicillin-resistant, hospital-associated *E. faecium* strains is a pre-requisite for successful establishment of VRE and further dissemination of vancomycin resistance among the hospital *E. faecium* population in general (Willems and Bonten 2007; Galloway-Pena et al., 2009; Willems and van Schaik W. 2009). To a larger or lesser extent, non-microbiological factors such as antibiotic consumption (particular classes and in general); "colonisation pressure", "understaffing", compliance with hand hygiene and other infection control measures also affect the role and number of enterococcal infections (Bonten et al., 1998; Cetinkaya et al., 2000; Murray 2000; Bonten et al., 2001; Panesso et al., 2010). Therefore, it might not come as a big surprise that despite having similar starting points and preconditions different countries experienced diverse trends in VRE prevalence. Already during the early and mid-1990s, epidemic clonal types of *E. faecium* were prevalent in hospitals in many countries, and this coincided in some European countries with a high prevalence of vancomycin resistance among *E. faecium* from animals and healthy volunteers linked to a widespread use of avoparcin as a growth promoter in commercial animal husbandry (Murray 1990; Murray 2000; Bonten et al., 2001; Panesso et al., 2010). However, VRE rates in clinical isolates increased in many countries and peaked only almost ten years later when glycopeptide resistance had already declined in the non-hospital reservoir. Retrospective epidemiological analyses in hospitals experiencing larger VRE outbreaks revealed that changes in specific procedures such as antibiotic policy, staffing, infection prevention and control regimes were, in some instances, significantly associated with increasing VRE rates, whereas in other settings this could not be shown. Increased VRE

---

[2] AFLP, Amplified-fragment length polymorphism; MLVA, Multiple Locus Variable number of tandem repeat Analysis; MLST, Multi-Locus Sequence Typing

prevalence is partly associated with spread of single, distinct epidemic clones or types (Klare et al., 2005; Top et al., 2007; Bonora et al., 2007; Werner et al., 2007c; Valdezate et al., 2009; Zhu et al., 2010; Johnson et al., 2010; Hsieh et al., 2010). In contrast, VRE outbreaks in single centres tend to be polyclonal suggesting a diverse population of hospital-acquired *E. faecium* strains and a highly mobile resistance determinant capable of spreading widely among suitable recipient strains (Yoo et al., 2006; Deplano et al., 2007; Kawalec et al., 2007; Borgmann et al., 2007; Werner et al., 2007c; Hsieh et al., 2009). Many facets of VRE and vancomycin resistance epidemiology are currently not fully understood and the question why vancomycin resistance is still mainly limited to *E. faecium* remains mainly unanswered (Garcia-Migura et al., 2007; Garcia-Migura et al., 2008; Werner et al., 2010b).

The main prevalent genotypes of acquired vancomycin resistance in enterococci worldwide are *vanA* and to a lesser extent *vanB*. The reservoir for *vanA/B* gene clusters is mainly in *E. faecium*; *vanA/B*-type resistant *E. faecalis* remain rare all over the world. Countries experiencing problems with increasing or significant higher rates of VRE always report about vancomycin-resistant *E. faecium*. Infections with members of other enterococcal species remain rare although also outbreaks with *vanA/B*-type resistant *E. faecalis*, *E. raffinosus* or *VanC-type E. gallinarum* were reported (Foglia et al., 2003; Kawalec et al., 2007; Neves et al., 2009; Shirano et al., 2010). In conclusion, the problem of VRE is mainly an issue of *vanA*-type vancomycin-resistant *E. faecium* (see the following).

6.1 Europe

Several national and European surveillance systems collect data on vancomycin resistance in enterococci. In some countries mandatory VRE surveillance is already established, in others coverage for the general population or selected settings is rather limited and the available data do not allow reliable statistical analyses and in some countries data are completely lacking. The most successful European antibiotic resistance surveillance scheme is the European Antimicrobial Resistance Surveillance System/network (EARSS/EARS-Net),[3] which was established in 1998 and is now funded by the European Centre for Disease Prevention and Control ECDC. EARS-Net collects data on antibiotic resistances in indicator bacteria exclusively from invasive (bloodstream) infections currently covering *Streptococcus pneumoniae*, *S. aureus*, *Escherichia coli*, *E. faecalis/E. faecium*, *Klebsiella pneumoniae* and *Pseudomonas aeruginosa*. In 2008 over 900 microbiological laboratories serving more than 1,500 hospitals from 33 countries provided susceptibility data from more than 700,000 invasive isolates. Inter-country comparison of collected data in the given setting reveals some drawbacks and limitations (not discussed here, see EARS reports and website). Accordingly, simple comparisons of surveillance data over time and between countries or even within single countries should be done carefully (see also chapter 4 in the EARS Annual Report 2008)(EARSS 2009). VRE surveillance within Europe has recently been reviewed and the reader is referred to this paper for any further details (Werner et al., 2008a). In the following only a short summary and, in addition, some new aspects to these previous reports are given.

---

[3] http://ecdc.europa.eu/en/activities/surveillance/EARS-Net/about_EARS-Net/Pages/about_networ k.aspx

VRE surveillance in the Nordic European countries, Norway, Denmark, Sweden, Finland and Iceland, is based on national public health programmes for containment of antimicrobial resistance, participation in EARS and in some countries case notification from laboratories and clinicians. The Nordic countries have traditionally had a low prevalence of antimicrobial resistance, and this is also true for VRE. Within the last years a recognisable reservoir of vancomycin resistance among animal enterococci was demonstrated despite the ban of using any antimicrobial growth promoter, especially avoparcin (Sorum et al., 2006; Nilsson et al., 2009a; Nilsson et al., 2009b). It is still unclear if and to what extent this reservoir influences the situation in the clinical setting. In Sweden, the situation has been stable with 18–53 cases of VRE infections and colonisations being reported annually between 2000 and 2007. However, the situation has changed rapidly with the predominant spread of a *vanB E. faecium* clone with 634 among 760 VRE cases described within a 20 months' period from 2007-2009 (Soderblom et al., 2010). General prevalence of VRE in a Swedish hospital during a post-outbreak situation was still low (Fang et al., 2010).

There is no single comprehensive surveillance scheme for monitoring VRE infections in the United Kingdom (UK). However, bacteraemia caused by VRE is monitored by four complementary surveillance programmes, with varying degrees of coverage and participation (Werner et al., 2008a). Numbers of VRE cases from invasive infections and general prevalence of vancomycin resistance in enterococci from the clinical setting is comparably high in relation to other European countries. Given the tremendous activities and partial success in reducing the MRSA burden in UK hospitals one might expect that these measures also lead to a reduction of VRE bacteraemia cases. Rates of vancomycin resistance among invasive *E. faecium* isolates varied between 33% (2005), 18% (2006), 21% (2007), 28% (2008), 13% (2009) (data from EARS-Net). The Department of Health mandatory glycopeptide-resistant enterococcal bacteraemia reporting scheme collects the total number of VRE bacteraemias in England each year. A supposed reduction in bacteraemia cases in both surveillance schemes conflicts with a possible reporting bias of participating hospitals and laboratories and it has to be shown that the supposed trends will be stable for the coming years[4]. The British Society for Antimicrobial Chemotherapy (BSAC) Bacteraemia Surveillance Programme reports data until 2008; however, a specific trend cannot be specified for "*E. faecium*" and "vancomycin resistance"[5].

Certain European countries (Netherlands, Denmark, Spain) showed a wide prevalence of hospital-associated clonal types of *E. faecium* but vancomycin resistance rates are still low (Oteo et al., 2007; Lester et al., 2008; Top et al., 2008b; Valdezate et al., 2009; Lester et al., 2009). In other countries rates of VRE remain at a comparably high rate such as Ireland and Portugal[5] (Novais et al., 2008; Morris-Downes et al., 2010). Decreasing rates were considered significant in countries like Italy, France, Israel and Greece; however, it has to be documented if these trends are indeed lasting and not biased by other, so far unknown factors (see EARS-Net data).

---

[4] http://www.hpa.org.uk/web/HPAwebFile/HPAweb_C/GGTSPU-vaccine-see.rki.de-11200-6823805-DAT/1278944284940

[5]   http://www.bsacsurv.org/mrsweb/bacteraemia?organism=E.%20faecium&antimicrobial=van&year=All&country=All&summary=Enzyme%20Production&formname=bsac_bacteraemia&submit=Search%20%28%20this%20tab%20%29

Molecular typing of clinical enterococci sent to the German Focal Laboratory for Enterococcus revealed a significant increase in the number of *vanB*-type *E. faecium* among vancomycin-resistant *E. faecium* prevalent in different German hospitals (2006: 53/302, 18%; 2007: 65/249, 26%; 2008: 95/298, 32%; 2009: 157/333, 52%; (Klare et al., 2010)). Preliminary findings direct to a similar trend in other European countries like Sweden (Soderblom et al., 2010; Fang et al., 2010). If this increased VanB-type prevalence is linked to a supposed reservoir of *vanB* among enterococcal or non-enterococcal intestinal colonizers (Stamper et al., 2007; Young et al., 2007; Graham et al., 2008; Usacheva et al., 2010; Bourdon et al., 2010; Werner et al., 2011c) or simply linked to an improved and better identification of low-level expressed VanB-type resistance (Pendle et al., 2008; Grabsch et al., 2008a; Grabsch et al., 2008b; Stamper et al., 2010) in relation to a reduced breakpoint as defined by EUCAST (EUCAST Clinical Breakpoint Table v. 1.1 2010-04-27)[6] remains to be elucidated in further studies.

6.2 Northern America

Canada and the USA illustrate two divergent scenarios concerning vancomycin resistance rates among enterococci. In Canada resistance rates are persistently low (Karlowsky et al., 1999; Zhanel et al., 2000; Nichol et al., 2006; Zhanel et al., 2008a; Zhanel et al., 2010b). Results of a recent CANWARD study performed in 2008 among 10 participating Canadian hospitals revealed 3.1% VRE among 320 clinical enterococcal isolates (Zhanel et al., 2010b). All 10 VRE were *vanA*-type *E. faecium*. VRE prevalence among Canadian ICU patients is low as well; VRE accounted for <1% (n= 17/ 4133) of all isolates and 6.7% (n= 17/255) of enterococcal isolates, majority of them (88%) possessed *vanA* (Zhanel et al., 2008b). Despite the low prevalence of the more common vancomycin resistance genotypes, a number of new and still rare vancomycin resistance genotypes of the *vanD*, *vanE*, *vanG* and *vanL* classes were identified in Canadian enterococci (Boyd et al., 2000; Van Caeseele et al., 2001; Boyd et al., 2002; Boyd et al., 2004; Boyd et al., 2006a; Boyd et al., 2008).

In contrast to the situation in Canada, vancomycin resistance among clinical enterococci from US medical centres is highly prevalent. It is mainly encoded by *vanA*-type resistance widely prevalent among hospital-associated clonal types of *E. faecium* (Karlowsky et al., 2004; Nichol et al., 2006). The rapid increase in vancomycin resistance among the *E. faecium* population in US hospitals in general and the intensive care setting especially after its first appearance within a 10 years' time span is a dramatic example of a fast growing resistance problem that nowadays neither can be controlled nor prevented or reversed. The obvious coincidence of a number of unfortunate circumstances and factors from either side, the health care setting (e. g., delayed compliance with infection control and prevention strategies; permission of oral vancomycin use) and the bacteria themselves (e. g., rapid spread of hospital-associated epidemic clones; vancomycin resistance genes in a stable and transferable genetic background) may have led to such a scenario (Martone 1998; Nichol et al., 2006). The Surveillance Network (TSN) collects data on blood culture isolates from patients from 268 US hospitals. Data for 2002 revealed in 67% vancomycin resistance among altogether 1.285 *E. faecium* isolates whereas the same resistance characteristics still remained

[6] http://www.eucast.org/fileadmin/src/media/PDFs/EUCAST_files/Disk_test_documents/EUCAST_b reakpoints_v1.1.pdf

rare with <5% among *E. faecalis* isolates (Karlowsky et al., 2004). Results of other studies revealed similar rates (Nichol et al., 2006; Deshpande et al., 2007). The overall situation is even impaired during the last years showing a rise in the total number of hospitalisations due to VRE infections (Ramsey and Zilberberg 2009). The Nationwide Inpatient Sample available through the Healthcare Costs and Utilization Project Website showed increased incidence of VRE infections from 3.2 to 6.5 between 2003 and 2006. An increased use of vancomycin to treat increasing numbers of MRSA and *Clostridium difficile* infections was one of the major drivers.

6.3 Latin America

In Latin America, prevalence of VRE is generally considered to be low with rates <5% among enterococci in general and before 2005 (Quinones Perez 2006); however, reliable data based on comprehensive studies or data sets were missing. Results of a recent SENTRY study revealed a recognizable change of vancomycin resistance rates among clinical enterococcal isolates from participating Latin American countries/hospitals increasing from 5 to 15.5% within 6 years (between 2003 and 2008). The most significant increase was demonstrated for Brazil with VRE rates rising from 7 to 31% (Sader et al., 2009). Considering that the majority of enterococcal isolates is *E. faecalis* which mainly remained susceptible to vancomycin, the increase of vancomycin resistance among *E. faecium* isolates seems even more dramatic based on the numbers specified. A molecular characterization of prospectively collected 732 enterococcal isolates from 2006 to 2008 from 32 hospitals in Colombia, Ecuador, Peru and Venezuela revealed vancomycin resistance in 6% of all isolates (Panesso et al., 2010). Considering only isolates of *E. faecium* (n= 111) prevalence of vancomycin resistance ranged from 24 to 48%; however, sample size per country was quite limited and a sampling bias cannot be excluded. Nevertheless, all vancomycin-resistant *E. faecium* were of the *vanA* genotype and represented hospital-associated strain types as determined by MLST (ST17, ST18, ST203, ST280 and others). Tn*5382-vanB2* encoded VanB type resistance was demonstrated to be linked to two epidemic clones; a ST201 *E. faecalis* and a ST64 *E. faecium* disseminated among 9 and 15 Chilean hospitals, respectively (Lopez et al., 2009).

6.4 Asia, Australia and New Zealand

VanB-type resistance is only highly prevalent in certain parts of the world, for instance, in Australia (Christiansen et al., 2004; Pearman 2006; Worth et al., 2008; Pendle et al., 2008; Johnson et al., 2010) or Singapore (Koh et al., 2006; Koh et al., 2009) where *vanB*-type vancomycin resistance among clinical *E. faecium* is more prevalent than the *vanA*-type. The reason(s) for this remain unknown and are not linked to a supposed larger reservoir of the *vanB* cluster in commensal intestinal colonizers (Padiglione et al., 2000), rates of which were similar in Australian, US-American and European studies (Stamper et al., 2007; Graham et al., 2008; Grabsch et al., 2008b; Bourdon et al., 2010; Werner et al., 2011c). A larger reservoir of *vanB*-type resistance in isolates from commercial animal farming associated with an avoparcin use is unlikely; avoparcin use was ceased in Australia in 2000 and Singapore has no significant agriculture at all thus excluding a distinct animal *vanB*-type VRE reservoir (see chapter 7). However, community carriage linked to a consumption of imported and contaminated food cannot be excluded. Studies performed in New Zealand described a supposed dissemination of *vanA*-type resistance among *E. faecalis* strains rather then *E. faecium* in a background of generally low level of vancomycin resistance (Manson et al., 2003a; Manson et al., 2003b). VRE epidemiology in other Australasian countries reflects a similar scenario as in Europe or Northern America with *vanA*-type resistance highly prevalent among *E. faecium*. Several studies performed during outbreaks in Taiwanese hospitals revealed a preferred prevalence of (hospital-associated) *vanA*-type vancomycin-resistant *E. faecium* strains (Hsieh et al., 2009; Hsieh et al., 2010). In South-Korean hospitals (and outside hospitals) *vanA*-genotype (VanB phenotype) *E. faecium* were widely prevalent (Ko et al., 2005; Shin et al., 2006; Park et al., 2008). Recent reports from China revealed also a preferred prevalence of *vanA*-type vancomycin resistance among clinical VRE (Zheng et al., 2007a; Zheng et al., 2007b; Zhu et al., 2009).

7. Vancomycin resistance among enterococci from farm animals, feedstuff and non-hospitalized humans and the environment

Surveillance of antimicrobial resistance among enterococci as commensal colonizers of food-producing animals became prominent during the early and mid 1990ies. At this time scientific and public awareness arose due to the argument that use of antimicrobial growth promoters, focused on the glycopeptide avoparcin, added to the feed of food animals in sub-inhibitory concentrations is capable of selecting antibiotic-resistant bacteria; here glycopeptide/vancomycin-resistant enterococci. Large studies were initiated when higher numbers of VRE were suspiciously found in environmental samples without any known reservoir in or link to use of glycopeptides in human medicine (Klare et al., 1993; Torres et al., 1994). Soon after, avoparcin, another glycopeptide class antibiotic used in animal husbandry as a feed additive (growth promoter) was identified to select VRE in the animal setting (Bates et al., 1994; Klare et al., 1995a; Klare et al., 1995b; Bates 1997). Consequently, meat samples from commercially raised animals were highly contaminated with VRE including samples of pork, beef, chicken and turkey (Klare et al., 1995a; Klare et al., 1995b; Schouten et al., 1997; Klein et al., 1998; Simonsen et al., 1998; Kruse et al., 1999). Samples from organic or private farms of smaller sizes that did not use avoparcin or feed additives at all were free of VRE (Klare et al., 1995b; Klare and Witte 1998). Following the food chain, VRE reached humans and were capable of colonizing the intestines of healthy people; in contrast, a small study in vegetarians showed no detectable VRE counts (Schouten et al., 1997; Van Den Bogaard et al., 1997; Stobberingh et al., 1999). Similar studies were performed all over Europe and data have already been reviewed in previous papers and book chapters and are thus not discussed in greater details here (Woodford et al., 1998; Klare and Witte 1998; Aarestrup et al., 2000b; Bonten et al., 2001; Klare et al., 2003). In countries within the EU, avoparcin was abandoned in Norway and Denmark in 1995, Germany 1996 and in the remaining EU countries in 1997. Studies performed in some European countries soon after identified a reduced prevalence of VRE, their numbers dropped qualitatively and quantitatively in samples from commercial animal farms, food samples and following the food chain in humans of the general population (Klare et al., 1999). However, studies from Denmark and Norway showed that other antimicrobial growth promoters may lead to a co-selection phenomenon and reduced VRE numbers were only documentable when other growth promoters like macrolides (spiramycin, tylosin) were also banned. The reason was a genetic linkage of both resistance determinants *erm*(B) and *vanA* on similar plasmids (Aarestrup 2000; Borgen et al., 2002). Based on the precautionary principle the European

Commission postponed the further use of four antimicrobial growth promoters with a supposed link (same antibiotic class) to antibiotics used in human medicine in 1998. This decision was confirmed in 2003 specifying the phasing out of all antimicrobial growth promoters within the EU [Regulation (EC) No. 1831/2003 on additives for use in animal nutrition]. However, VRE counts did not drop to zero. Studies in animal farms performed several years after the ban of several growth promoters including avoparcin revealed a permanent reservoir of VRE (Borgen et al., 2000; Borgen et al., 2001; Ghidan et al., 2008). Recent studies performed in Swedish animal farms still highlighted a considerable reservoir of VRE (Nilsson et al., 2009b). Sweden banned avoparcin and other growth promoters already in 1986 and VRE prevalence among the clinical setting as well as the general population was and still is very low but somehow widely found in sewage (Sahlstrom et al., 2009). Phenotypic and genotypic characterization of the sewage VRE identified for the majority of them (a) species *E. faecium* and (b) the *vanB*-type. PFGE analysis revealed different strains prevalent over the study period. This finding is especially noticeable since a few years later rates of VanB-type *E. faecium* increased in certain Swedish hospitals (Soderblom et al., 2010; Fang et al., 2010).

Outside Europe similar scenarios of VRE epidemiology were described. In Korea, VRE were still prevalent in livestock samples four years after banning avoparcin (Lim et al., 2006). VRE were isolated from 17% of the chicken samples (n= 57 strains from 342 meat samples) and 2% of the pig samples (4 from 214 fecal samples) whereas no VRE were isolated from 110 bovine samples. All the 61 VRE isolates were *vanA*-type *E. faecium*. A study performed in Japan three years after the ban of avoparcin (1997) did not identify any VRE among 515 fresh faecal samples from 178 beef cattle, 179 pig and 158 broiler chicken farms representing all 47 Japanese prefectures (Kojima et al., 2010) whereas in 1996, one year before the ban, 3% (8/263) of enterococci tested were vancomycin-resistant (Yoshimura et al., 1998). However, in these two studies it was only screened for enterococci in general and subsequently resistances were determined. So it cannot be ruled out that samples contained VRE but at lower numbers then statistically recognizable with the described non-selective screening strategy. Avoparcin use was banned in Taiwan in 2000. A nationwide surveillance was initiated to study VRE prevalence on chicken farms from 2000 to 2003 (Lauderdale et al., 2007). VRE were still identified, but counts dropped in a quantitative manner, only 8.8% (n= 7/80) of the chicken farms surveyed harboured VRE in 2003 compared with 25% (15/60) in 2000. Interestingly, majority were vancomycin-resistant *E. faecalis* (see below). This reflects a somehow different VRE epidemiology than in the rest of the world; similar to Australia where *vanB*-type *E. faecium* and *vanA*-type *E. faecalis* predominate (Worth et al., 2008; Johnson et al., 2010). In Australia, the general scenario appears to be different; a larger reservoir of VRE outside the clinical setting could not be identified despite an ongoing high use of avoparcin. For instance, prevalence rates of VRE in the general population were extremely low (0,2%), the two identified VRE among 1085 community specimens were *vanB*-type *E. faecium* (Padiglione et al., 2000).

In the US, avoparcin has never been used as a feed additive, a reservoir for VRE outside the clinical setting could not be identified when screening samples from various animal farms, meat, environmental sources and stool samples from healthy people during this time (Coque et al., 1996; McDonald et al., 1997; Martone 1998). However, situation changed the last years and vancomycin resistance was prevalent among 6 of 55 pig samples investigated in 2008 (Donabedian et al., 2010).

8. Localization and spread of *vanA*- and *vanB*-type resistance

Vancomycin resistance in animal, human commensal and environmental sources is mostly encoded by *vanA*-type resistance clusters and its reservoir is in isolates of *E. faecium*; thus it reflects the same situation as in the clinical setting in most parts of the world. Exchange of resistant strains among different ecosystems is less probable due to the supposed ecovar association, especially among hospital-associated *E. faecium* strains (see chapter 5), although dissemination across host barriers of vancomycin- and multi-resistant enterococci was described anecdotally, especially for the less strongly host-adapted *E. faecalis* strains (Manson et al., 2003a; Manson et al., 2003b; Manson et al., 2004; Agerso et al., 2008; Larsen et al., 2010; Hammerum et al., 2010; Freitas et al., 2011a). Vancomycin resistance among enterococci most probably spreads via a dissemination of mobile genetic elements of variants of the *vanA*-type element Tn*1546* mostly located on mobilizable or conjugative plasmids (Sletvold et al., 2007; Novais et al., 2008; Sletvold et al., 2008; Freitas et al., 2009; Rosvoll et al., 2009; Sletvold et al., 2010; Laverde Gomez et al., 2011; Werner et al., 2011b; Freitas et al., 2011b). In vitro transfer of *vanA* plasmids has been determined in a number of studies (Werner et al., 1997; van den Braak et al., 1998; Werner et al., 2010b) and transfer in vivo in digestive tracts of animals and human volunteers was also shown (Moubareck et al., 2003; Lester et al., 2006; Lester and Hammerum 2010). Transfer rates under natural conditions may be higher than determined in vitro (Dahl et al., 2007).

Molecular studies revealed a tremendous number of deletions, insertions, and modifications of the original Tn*1546*-like structure in different not epidemiologically linked VRE leading to a wide diversity of various Tn*1546* subtypes (van den Braak et al., 1998; Willems et al., 1999; Huh et al., 2004; Werner et al., 2006; Lim et al., 2006; Yoo et al., 2006). Despite its high diversity, identical cluster types were identified among clinical human and animal commensal and environmental strains suggesting a common reservoir and exchange of its mobile elements via conjugative plasmids or as part of larger mobile genomic islands in European, Asian and Australian studies (van den Braak et al., 1998; Jensen et al., 1998; Willems et al., 1999; Werner et al., 2006; Jung et al., 2007). Garcia-Migura and co-workers identified a hot spot for integration of Tn*1546*-like elements and it could be speculated if this integration site is more prevalent among plasmids and is the reason for the preferred prevalence of *vanA* clusters on specific plasmids (Garcia-Migura et al., 2008). Results of a recent study about horizontal transferability of *vanA* plasmids among enterococci, other lactic acid bacteria and bifidobacteria revealed a preferred transfer into and a possible host restriction within the species *E. faecium* (Werner et al., 2010b). In contrast, *vanB*-type elements preferably integrate into the chromosome, but are mobile as part of integrative and conjugative elements ICE (Paulsen et al., 2003; Hegstad et al., 2010). Occasionally *vanB* resides on (transferable) plasmids (Rice et al., 1998; Zheng et al., 2009); as noticed recently associated with larger VanB-type VRE outbreaks (Sivertsen et al., 2011; Bjorkeng et al., 2011). Many surveillance studies failed to recognize a considerable reservoir of *vanB* among enterococcal colonizers in animals and humans, whereas recent real-time based studies targeting *vanB* or improved methods of detection revealed a considerable reservoir among intestinal colonizers, maybe also non-enterococcal bacteria (see above). In general, the supposed low expression of vancomycin resistance among *vanB* strains may have lead to an underestimation of its general prevalence, since in many screening studies comparably high vancomycin concentrations were used to select VRE (Poole et al., 2005; Hershberger et al., 2005). Rates of clinical *vanB*-type VRE are increasing, at least in some European countries during last years (Johnson et al., 2010; Soderblom et al., 2010; Bourdon et al., 2011) and a link to a supposed reservoir outside the clinical setting, for instance, among mammal intestinal colonizers is discussed also in areas where *vanB*-type vancomycin resistance is more prevalent (Christiansen et al., 2004; Johnson et al., 2010).

9. Genereal conclusion

Vancomycin resistance in enterococci has established as an important health care problem worldwide. Eight genotypes of acquired vancomycin resistance in enterococci are known. The *vanA*-type resistance encoded by transposon Tn*1546* and Tn*1546*-derived elements is the most prevalent resistance determinant followed by *vanB*-type clusters which are mainly part of integrative and conjugative elements (ICE) mostly residing within the chromosome. The main *van* genotype reservoir is in *E. faecium*. Prevalence of VRE among the clinical setting varies in different parts of the world. Their increased incidence is linked to characteristic predisposing factors in affected patients but also to the bacteria themselves. The latter concerns a preferred spread of hospital-associated strain types among health care settings. These strains differ from commensal strains by their core genomes (different MLST types and clonal complexes) and an additional genomic content including specific (resistance) plasmids. However, countries and institutions having similar pre-conditions may experience different developments and changes in VRE prevalence are multifactorial and cannot be simply addressed to or predicted from specific factors and circumstances. VRE and their resistance determinants are still prevalent among commercial animal husbandry despite the glycopeptide avoparcin and other antimicrobial substances were banned for growth promotion in many parts of the world. Their role to feed the (vancomycin) resistance gene pool of hospital-associated strain types remains to be elucidated in further studies.

10. References

Aarestrup, F.M., 2000. Characterization of glycopeptide-resistant enterococcus faecium (GRE) from broilers and pigs in Denmark: genetic evidence that persistence of GRE in pig herds is associated with coselection by resistance to macrolides. J. Clin. Microbiol. 38, 2774-2777.

Aarestrup, F.M., Agerso, Y., Gerner-Smidt, P., Madsen, M., Jensen, L.B., 2000a. Comparison of antimicrobial resistance phenotypes and resistance genes in Enterococcus faecalis and Enterococcus faecium from humans in the community, broilers, and pigs in Denmark. Diagn. Microbiol. Infect. Dis. 37, 127-137.

Aarestrup, F.M., Bager, F., Andersen, J.S., 2000b. Association between the use of avilamycin for growth promotion and the occurrence of resistance among Enterococcus faecium from broilers: epidemiological study and changes over time. Microb. Drug Resist. 6, 71-75.

Abadia Patino, L., Christiansen, K., Bell, J., Courvalin, P., Perichon, B., 2004. VanE-type vancomycin-resistant Enterococcus faecalis clinical isolates from Australia. Antimicrob. Agents Chemother. 48, 4882-4885.

Abadia Patino, L., Courvalin, P., Perichon, B., 2002. vanE gene cluster of vancomycin-resistant Enterococcus faecalis BM4405. J. Bacteriol. 184, 6457-6464.

Agerso, Y., Lester, C.H., Porsbo, L.J., Orsted, I., Emborg, H.D., Olsen, K.E., Jensen, L.B., Heuer, O.E., Frimodt-Moller, N., Aarestrup, F.M., Hammerum, A.M., 2008. Vancomycin-resistant Enterococcus faecalis isolates from a Danish patient and two healthy human volunteers are possibly related to isolates from imported turkey meat. J. Antimicrob. Chemother. 62, 844-845.

Agerso, Y., Pedersen, A.G., Aarestrup, F.M., 2006. Identification of Tn5397-like and Tn916-like transposons and diversity of the tetracycline resistance gene tet(M) in enterococci from humans, pigs and poultry. J. Antimicrob. Chemother. 57, 832-839.

Arias, C.A., Courvalin, P., Reynolds, P.E., 2000. vanC cluster of vancomycin-resistant Enterococcus gallinarum BM4174. Antimicrob. Agents Chemother. 44, 1660-1666.

Arias, C.A., Martin-Martinez, M., Blundell, T.L., Arthur, M., Courvalin, P., Reynolds, P.E., 1999. Characterization and modelling of VanT: a novel, membrane-bound, serine racemase from vancomycin-resistant Enterococcus gallinarum BM4174. Mol. Microbiol. 31, 1653-1664.

Arias, C.A., Murray, B.E., 2008. Emergence and management of drug-resistant enterococcal infections. Expert. Rev. Anti. Infect. Ther. 6, 637-655.

Arsene, S., Leclercq, R., 2007. Role of a qnr-like gene in the intrinsic resistance of Enterococcus faecalis to fluoroquinolones. Antimicrob. Agents Chemother. 51, 3254-3258.

Arthur, M., Depardieu, F., Gerbaud, G., Galimand, M., Leclercq, R., Courvalin, P., 1997. The VanS sensor negatively controls VanR-mediated transcriptional activation of glycopeptide resistance genes of Tn1546 and related elements in the absence of induction. J. Bacteriol. 179, 97-106.

Arthur, M., Molinas, C., Depardieu, F., Courvalin, P., 1993. Characterization of Tn1546, a Tn3-related transposon conferring glycopeptide resistance by synthesis of depsipeptide peptidoglycan precursors in Enterococcus faecium BM4147. J. Bacteriol. 175, 117-127.

Arthur, M., Quintiliani, R., Jr., 2001. Regulation of VanA- and VanB-type glycopeptide resistance in enterococci. Antimicrob. Agents Chemother. 45, 375-381.

Ballard, S.A., Grabsch, E.A., Johnson, P.D., Grayson, M.L., 2005a. Comparison of three PCR primer sets for identification of vanB gene carriage in feces and correlation with carriage of vancomycin-resistant enterococci: interference by vanB-containing anaerobic bacilli. Antimicrob. Agents Chemother. 49, 77-81.

Ballard, S.A., Pertile, K.K., Lim, M., Johnson, P.D., Grayson, M.L., 2005b. Molecular characterization of vanB elements in naturally occurring gut anaerobes. Antimicrob. Agents Chemother. 49, 1688-1694.

Baptista, M., Rodrigues, P., Depardieu, F., Courvalin, P., Arthur, M., 1999. Single-cell analysis of glycopeptide resistance gene expression in teicoplanin-resistant mutants of a VanB-type Enterococcus faecalis. Mol. Microbiol. 32, 17-28.

Batchelor, M., Zhou, D., Cooper, M.A., Abell, C., Rayment, T., 2010. Vancomycin dimer formation between analogues of bacterial peptidoglycan surfaces probed by force spectroscopy. Org. Biomol. Chem. 8, 1142-1148.

Bates, J., 1997. Epidemiology of vancomycin-resistant enterococci in the community and the relevance of farm animals to human infection. J. Hosp. Infect. 37, 89-101.

Bates, J., Jordens, J.Z., Griffiths, D.T., 1994. Farm animals as a putative reservoir for vancomycin-resistant enterococcal infection in man. J. Antimicrob. Chemother. 34, 507-514.

Bischoff, K., Jacob, J., 1996. [The sat4 streptothricin acetyltransferase gene of Campylobacter coli: its distribution in the environment and use as epidemiological marker]. Zentralbl. Hyg. Umweltmed. 198, 241-257.

Bjorkeng, E., Rasmussen, G., Sundsfjord, A., Sjoberg, L., Hegstad, K., Soderquist, B., 2011. Clustering of polyclonal VanB-type vancomycin-resistant Enterococcus faecium in a low-endemic area was associated with CC17-genogroup strains harbouring transferable vanB2-Tn5382 and pRUM-like repA containing plasmids with axe-txe plasmid addiction systems. APMIS 119, 247-258.

Boguslawska, J., Zycka-Krzesinska, J., Wilcks, A., Bardowski, J., 2009. Intra- and interspecies conjugal transfer of Tn916-like elements from Lactococcus lactis in vitro and in vivo. Appl. Environ. Microbiol. 75, 6352-6360.

Bonora, M.G., Ligozzi, M., Luzzani, A., Solbiati, M., Stepan, E., Fontana, R., 2006. Emergence of linezolid resistance in Enterococcus faecium not dependent on linezolid treatment. Eur. J. Clin. Microbiol. Infect. Dis. 25, 197-198.

Bonora, M.G., Olioso, D., Lo, C.G., Fontana, R., 2007. Phylogenetic analysis of vancomycin-resistant Enterococcus faecium genotypes associated with outbreaks or sporadic infections in Italy. Microb. Drug Resist. 13, 171-177.

Bonten, M.J., Slaughter, S., Ambergen, A.W., Hayden, M.K., van, V.J., Nathan, C., Weinstein, R.A., 1998. The role of "colonization pressure" in the spread of vancomycin-resistant enterococci: an important infection control variable. Arch. Intern. Med. 158, 1127-1132.

Bonten, M.J., Willems, R., Weinstein, R.A., 2001. Vancomycin-resistant enterococci: why are they here, and where do they come from? The Lancet Infectious Diseases 1, 314-325.

Borgen, K., Simonsen, G.S., Sundsfjord, A., Wasteson, Y., Olsvik, O., Kruse, H., 2000. Continuing high prevalence of VanA-type vancomycin-resistant enterococci on Norwegian poultry farms three years after avoparcin was banned. J. Appl. Microbiol. 89, 478-485.

Borgen, K., Sorum, M., Wasteson, Y., Kruse, H., 2001. VanA-type vancomycin-resistant enterococci (VRE) remain prevalent in poultry carcasses 3 years after avoparcin was banned. Int. J. Food Microbiol. 64, 89-94.

Borgen, K., Sorum, M., Wasteson, Y., Kruse, H., Oppegaard, H., 2002. Genetic linkage between erm(B) and vanA in Enterococcus hirae of poultry origin. Microb. Drug Resist. 8, 363-368.

Borgmann, S., Schulte, B., Wolz, C., Gruber, H., Werner, G., Goerke, C., Klare, I., Beyser, K., Heeg, P., Autenrieth, I.B., 2007. Discrimination between epidemic and non-epidemic glycopeptide-resistant E. faecium in a post-outbreak situation. J. Hosp. Infect. 67, 49-55.

Boumghar-Bourtchai, L., Dhalluin, A., Malbruny, B., Galopin, S., Leclercq, R., 2009. Influence of recombination on development of mutational resistance to linezolid in Enterococcus faecalis JH2-2. Antimicrob. Agents Chemother. AAC-

Bourdon, N., Berenger, R., Lepoultier, R., Mouet, A., Lesteven, C., Borgey, F., Fines-Guyon, M., Leclercq, R., Cattoir, V., 2010. Rapid detection of vancomycin-resistant enterococci from rectal swabs by the Cepheid Xpert vanA/vanB assay. Diagn. Microbiol. Infect. Dis. 67, 291-293.

Bourdon, N., Fines-Guyon, M., Thiolet, J.M., Maugat, S., Coignard, B., Leclercq, R., Cattoir, V., 2011. Changing trends in vancomycin-resistant enterococci in French hospitals, 2001-08. J. Antimicrob. Chemother. 66, 713-721.

Bourgeois-Nicolaos, N., Massias, L., Couson, B., Butel, M.J., Andremont, A., Doucet-
    Populaire, F., 2007. Dose dependence of emergence of resistance to linezolid in
    Enterococcus faecalis in vivo. J Infect Dis 195, 1480-1488.
Boyd, D.A., Cabral, T., Van, C.P., Wylie, J., Mulvey, M.R., 2002. Molecular characterization
    of the vanE gene cluster in vancomycin-resistant Enterococcus faecalis N00-410
    isolated in Canada. Antimicrob. Agents Chemother. 46, 1977-1979.
Boyd, D.A., Conly, J., Dedier, H., Peters, G., Robertson, L., Slater, E., Mulvey, M.R., 2000.
    Molecular characterization of the vanD gene cluster and a novel insertion element
    in a vancomycin-resistant enterococcus isolated in Canada. J. Clin. Microbiol. 38,
    2392-2394.
Boyd, D.A., Du, T., Hizon, R., Kaplen, B., Murphy, T., Tyler, S., Brown, S., Jamieson, F.,
    Weiss, K., Mulvey, M.R., 2006a. VanG-type vancomycin-resistant Enterococcus
    faecalis strains isolated in Canada. Antimicrob. Agents Chemother. 50, 2217-2221.
Boyd, D.A., Kibsey, P., Roscoe, D., Mulvey, M.R., 2004. Enterococcus faecium N03-0072
    carries a new VanD-type vancomycin resistance determinant: characterization of
    the VanD5 operon. J. Antimicrob. Chemother. 54, 680-683.
Boyd, D.A., Miller, M.A., Mulvey, M.R., 2006b. Enterococcus gallinarum N04-0414 harbors a
    VanD-type vancomycin resistance operon and does not contain a D-alanine:D-
    alanine 2 (ddl2) gene. Antimicrob. Agents Chemother. 50, 1067-1070.
Boyd, D.A., Willey, B.M., Fawcett, D., Gillani, N., Mulvey, M.R., 2008. Molecular
    characterization of Enterococcus faecalis N06-0364 with low-level vancomycin
    resistance harboring a novel D-Ala-D-Ser gene cluster, vanL. Antimicrob. Agents
    Chemother. 52, 2667-2672.
Canton, R., Ruiz-Garbajosa, P., Chaves, R.L., Johnson, A.P., 2010. A potential role for
    daptomycin in enterococcal infections: what is the evidence? J. Antimicrob.
    Chemother. 65, 1126-1136.
Carias, L.L., Rudin, S.D., Donskey, C.J., Rice, L.B., 1998. Genetic linkage and cotransfer of a
    novel, vanB-containing transposon (Tn5382) and a low-affinity penicillin-binding
    protein 5 gene in a clinical vancomycin-resistant Enterococcus faecium isolate. J.
    Bacteriol. 180, 4426-4434.
Casadewall, B., Courvalin, P., 1999. Characterization of the vanD Glycopeptide Resistance
    Gene Cluster from Enterococcus faecium BM4339. J. Bacteriol. 181, 3644-3648.
Casetta, A., Hoi, A.B., de, C.G., Horaud, T., 1998. Diversity of structures carrying the high-
    level gentamicin resistance gene (aac6-aph2) in Enterococcus faecalis strains
    isolated in France. Antimicrob. Agents Chemother. 42, 2889-2892.
Cetinkaya, Y., Falk, P., Mayhall, C.G., 2000. Vancomycin-resistant enterococci. Clin.
    Microbiol. Rev. 13, 686-707.
Chang, S., Sievert, D.M., Hageman, J.C., Boulton, M.L., Tenover, F.C., Downes, F.P., Shah, S.,
    Rudrik, J.T., Pupp, G.R., Brown, W.J., Cardo, D., Fridkin, S.K., the Vancomycin-
    Resistant Staphylococcus aureus Investigative Team, 2003. Infection with
    vancomycin-resistant Staphylococcus aureus containing the vanA resistance gene.
    N Engl J Med 348, 1342-1347.
Christiansen, K.J., Tibbett, P.A., Beresford, W., Pearman, J.W., Lee, R.C., Coombs, G.W., Kay,
    I.D., O'Brien, F.G., Palladino, S., Douglas, C.R., Montgomery, P.D., Orrell, T.,
    Peterson, A.M., Kosaras, F.P., Flexman, J.P., Heath, C.H., McCullough, C.A., 2004.
    Eradication of a large outbreak of a single strain of vanB vancomycin-resistant

Enterococcus faecium at a major Australian teaching hospital. Infect. Control Hosp. Epidemiol. 25, 384-390.

Clark, N.C., Weigel, L.M., Patel, J.B., Tenover, F.C., 2005. Comparison of Tn1546-like elements in vancomycin-resistant Staphylococcus aureus isolates from Michigan and Pennsylvania. Antimicrob. Agents Chemother. 49, 470-472.

Coque, T.M., Tomayko, J.F., Ricke, S.C., Okhyusen, P.C., Murray, B.E., 1996. Vancomycin-resistant enterococci from nosocomial, community, and animal sources in the United States. Antimicrob. Agents Chemother. 40, 2605-2609.

Courvalin, P., 2005. Genetics of glycopeptide resistance in gram-positive pathogens. Int. J. Med. Microbiol. 294, 479-486.

Courvalin, P., 2006. Vancomycin resistance in gram-positive cocci. Clin. Infect. Dis. 42 Suppl 1, S25-S34.

Cui, L., Lian, J.Q., Neoh, H.M., Reyes, E., Hiramatsu, K., 2005. DNA microarray-based identification of genes associated with glycopeptide resistance in Staphylococcus aureus. Antimicrob. Agents Chemother. 49, 3404-3413.

Dahl, K.H., Mater, D.D., Flores, M.J., Johnsen, P.J., Midtvedt, T., Corthier, G., Sundsfjord, A., 2007. Transfer of plasmid and chromosomal glycopeptide resistance determinants occurs more readily in the digestive tract of mice than in vitro and exconjugants can persist stably in vivo in the absence of glycopeptide selection. J. Antimicrob. Chemother. 59, 478-486.

Dahl, K.H., Rokenes, T.P., Lundblad, E.W., Sundsfjord, A., 2003. Nonconjugative transposition of the vanB-containing Tn5382-like element in Enterococcus faecium. Antimicrob. Agents Chemother. 47, 786-789.

Dahl, K.H., Sundsfjord, A., 2003. Transferable vanB2 Tn5382-containing elements in fecal streptococcal strains from veal calves. Antimicrob. Agents Chemother. 47, 2579-2583.

David, V., Bozdogan, B., Mainardi, J.L., Legrand, R., Gutmann, L., Leclercq, R., 2004. Mechanism of intrinsic resistance to vancomycin in Clostridium innocuum NCIB 10674. J. Bacteriol. 186, 3415-3422.

de Vries, L.E., Christensen, H., Skov, R.L., Aarestrup, F.M., Agerso, Y., 2009. Diversity of the tetracycline resistance gene tet(M) and identification of Tn916- and Tn5801-like (Tn6014) transposons in Staphylococcus aureus from humans and animals. J. Antimicrob. Chemother. 64, 490-500.

Deghorain, M., Goffin, P., Fontaine, L., Mainardi, J.L., Daniel, R., Errington, J., Hallet, B., Hols, P., 2007. Selectivity for D-lactate incorporation into the peptidoglycan precursors of Lactobacillus plantarum: role of Aad, a VanX-like D-alanyl-D-alanine dipeptidase. J. Bacteriol. 189, 4332-4337.

Depardieu, F., Bonora, M.G., Reynolds, P.E., Courvalin, P., 2003a. The vanG glycopeptide resistance operon from Enterococcus faecalis revisited. Mol. Microbiol. 50, 931-948.

Depardieu, F., Foucault, M.L., Bell, J., Dubouix, A., Guibert, M., Lavigne, J.P., Levast, M., Courvalin, P., 2009. New combinations of mutations in VanD-Type vancomycin-resistant Enterococcus faecium, Enterococcus faecalis, and Enterococcus avium strains. Antimicrob. Agents Chemother. 53, 1952-1963.

Depardieu, F., Reynolds, P.E., Courvalin, P., 2003b. VanD-type vancomycin-resistant Enterococcus faecium 10/96A. Antimicrob. Agents Chemother. 47, 7-18.

Depardieu, F., Kolbert, M., Pruul, H., Bell, J., Courvalin, P., 2004. vanD-Type vancomycin-resistant Enterococcus faecium and Enterococcus faecalis. Antimicrob. Agents Chemother. 48, 3892-3904.

Deplano, A., Denis, O., Nonhoff, C., Rost, F., Byl, B., Jacobs, F., Vankerckhoven, V., Goossens, H., Struelens, M.J., 2007. Outbreak of hospital-adapted clonal complex-17 vancomycin-resistant Enterococcus faecium strain in a haematology unit: role of rapid typing for early control. J. Antimicrob. Chemother. 60, 849-854.

Derbise, A., Aubert, S., El, S.N., 1997. Mapping the regions carrying the three contiguous antibiotic resistance genes aadE, sat4, and aphA-3 in the genomes of staphylococci. Antimicrob. Agents Chemother. 41, 1024-1032.

Derbise, A., Dyke, K.G., El Solh, N., 1996. Characterization of a Staphylococcus aureus transposon, Tn5405, located within Tn5404 and carrying the aminoglycoside resistance genes, aphA-3 and aadE. Plasmid 35, 174-188.

Deshpande, L.M., Fritsche, T.R., Moet, G.J., Biedenbach, D.J., Jones, R.N., 2007. Antimicrobial resistance and molecular epidemiology of vancomycin-resistant enterococci from North America and Europe: a report from the SENTRY antimicrobial surveillance program. Diagn. Microbiol. Infect. Dis. 58, 163-170.

Domingo, M.C., Huletsky, A., Boissinot, M., Bernard, K.A., Picard, F.J., Bergeron, M.G., 2008. Ruminococcus gauvreauii sp. nov., a glycopeptide-resistant species isolated from a human faecal specimen. Int. J. Syst. Evol. Microbiol. 58, 1393-1397.

Domingo, M.C., Huletsky, A., Giroux, R., Boissinot, K., Picard, F.J., Lebel, P., Ferraro, M.J., Bergeron, M.G., 2005. High prevalence of glycopeptide resistance genes vanB, vanD, and vanG not associated with enterococci in human fecal flora. Antimicrob. Agents Chemother. 49, 4784-4786.

Domingo, M.C., Huletsky, A., Giroux, R., Picard, F.J., Bergeron, M.G., 2007. vanD and vanG-Like gene clusters in a Ruminococcus species isolated from human bowel flora. Antimicrob. Agents Chemother. 51, 4111-4117.

Donabedian, S.M., Perri, M.B., Abdujamilova, N., Gordoncillo, M.J., Naqvi, A., Reyes, K.C., Zervos, M.J., Bartlett, P., 2010. Characterization of vancomycin-resistant Enterococcus faecium isolated from swine in three Michigan counties. J. Clin. Microbiol.

Donskey, C.J., 2004. The role of the intestinal tract as a reservoir and source for transmission of nosocomial pathogens. Clin. Infect. Dis. 39, 219-226.

Dutta, I., Reynolds, P.E., 2002. Biochemical and genetic characterization of the vanC-2 vancomycin resistance gene cluster of Enterococcus casseliflavus ATCC 25788. Antimicrob. Agents Chemother. 46, 3125-3132.

EARSS, 2009. EARSS Annual report 2008. EARSS Annual report 2008 10, 1-180.

Facklam, R.R., Carvalho, M.d.G.S., Teixeira, L.M., 2002. History, taxonomy, biochemical characteristics, and antibiotic susceptibility testing of enterococci. In: Gilmore, M.S. (Eds), The enterococci: Pathogenesis, molecular biology, and antibiotic resistance. ASM Press, Washington, D.C., pp. 1-54.

Fang, H., Nord, C.E., Ullberg, M., 2010. Screening for vancomycin-resistant enterococci: results of a survey in Stockholm. APMIS 118, 413-417.

Fines, M., Perichon, B., Reynolds, P., Sahm, D.F., Courvalin, P., 1999. VanE, a new type of acquired glycopeptide resistance in Enterococcus faecalis BM4405. Antimicrob. Agents Chemother. 43, 2161-2164.

Finks, J., Wells, E., Dyke, T.L., Husain, N., Plizga, L., Heddurshetti, R., Wilkins, M., Rudrik, J., Hageman, J., Patel, J., Miller, C., 2009. Vancomycin-resistant Staphylococcus aureus, Michigan, USA, 2007. Emerg. Infect. Dis. 15, 943-945.

Fischer, A., Yang, S.J., Bayer, A.S., Vaezzadeh, A.R., Herzig, S., Stenz, L., Girard, M., Sakoulas, G., Scherl, A., Yeaman, M.R., Proctor, R.A., Schrenzel, J., Francois, P., 2011. Daptomycin resistance mechanisms in clinically derived Staphylococcus aureus strains assessed by a combined transcriptomics and proteomics approach. J. Antimicrob. Chemother. 66, 1696-1711.

Foglia, G., Del, G.M., Vignaroli, C., Bagnarelli, P., Varaldo, P.E., Pantosti, A., Biavasco, F., 2003. Molecular analysis of Tn1546-like elements mediating high-level vancomycin resistance in Enterococcus gallinarum. J. Antimicrob. Chemother. 52, 772-775.

Foucault, M.L., Courvalin, P., Grillot-Courvalin, C., 2009. Fitness cost of VanA-type vancomycin resistance in methicillin-resistant Staphylococcus aureus. Antimicrob. Agents Chemother. 53, 2354-2359.

Foucault, M.L., Depardieu, F., Courvalin, P., Grillot-Courvalin, C., 2010. Inducible expression eliminates the fitness cost of vancomycin resistance in enterococci. Proc. Natl. Acad. Sci. U. S. A 107, 16964-16969.

Fraimow, H., Knob, C., Herrero, I.A., Patel, R., 2005. Putative VanRS-like two-component regulatory system associated with the inducible glycopeptide resistance cluster of Paenibacillus popilliae. Antimicrob. Agents Chemother. 49, 2625-2633.

Freitas, A.R., Coque, T.M., Novais, C., Hammerum, A.M., Lester, C.H., Zervos, M.J., Donabedian, S., Jensen, L.B., Francia, M.V., Baquero, F., Peixe, L., 2011b. Human and swine hosts share vancomycin-resistant Enterococcus faecium CC17 and CC5 and Enterococcus faecalis CC2 clonal clusters harboring Tn1546 on indistinguishable plasmids. J. Clin. Microbiol. 49, 925-931.

Freitas, A.R., Coque, T.M., Novais, C., Hammerum, A.M., Lester, C.H., Zervos, M.J., Donabedian, S., Jensen, L.B., Francia, M.V., Baquero, F., Peixe, L., 2011a. Human and swine hosts share vancomycin-resistant Enterococcus faecium CC17 and CC5 and Enterococcus faecalis CC2 clonal clusters harboring Tn1546 on indistinguishable plasmids. J. Clin. Microbiol. 49, 925-931.

Freitas, A.R., Novais, C., Ruiz-Garbajosa, P., Coque, T.M., Peixe, L., 2009. Clonal expansion within clonal complex 2 and spread of vancomycin-resistant plasmids among different genetic lineages of Enterococcus faecalis from Portugal. J. Antimicrob. Chemother. 63, 1104-1111.

Galloway-Pena, J.R., Nallapareddy, S.R., Arias, C.A., Eliopoulos, G.M., Murray, B.E., 2009. Analysis of clonality and antibiotic resistance among early clinical isolates of Enterococcus faecium in the United States. J. Infect. Dis. 15, 1566-1573.

Galloway-Pena, J.R., Rice, L.B., Murray, B.E., 2011. Analysis of PBP5 of early U.S. isolates of Enterococcus faecium: Sequence variation alone does not explain increasing ampicillin resistance over time. Antimicrob. Agents Chemother. 55, 3272-3277.

Garcia-Migura, L., Hasman, H., Svendsen, C., Jensen, L.B., 2008. Relevance of hot spots in the evolution and transmission of Tn1546 in glycopeptide-resistant Enterococcus faecium (GREF) from broiler origin. J. Antimicrob. Chemother. 62, 681-687.

Garcia-Migura, L., Liebana, E., Jensen, L.B., 2007. Transposon characterization of vancomycin-resistant Enterococcus faecium (VREF) and dissemination of resistance associated with transferable plasmids. J. Antimicrob. Chemother. 60, 263-268.

Gfeller, K.Y., Roth, M., Meile, L., Teuber, M., 2003. Sequence and genetic organization of the 19.3-kb erythromycin- and dalfopristin-resistance plasmid pLME300 from Lactobacillus fermentum ROT1. Plasmid 50, 190-201.

Ghidan, A., Kaszanyitzky, E.J., Dobay, O., Nagy, K., Amyes, S.G., Rozgonyi, F., 2008. Distribution and genetic relatedness of vancomycin-resistant enterococci (VRE) isolated from healthy slaughtered chickens in Hungary from 2001 to 2004. Acta Vet. Hung. 56, 13-25.

Goffin, P., Deghorain, M., Mainardi, J.L., Tytgat, I., Champomier-Verges, M.C., Kleerebezem, M., Hols, P., 2005. Lactate racemization as a rescue pathway for supplying D-lactate to the cell wall biosynthesis machinery in Lactobacillus plantarum. J. Bacteriol. 187, 6750-6761.

Grabsch, E.A., Chua, K., Xie, S., Byrne, J., Ballard, S.A., Ward, P.B., Grayson, M.L., 2008a. Improved detection of vanB2-containing Enterococcus faecium with vancomycin susceptibility by Etest using oxgall supplementation. J. Clin. Microbiol. 46, 1961-1964.

Grabsch, E.A., Ghaly-Derias, S., Gao, W., Howden, B.P., 2008b. Comparative study of selective chromogenic (chromID VRE) and bile esculin agars for isolation and identification of vanB-containing vancomycin-resistant enterococci from feces and rectal swabs. J. Clin. Microbiol. 46, 4034-4036.

Graham, M., Ballard, S.A., Grabsch, E.A., Johnson, P.D.R., Grayson, M.L., 2008. High rates of fecal carriage of nonenterococcal vanB in both children and adults. Antimicrob. Agents Chemother. 52, 1195-1197.

Guardabassi, L., Christensen, H., Hasman, H., Dalsgaard, A., 2004. Members of the genera Paenibacillus and Rhodococcus harbor genes homologous to enterococcal glycopeptide resistance genes vanA and vanB. Antimicrob. Agents Chemother. 48, 4915-4918.

Guardabassi, L., Agerso, Y., 2006. Genes homologous to glycopeptide resistance vanA are widespread in soil microbial communities. FEMS Microbiology Letters 259, 221-225.

Guardabassi, L., Perichon, B., van Heijenoort, J., Blanot, D., Courvalin, P., 2005. Glycopeptide resistance vanA operons in Paenibacillus strains isolated from soil. Antimicrob. Agents Chemother. 49, 4227-4233.

Haenni, M., Saras, E., Chatre, P., Meunier, D., Martin, S., Lepage, G., Menard, M.F., Lebreton, P., Rambaud, T., Madec, J.Y., 2009. vanA in Enterococcus faecium, Enterococcus faecalis, and Enterococcus casseliflavus detected in French cattle. Foodborne. Pathog. Dis. 6, 1107-1111.

Hallgren, A., Saeedi, B., Nilsson, M., Monstein, H.J., Isaksson, B., Hanberger, H., Nilsson, L.E., 2003. Genetic relatedness among Enterococcus faecalis with transposon-mediated high-level gentamicin resistance in Swedish intensive care units. J. Antimicrob. Chemother. 52, 162-167.

Hammerum, A.M., Lester, C.H., Heuer, O.E., 2010. Antimicrobial-resistant enterococci in animals and meat: a human health hazard? Foodborne. Pathog. Dis. 7, 1137-1146.

Hegstad, K., Mikalsen, T., Coque, T.M., Werner, G., Sundsfjord, A., 2010. Mobile genetic elements and their contribution to the emergence of antimicrobial resistant Enterococcus faecalis and Enterococus faecium. Clin. Microbiol. Infect. 16, 541-554.

Heikens, E., van Schaik, W., Leavis, H.L., Bonten, M.J.M., Willems, R.J.L., 2008. Identification of a novel genomic island specific to hospital-acquired clonal complex 17 Enterococcus faecium isolates. Appl. Environ. Microbiol. 74, 7094-7097.

Hendrickx, A.P., Willems, R.J., Bonten, M.J., van, S.W., 2009. LPxTG surface proteins of enterococci. Trends Microbiol. 17, 423-430.

Hendrickx, A.P.A., Bonten, M.J.M., van Luit-Asbroek, M., Schapendonk, C.M.E., Kragten, A.H.M., Willems, R.J.L., 2008. Expression of two distinct types of pili by a hospital-acquired Enterococcus faecium isolate. Microbiology 154, 3212-3223.

Hendrickx, A.P.A., Van Wamel, W.J.B., Posthuma, G., Bonten, M.J.M., Willems, R.J.L., 2007. Five genes encoding surface exposed LPXTG proteins are enriched in hospital-adapted Enterococcus faecium Clonal Complex-17 isolates. J. Bacteriol. 189, 8321-8332.

Hershberger, E., Oprea, S.F., Donabedian, S.M., Perri, M., Bozigar, P., Bartlett, P., Zervos, M.J., 2005. Epidemiology of antimicrobial resistance in enterococci of animal origin. J. Antimicrob. Chemother. 55, 127-130.

Hooper, D.C., 2002. Fluoroquinolone resistance among Gram-positive cocci. The Lancet Infectious Diseases 2, 530-538.

Horinouchi, S., Weisblum, B., 1980. Posttranscriptional modification of mRNA conformation: mechanism that regulates erythromycin-induced resistance. Proc. Natl. Acad. Sci. U. S. A 77, 7079-7083.

Horodniceanu, T., Bougueleret, L., El-Solh, N., Bieth, G., Delbos, F., 1979. High-level, plasmid-borne resistance to gentamicin in Streptococcus faecalis subsp. zymogenes. Antimicrob. Agents Chemother. 16, 686-689.

Howden, B.P., Davies, J.K., Johnson, P.D., Stinear, T.P., Grayson, M.L., 2010. Reduced vancomycin susceptibility in Staphylococcus aureus, including vancomycin-intermediate and heterogeneous vancomycin-intermediate strains: resistance mechanisms, laboratory detection, and clinical implications. Clin. Microbiol. Rev. 23, 99-139.

Hsieh, Y.C., Lee, W.S., Ou, T.Y., Hsueh, P.R., 2010. Clonal spread of CC17 vancomycin-resistant Enterococcus faecium with multilocus sequence type 78 (ST78) and a novel ST444 in Taiwan. Eur. J. Clin. Microbiol. Infect. Dis. 29, 25-30.

Hsieh, Y.C., Ou, T.Y., Teng, S.O., Lee, W.C., Lin, Y.C., Wang, J.T., Chang, S.C., Lee, W.S., 2009. Vancomycin-resistant enterococci in a tertiary teaching hospital in Taiwan. J. Microbiol. Immunol. Infect. 42, 63-68.

Huh, J.Y., Lee, W.G., Lee, K., Shin, W.S., Yoo, J.H., 2004. Distribution of insertion sequences associated with Tn1546-like elements among Enterococcus faecium isolates from patients in Korea. J. Clin. Microbiol. 42, 1897-1902.

Jackson, C.R., Fedorka-Cray, P.J., Barrett, J.B., Ladely, S.R., 2004. Genetic relatedness of high-level aminoglycoside-resistant enterococci isolated from poultry carcasses. Avian Dis. 48, 100-107.

Jackson, C.R., Fedorka-Cray, P.J., Barrett, J.B., Ladely, S.R., 2005. High-level aminoglycoside resistant enterococci isolated from swine. Epidemiol. Infect. 133, 367-371.

Jacob, J., Evers, S., Bischoff, K., Carlier, C., Courvalin, P., 1994. Characterization of the sat4 gene encoding a streptothricin acetyltransferase in Campylobacter coli BE/G4. FEMS Microbiol. Lett. 120, 13-17.

Jacoby, G.A., 2005. Mechanisms of resistance to quinolones. Clin. Infect. Dis. 41 Suppl 2, S120-S126.

Jasni, A.S., Mullany, P., Hussain, H., Roberts, A.P., 2010. Demonstration of conjugative transposon (Tn5397)-mediated horizontal gene transfer between Clostridium difficile and Enterococcus faecalis. Antimicrob. Agents Chemother. 54, 4924-4926.

Jensen, L.B., Ahrens, P., Dons, L., Jones, R.N., Hammerum, A.M., Aarestrup, F.M., 1998. Molecular analysis of Tn1546 in Enterococcus faecium isolated from animals and humans. J. Clin. Microbiol. 36, 437-442.

Johnson, P.D., Ballard, S.A., Grabsch, E.A., Stinear, T.P., Seemann, T., Young, H.L., Grayson, M.L., Howden, B.P., 2010. A sustained hospital outbreak of vancomycin-resistant Enterococcus faecium bacteremia due to emergence of vanB E. faecium sequence type 203. J. Infect. Dis. 202, 1278-1286.

Jones, R.N., Deshpande, L.M., 2004. Are Enterococcus faecalis strains with vat(E) in poultry a reservoir for human streptogramin resistance? vat(E) occurrence in human enterococcal bloodstream infections in North America (SENTRY Antimicrobial Surveillance Program, 2002). Antimicrob. Agents Chemother. 48, 360-361.

Jung, W.K., Lim, J.Y., Kwon, N.H., Kim, J.M., Hong, S.K., Koo, H.C., Kim, S.H., Park, Y.H., 2007. Vancomycin-resistant enterococci from animal sources in Korea. Int. J. Food Microbiol. 113, 102-107.

Jung, Y.H., Shin, E.S., Kim, O., Yoo, J.S., Lee, K.M., Yoo, J.I., Chung, G.T., Lee, Y.S., 2010. Characterization of two newly identified genes, vgaD and vatG, conferring resistance to streptogramin A in Enterococcus faecium. Antimicrob. Agents Chemother. 54, 4744-4749.

JUREEN, R., MOHN, S.C., Harthug, S., HAARR, L., LANGELAND, N., 2004. Role of penicillin-binding protein 5 C-terminal amino acid substitutions in conferring ampicillin resistance in Norwegian clinical strains of Enterococcus faecium. APMIS 112, 291-298.

Karlowsky, J.A., Jones, M.E., Draghi, D.C., Thornsberry, C., Sahm, D.F., Volturo, G.A., 2004. Prevalence and antimicrobial susceptibilities of bacteria isolated from blood cultures of hospitalized patients in the United States in 2002. Ann. Clin. Microbiol. Antimicrob. 3, 7-

Karlowsky, J.A., Zhanel, G.G., Hoban, D.J., 1999. Vancomycin-resistant enterococci (VRE) colonization of high-risk patients in tertiary care Canadian hospitals. Canadian VRE Surveillance Group. Diagn. Microbiol. Infect. Dis. 35, 1-7.

Kawalec, M., Gniadkowski, M., Kedzierska, J., Skotnicki, A., Fiett, J., Hryniewicz, W., 2001b. Selection of a teicoplanin-resistant Enterococcus faecium mutant during an outbreak caused by vancomycin-resistant enterococci with the vanB phenotype. J. Clin. Microbiol. 39, 4274-4282.

Kawalec, M., Gniadkowski, M., Kedzierska, J., Skotnicki, A., Fiett, J., Hryniewicz, W., 2001a. Selection of a teicoplanin-resistant Enterococcus faecium mutant during an outbreak caused by vancomycin-resistant enterococci with the vanB phenotype. J. Clin. Microbiol. 39, 4274-4282.

Kawalec, M., Kedzierska, J., Gajda, A., Sadowy, E., Wegrzyn, J., Naser, S., Skotnicki, A.B., Gniadkowski, M., Hryniewicz, W., 2007. Hospital outbreak of vancomycin-resistant enterococci caused by a single clone of Enterococcus raffinosus and several clones of Enterococcus faecium. Clinical Microbiology and Infection 13, 893-901.

Kerr, I.D., Reynolds, E.D., Cove, J.H., 2005. ABC proteins and antibiotic drug resistance: is it all about transport? Biochem. Soc. Trans. 33, 1000-1002.

Klare, I., Badstubner, D., Konstabel, C., Bohme, G., Claus, H., Witte, W., 1999. Decreased incidence of VanA-type vancomycin-resistant enterococci isolated from poultry meat and from fecal samples of humans in the community after discontinuation of avoparcin usage in animal husbandry. Microb. Drug Resist. 5, 45-52.

Klare, I., Heier, H., Claus, H., Bohme, G., Marin, S., Seltmann, G., Hakenbeck, R., Antanassova, V., Witte, W., 1995a. Enterococcus faecium strains with vanA-mediated high-level glycopeptide resistance isolated from animal foodstuffs and fecal samples of humans in the community. Microb. Drug Resist. 1, 265-272.

Klare, I., Heier, H., Claus, H., Reissbrodt, R., Witte, W., 1995b. vanA-mediated high-level glycopeptide resistance in Enterococcus faecium from animal husbandry. FEMS Microbiol. Lett. 125, 165-171.

Klare, I., Heier, H., Claus, H., Witte, W., 1993. Environmental strains of Enterococcus faecium with inducible high-level resistance to glycopeptides. FEMS Microbiol. Lett. 106, 23-29.

Klare, I., Konstabel, C., Badstübner, D., Werner, G., Witte, W., 2003. Occurrence and spread of antibiotic resistances in Enterococcus faecium. Int. J. Food Microbiol. 88, 269-290.

Klare, I., Konstabel, C., Mueller-Bertling, S., Werner, G., Strommenger, B., Kettlitz, C., Borgmann, S., Schulte, B., Jonas, D., Serr, A., Fahr, A., Eigner, U., Witte, W., 2005. Spread of ampicillin/vancomycin-resistant Enterococcus faecium of the epidemic-virulent clonal complex-17 carrying the genes esp and hyl in German hospitals. European Journal of Clinical Microbiology & Infectious Diseases 24, 815-825.

Klare, I., Werner, G., Witte, W., 2010. Enterococci with vancomycin resistance from German hospitals in 2008/2009 (German). Epidemiologisches Bulletin 2010, 427-437.

Klare, I., Witte, W., 1998. VRE: animal reservoirs and food. In: Brun-Buisson, C., Eliopoulos, G.M., Leclercq, R. (Eds), Bacterial resistance to glycopeptides. Flammarion Médecine-Sciences, Paris, pp. 83-93.

Klein, G., Pack, A., Reuter, G., 1998. Antibiotic resistance patterns of enterococci and occurrence of vancomycin-resistant enterococci in raw minced beef and pork in Germany. Appl. Environ. Microbiol. 64, 1825-1830.

Ko, K.S., Baek, J.Y., Lee, J.Y., Oh, W.S., Peck, K.R., Lee, N., Lee, W.G., Lee, K., Song, J.H., 2005. Molecular characterization of vancomycin-resistant Enterococcus faecium isolates from Korea. J. Clin. Microbiol. 43, 2303-2306.

Koh, T.H., Hsu, L.Y., Chiu, L.L., Lin, R.V.T.P., 2006. Emergence of epidemic clones of vancomycin-resistant Enterococcus faecium in Singapore. Journal of Hospital Infection 63, 234-236.

Koh, T.H., Low, B.S., Leo, N., Hsu, L.Y., Lin, R.T., Krishnan, P., Chan, D., Nadarajah, M., Toh, S.L., Ong, K.H., 2009. Molecular epidemiology of vancomycin-resistant enterococci in Singapore. Pathology 41, 676-680.

Kojima, A., Morioka, A., Kijima, M., Ishihara, K., Asai, T., Fujisawa, T., Tamura, Y., Takahashi, T., 2010. Classification and antimicrobial susceptibilities of enterococcus species isolated from apparently healthy food-producing animals in Japan. Zoonoses. Public Health 57, 137-141.

Kruse, H., Johansen, B.K., Rorvik, L.M., Schaller, G., 1999. The use of avoparcin as a growth promoter and the occurrence of vancomycin-resistant Enterococcus species in Norwegian poultry and swine production. Microb. Drug Resist. 5, 135-139.

Kuzin, A.P., Sun, T., Jorczak-Baillass, J., Healy, V.L., Walsh, C.T., Knox, J.R., 2000. Enzymes of vancomycin resistance: the structure of D-alanine-D-lactate ligase of naturally resistant Leuconostoc mesenteroides. Structure. 8, 463-470.

Kwong, S.M., Lim, R., Lebard, R.J., Skurray, R.A., Firth, N., 2008. Analysis of the pSK1 replicon, a prototype from the staphylococcal multiresistance plasmid family. Microbiology 154, 3084-3094.

Larsen, J., Schonheyder, H.C., Lester, C.H., Olsen, S.S., Porsbo, L.J., Garcia-Migura, L., Jensen, L.B., Bisgaard, M., Hammerum, A.M., 2010. Porcine-origin gentamicin-resistant Enterococcus faecalis in Humans, Denmark. Emerg. Infect. Dis. 16, 682-684.

Lauderdale, T.L., Shiau, Y.R., Wang, H.Y., Lai, J.F., Huang, I.W., Chen, P.C., Chen, H.Y., Lai, S.S., Liu, Y.F., Ho, M., 2007. Effect of banning vancomycin analogue avoparcin on vancomycin-resistant enterococci in chicken farms in Taiwan. Environmental Microbiology 9, 819-823.

Launay, A., Ballard, S.A., Johnson, P.D.R., Grayson, M.L., Lambert, T., 2006. Transfer of vancomycin resistance transposon Tn1549 from Clostridium symbiosum to Enterococcus spp. in the gut of gnotobiotic mice. Antimicrob. Agents Chemother. 50, 1054-1062.

Laverde Gomez, J.A., van, S.W., Freitas, A.R., Coque, T.M., Weaver, K.E., Francia, M.V., Witte, W., Werner, G., 2010. A multiresistance megaplasmid pLG1 bearing a hyl(Efm) genomic island in hospital Enterococcus faecium isolates. Int. J. Med. Microbiol.

Laverde Gomez, J.A., van, S.W., Freitas, A.R., Coque, T.M., Weaver, K.E., Francia, M.V., Witte, W., Werner, G., 2011. A multiresistance megaplasmid pLG1 bearing a hylEfm genomic island in hospital Enterococcus faecium isolates. Int. J. Med. Microbiol. 301, 165-175.

Leavis, H.L., Willems, R.J., van Wamel, W.J., Schuren, F.H., Caspers, M.P., Bonten, M.J., 2007. Insertion sequence-driven diversification creates a globally dispersed emerging multiresistant subspecies of E. faecium. PLoS. Pathog. 3, e7-75.

Leavis, H.L., Willems, R.J.L., Top, J., Bonten, M.J.M., 2006. High-Level ciprofloxacin resistance from point mutations in gyrA and parC confined to global hospital-adapted clonal lineage CC17 of Enterococcus faecium. J. Clin. Microbiol. 44, 1059-1064.

Leclercq, R., Derlot, E., Duval, J., Courvalin, P., 1988. Plasmid-mediated resistance to vancomycin and teicoplanin in Enterococcus faecium. N. Engl. J. Med. 319, 157-161.

Leclercq, R., Derlot, E., Weber, M., Duval, J., Courvalin, P., 1989. Transferable vancomycin and teicoplanin resistance in Enterococcus faecium. Antimicrob. Agents Chemother. 33, 10-15.

Lee, S.Y., Park, K.G., Lee, G.D., Park, J.J., Park, Y.J., 2010. Comparison of Seeplex VRE detection kit with ChromID VRE agar for detection of vancomycin-resistant enterococci in rectal swab specimens. Ann. Clin. Lab Sci. 40, 163-166.

Lester, C.H., Hammerum, A.M., 2010. Transfer of vanA from an Enterococcus faecium isolate of chicken origin to a CC17 E. faecium isolate in the intestine of cephalosporin-treated mice. J. Antimicrob. Chemother. 65, 1534-1536.

Lester, C.H., Olsen, S.S., Schonheyder, H.C., Hansen, D.S., Tvede, M., Holm, A., Arpi, M., Friis-Moller, A., Jensen, K.T., Kemp, M., Hammerum, A.M., 2009. Typing of vancomycin-resistant enterococci obtained from patients at Danish hospitals and detection of a genomic island specific to CC17 Enterococcus faecium. Int. J. Antimicrob. Agents 35, 312-314.

Lester, C.H., Sandvang, D., Olsen, S.S., Schonheyder, H.C., Jarlov, J.O., Bangsborg, J., Hansen, D.S., Jensen, T.G., Frimodt-Moller, N., Hammerum, A.M., 2008. Emergence of ampicillin-resistant Enterococcus faecium in Danish hospitals. J. Antimicrob. Chemother. 62, 1203-1206.

Lester, C.H., Frimodt-Moller, N., Sorensen, T.L., Monnet, D.L., Hammerum, A.M., 2006. In vivo transfer of the vanA resistance gene from an Enterococcus faecium isolate of animal origin to an E. faecium isolate of human origin in the intestines of human volunteers. Antimicrob. Agents Chemother. 50, 596-599.

Lim, S.K., Kim, T.S., Lee, H.S., Nam, H.M., Joo, Y.S., Koh, H.B., 2006. Persistence of vanA-type Enterococcus faecium in Korean livestock after ban on avoparcin. Microbial Drug Resistance 12, 136-139.

Lobritz, M., Hutton-Thomas, R., Marshall, S., Rice, L.B., 2003. Recombination proficiency influences frequency and locus of mutational resistance to linezolid in Enterococcus faecalis. Antimicrob. Agents Chemother. 47, 3318-3320.

Lopez, M., Hormazabal, J.C., Maldonado, A., Saavedra, G., Baquero, F., Silva, J., Torres, C., Del, C.R., 2009. Clonal dissemination of Enterococcus faecalis ST201 and Enterococcus faecium CC17-ST64 containing Tn5382-vanB2 among 16 hospitals in Chile. Clin. Microbiol. Infect. 15, 586-588.

Mahbub, A.M., Kobayashi, N., Ishino, M., Sumi, A., Kobayashi, K., Uehara, N., Watanabe, N., 2005. Detection of a novel aph(2") allele (aph[2"]-Ie) conferring high-level gentamicin resistance and a spectinomycin resistance gene ant(9)-Ia (aad 9) in clinical isolates of enterococci. Microb. Drug Resist. 11, 239-247.

Mak, A., Miller, M.A., Chong, G., Monczak, Y., 2009. Comparison of PCR and culture for screening of vancomycin-resistant Enterococci: highly disparate results for vanA and vanB. J. Clin. Microbiol. 47, 4136-4137.

Mammina, C., Di Noto, A.M., Costa, A., Nastasi, A., 2005. VanB-VanC1 Enterococcus gallinarum, Italy. Emerg. Infect. Dis. 11, 1491-1492.

Manson, J.M., Keis, S., Smith, J.M., Cook, G.M., 2003a. Characterization of a vancomycin-resistant Enterococcus faecalis (VREF) isolate from a dog with mastitis: further evidence of a clonal lineage of VREF in New Zealand. J. Clin. Microbiol. 41, 3331-3333.

Manson, J.M., Smith, J.M., Cook, G.M., 2004. Persistence of vancomycin-resistant enterococci in New Zealand broilers after discontinuation of avoparcin use. Appl. Environ. Microbiol. 70, 5764-5768.

Manson, J.M., Keis, S., Smith, J.M.B., Cook, G.M., 2003b. A clonal lineage of VanA-type Enterococcus faecalis predominates in vancomycin-resistant enterococci isolated in New Zealand. Antimicrob. Agents Chemother. 47, 204-210.

Marner, E.S., Wolk, D.M., Carr, J., Hewitt, C., Dominguez, L.L., Kovacs, T., Johnson, D.R., Hayden, R.T., 2011. Diagnostic accuracy of the Cepheid GeneXpert vanA/vanB assay ver. 1.0 to detect the vanA and vanB vancomycin resistance genes in Enterococcus from perianal specimens. Diagn. Microbiol. Infect. Dis. 69, 382-389.

Marshall, C.G., Broadhead, G., Leskiw, B.K., Wright, G.D., 1997. D-Ala-D-Ala ligases from glycopeptide antibiotic-producing organisms are highly homologous to the enterococcal vancomycin-resistance ligases VanA and VanB. Proc. Natl. Acad. Sci. U. S. A 94, 6480-6483.

Marshall, C.G., Lessard, I.A., Park, I., Wright, G.D., 1998. Glycopeptide antibiotic resistance genes in glycopeptide-producing organisms. Antimicrob. Agents Chemother. 42, 2215-2220.

Marshall, S.H., Donskey, C.J., Hutton-Thomas, R., Salata, R.A., Rice, L.B., 2002. Gene dosage and linezolid resistance in Enterococcus faecium and Enterococcus faecalis. Antimicrob. Agents Chemother. 46, 3334-3336.

Martel, A., Devriese, L.A., Decostere, A., Haesebrouck, F., 2003. Presence of macrolide resistance genes in streptococci and enterococci isolated from pigs and pork carcasses. Int. J. Food Microbiol. 84, 27-32.

Martone, W.J., 1998. Spread of vancomycin-resistant enterococci: why did it happen in the United States? Infect. Control Hosp. Epidemiol. 19, 539-545.

McBride, S.M., Fischetti, V.A., Leblanc, D.J., Moellering, R.C., Jr., Gilmore, M.S., 2007. Genetic diversity among Enterococcus faecalis. PLoS. ONE. 2, e582-

McDonald, L.C., Kuehnert, M.J., Tenover, F.C., Jarvis, W.R., 1997. Vancomycin-resistant enterococci outside the health-care setting: prevalence, sources, and public health implications. Emerg. Infect. Dis. 3, 311-317.

McKessar, S.J., Berry, A.M., Bell, J.M., Turnidge, J.D., Paton, J.C., 2000. Genetic characterization of vanG, a novel vancomycin resistance locus of Enterococcus faecalis. Antimicrob. Agents Chemother. 44, 3224-3228.

Mevius, D., Devriese, L., Butaye, P., Vandamme, P., Verschure, M., Veldman, K., 1998. Isolation of glycopeptide resistant Streptococcus gallolyticus strains with vanA, vanB, and both vanA and vanB genotypes from faecal samples of veal calves in The Netherlands. J. Antimicrob. Chemother. 42, 275-276.

Meziane-Cherif, D., Saul, F.A., Moubareck, C., Weber, P., Haouz, A., Courvalin, P., Perichon, B., 2010. Molecular basis of vancomycin dependence in VanA-type Staphylococcus aureus VRSA-9. J. Bacteriol. 192, 5465-5471.

Min, Y.H., Kwon, A.R., Yoon, J.M., Yoon, E.J., Shim, M.J., Choi, E.C., 2008. Molecular analysis of constitutive mutations in ermB and ermA selected in vitro from inducibly MLSB-resistant enterococci. Arch. Pharm. Res. 31, 377-380.

Moore, I.F., Hughes, D.W., Wright, G.D., 2005. Tigecycline is modified by the flavin-dependent monooxygenase TetX. Biochemistry 44, 11829-11835.

Morris-Downes, M., Smyth, E.G., Moore, J., Thomas, T., Fitzpatrick, F., Walsh, J., Caffrey, V., Morris, A., Foley, S., Humphreys, H., 2010. Surveillance and endemic vancomycin-resistant enterococci: some success in control is possible. J. Hosp. Infect. 75, 228-233.

Moubareck, C., Bourgeois, N., Courvalin, P., Doucet-Populaire, F., 2003. Multiple antibiotic resistance gene transfer from animal to human enterococci in the digestive tract of gnotobiotic mice. Antimicrob. Agents Chemother. 47, 2993-2996.

Moubareck, C., Meziane-Cherif, D., Courvalin, P., Perichon, B., 2009. VanA-type Staphylococcus aureus strain VRSA-7 is partially dependent on vancomycin for growth. Antimicrob. Agents Chemother. 53, 3657-3663.

Murray, B.E., 1990. The life and times of the Enterococcus. Clin. Microbiol. Rev. 3, 46-65.

Murray, B.E., 2000. Vancomycin-resistant enterococcal infections. N. Engl. J. Med. 342, 710-721.

Nallapareddy, S.R., Singh, K.V., Okhuysen, P.C., Murray, B.E., 2008. A functional collagen adhesin gene, acm, in clinical isolates of Enterococcus faecium correlates with the recent success of this emerging nosocomial pathogen. Infect. Immun. 76, 4110-4119.

Nallapareddy, S.R., Wenxiang, H., Weinstock, G.M., Murray, B.E., 2005. Molecular characterization of a widespread, pathogenic, and antibiotic resistance-receptive Enterococcus faecalis lineage and dissemination of its putative pathogenicity island. J. Bacteriol. 187, 5709-5718.

Nannini, E., Murray, B.E., Arias, C.A., 2010. Resistance or decreased susceptibility to glycopeptides, daptomycin, and linezolid in methicillin-resistant Staphylococcus aureus. Curr. Opin. Pharmacol. 10, 516-521.

Naser, S.M., Vancanneyt, M., Hoste, B., Snauwaert, C., Vandemeulebroecke, K., Swings, J., 2006b. Reclassification of Enterococcus flavescens Pompei et al. 1992 as a later synonym of Enterococcus casseliflavus (ex Vaughan et al. 1979) Collins et al. 1984 and Enterococcus saccharominimus Vancanneyt et al. 2004 as a later synonym of Enterococcus italicus Fortina et al. 2004. Int. J. Syst. Evol. Microbiol. 56, 413-416.

Naser, S.M., Vancanneyt, M., Hoste, B., Snauwaert, C., Vandemeulebroecke, K., Swings, J., 2006a. Reclassification of Enterococcus flavescens Pompei et al. 1992 as a later synonym of Enterococcus casseliflavus (ex Vaughan et al. 1979) Collins et al. 1984 and Enterococcus saccharominimus Vancanneyt et al. 2004 as a later synonym of Enterococcus italicus Fortina et al. 2004. Int. J. Syst. Evol. Microbiol. 56, 413-416.

Neves, F.P., Ribeiro, R.L., Duarte, R.S., Teixeira, L.M., Merquior, V.L., 2009. Emergence of the vanA genotype among Enterococcus gallinarum isolates colonising the intestinal tract of patients in a university hospital in Rio de Janeiro, Brazil. Int. J. Antimicrob. Agents 33, 211-215.

Nichol, K.A., Sill, M., Laing, N.M., Johnson, J.L., Hoban, D.J., Zhanel, G.G., 2006. Molecular epidemiology of urinary tract isolates of vancomycin-resistant Enterococcus faecium from North America. International Journal of Antimicrobial Agents 27, 392-396.

Nilsson, O., Greko, C., Bengtsson, B., 2009a. Environmental contamination by vancomycin resistant enterococci (VRE) in Swedish broiler production. Acta Vet. Scand. 51, 49-

Nilsson, O., Greko, C., Top, J., Franklin, A., Bengtsson, B., 2009b. Spread without known selective pressure of a vancomycin-resistant clone of Enterococcus faecium among broilers. J. Antimicrob. Chemother. 63, 868-872.

Noble, W.C., Virani, Z., Cree, R.G., 1992. Co-transfer of vancomycin and other resistance genes from Enterococcus faecalis NCTC 12201 to Staphylococcus aureus. FEMS Microbiol. Lett. 72, 195-198.

Novais, C., Freitas, A.R., Sousa, J.C., Baquero, F., Coque, T.M., Peixe, L.V., 2008. Diversity of Tn1546 and its role in the dissemination of vancomycin-resistant enterococci in Portugal. Antimicrob. Agents Chemother. 52, 1001-1008.

Novick, R.P., Murphy, E., 1985. MLS-resistance determinants in Staphylococcus aureus and their molecular evolution. J. Antimicrob. Chemother. 16 Suppl A, 101-110.

Onodera, Y., Okuda, J., Tanaka, M., Sato, K., 2002. Inhibitory activities of quinolones against DNA gyrase and topoisomerase IV of Enterococcus faecalis. Antimicrob. Agents Chemother. 46, 1800-1804.

Oteo, J., Cuevas, O., Navarro, C., Aracil, B., Campos, J., on behalf of the Spanish Group of 'The European Antimicrobial Resistance Surveillance System' (EARSS), 2007. Trends in antimicrobial resistance in 3469 enterococci isolated from blood (EARSS experience 2001-06, Spain): increasing ampicillin resistance in Enterococcus faecium. J. Antimicrob. Chemother. 59, 1044-1045.

Oyamada, Y., Ito, H., Fujimoto, K., Asada, R., Niga, T., Okamoto, R., Inoue, M., Yamagishi, J.i., 2006a. Combination of known and unknown mechanisms confers high-level resistance to fluoroquinolones in Enterococcus faecium. J Med Microbiol 55, 729-736.

Oyamada, Y., Ito, H., Inoue, M., Yamagishi, J.i., 2006b. Topoisomerase mutations and efflux are associated with fluoroquinolone resistance in Enterococcus faecalis. J Med Microbiol 55, 1395-1401.

Padiglione, A.A., Grabsch, E.A., Olden, D., Hellard, M., Sinclair, M.I., Fairley, C.K., Grayson, M.L., 2000. Fecal colonization with vancomycin-resistant enterococci in Australia. Emerg. Infect. Dis. 6, 534-536.

Pai, M.P., Rodvold, K.A., Schreckenberger, P.C., Gonzales, R.D., Petrolatti, J.M., Quinn, J.P., 2002. Risk factors associated with the development of infection with linezolid- and vancomycin-resistant Enterococcus faecium. Clin. Infect. Dis. 35, 1269-1272.

Palmer, K.L., Carniol, K., Manson, J.M., Heiman, D., Shea, T., Young, S., Zeng, Q., Gevers, D., Feldgarden, M., Birren, B., Gilmore, M.S., 2010. High-quality draft genome sequences of 28 Enterococcus sp. isolates. J. Bacteriol. 192, 2469-2470.

Panesso, D., badia-Patino, L., Vanegas, N., Reynolds, P.E., Courvalin, P., Arias, C.A., 2005. Transcriptional analysis of the vanC cluster from Enterococcus gallinarum strains with constitutive and inducible vancomycin resistance. Antimicrob. Agents Chemother. 49, 1060-1066.

Panesso, D., Reyes, J., Rincon, S., Diaz, L., Galloway-Pena, J., Zurita, J., Carrillo, C., Merentes, A., Guzman, M., Adachi, J.A., Murray, B.E., Arias, C.A., 2010. Molecular epidemiology of vancomycin-resistant Enterococcus faecium: a prospective, multicenter study in South American hospitals. J. Clin. Microbiol. 48, 1562-1569.

Park, I.J., Lee, W.G., Lim, Y.A., Cho, S.R., 2007. Genetic rearrangements of Tn1546-like elements in vancomycin-resistant Enterococcus faecium isolates collected from hospitalized patients over a seven-year period. J. Clin. Microbiol. 45, 3903-3908.

Park, I.J., Lee, W.G., Shin, J.H., Lee, K.W., Woo, G.J., 2008. VanB phenotype-vanA genotype Enterococcus faecium with heterogeneous expression of teicoplanin resistance. J. Clin. Microbiol. 46, 3091-3093.

Patel, R., 2000. Enterococcal-type glycopeptide resistance genes in non-enterococcal organisms. FEMS Microbiol. Lett. 185, 1-7.

Patel, R., Piper, K., Cockerill, F.R., III, Steckelberg, J.M., Yousten, A.A., 2000. The biopesticide Paenibacillus popilliae has a vancomycin resistance gene cluster homologous to the enterococcal VanA vancomycin resistance gene cluster. Antimicrob. Agents Chemother. 44, 705-709.

Paulsen, I.T., Banerjei, L., Myers, G.S., Nelson, K.E., Seshadri, R., Read, T.D., Fouts, D.E., Eisen, J.A., Gill, S.R., Heidelberg, J.F., Tettelin, H., Dodson, R.J., Umayam, L., Brinkac, L., Beanan, M., Daugherty, S., DeBoy, R.T., Durkin, S., Kolonay, J., Madupu, R., Nelson, W., Vamathevan, J., Tran, B., Upton, J., Hansen, T., Shetty, J., Khouri, H., Utterback, T., Radune, D., Ketchum, K.A., Dougherty, B.A., Fraser, C.M., 2003. Role of mobile DNA in the evolution of vancomycin-resistant Enterococcus faecalis. Science 299, 2071-2074.

Pearman, J.W., 2006. 2004 Lowbury Lecture: the Western Australian experience with vancomycin-resistant enterococci - from disaster to ongoing control. Journal of Hospital Infection 63, 14-26.

Pendle, S., Jelfs, P., Olma, T., Su, Y., Gilroy, N., Gilbert, G.L., 2008. Difficulties in detection and identification of Enterococcus faecium with low-level inducible resistance to vancomycin, during a hospital outbreak. Clin. Microbiol. Infect. 14, 853-857.

Perichon, B., Courvalin, P., 2004. Heterologous expression of the enterococcal vanA operon in methicillin-resistant Staphylococcus aureus. Antimicrob. Agents Chemother. 48, 4281-4285.

Perichon, B., Courvalin, P., 2006. Synergism between beta-lactams and glycopeptides against VanA-type Methicillin-Resistant Staphylococcus aureus and heterologous expression of the vanA operon. Antimicrob. Agents Chemother. 50, 3622-3630.

Poole, T.L., Hume, M.E., Campbell, L.D., Scott, H.M., Alali, W.Q., Harvey, R.B., 2005. Vancomycin-resistant Enterococcus faecium strains isolated from community wastewater from a semiclosed agri-food system in Texas. Antimicrob. Agents Chemother. 49, 4382-4385.

Poyart, C., Pierre, C., Quesne, G., Pron, B., Berche, P., Trieu-Cuot, P., 1997. Emergence of vancomycin resistance in the genus Streptococcus: characterization of a vanB transferable determinant in Streptococcus bovis. Antimicrob. Agents Chemother. 41, 24-29.

Prystowsky, J., Siddiqui, F., Chosay, J., Shinabarger, D.L., Millichap, J., Peterson, L.R., Noskin, G.A., 2001. Resistance to linezolid: characterization of mutations in rRNA and comparison of their occurrences in vancomycin-resistant enterococci. Antimicrob. Agents Chemother. 45, 2154-2156.

Qi, C., Zheng, X., Obias, A., Scheetz, M.H., Malczynski, M., Warren, J.R., 2006. Comparison of testing methods for detection of decreased linezolid susceptibility due to G2576T mutation of the 23S rRNA gene in Enterococcus faecium and Enterococcus faecalis. J. Clin. Microbiol. 44, 1098-1100.

Quinones Perez, D., 2006. Epidemiology of antimicrobial resistance in Enterococcus spp. from Cuba and other Latin American countries. In: Kobayashi, N. (Eds), Drug resistance of enterococci: Epidemiology and molecular mechanisms. Research Signpost, Kerala, India, pp. 1-20.

Rahim, S., Pillai, S.K., Gold, H.S., Venkataraman, L., Inglima, K., Press, R.A., 2003. Linezolid-resistant, vancomycin-resistant Enterococcus faecium infection in patients without prior exposure to linezolid. Clin. Infect. Dis. 36, E146-E148.

Ramsey, A.M., Zilberberg, M.D., 2009. Secular trends of hospitalization with vancomycin-resistant enterococcus infection in the United States, 2000-2006. Infect. Control Hosp. Epidemiol. 30, 184-186.

Reynolds, E., Cove, J.H., 2005. Enhanced resistance to erythromycin is conferred by the enterococcal msrC determinant in Staphylococcus aureus. J. Antimicrob. Chemother. 55, 260-264.

Reynolds, E., Ross, J.I., Cove, J.H., 2003. Msr(A) and related macrolide/streptogramin resistance determinants: incomplete transporters? Int. J. Antimicrob. Agents 22, 228-236.

Reynolds, P.E., Arias, C.A., Courvalin, P., 1999. Gene vanXYC encodes D,D -dipeptidase (VanX) and D,D-carboxypeptidase (VanY) activities in vancomycin-resistant Enterococcus gallinarum BM4174. Mol. Microbiol. 34, 341-349.

Reynolds, P.E., Courvalin, P., 2005. Vancomycin resistance in enterococci due to synthesis of precursors terminating in D-alanyl-D-serine. Antimicrob. Agents Chemother. 49, 21-25.

Rice, L.B., 2006. Antimicrobial resistance in gram-positive bacteria. Am. J. Infect. Control 34, S11-S19.

Rice, L.B., Carias, L.L., Donskey, C.L., Rudin, S.D., 1998. Transferable, plasmid-mediated vanB-type glycopeptide resistance in Enterococcus faecium. Antimicrob. Agents Chemother. 42, 963-964.

Rice, L.B., Carias, L.L., Marshall, S., Rudin, S.D., Hutton-Thomas, R., 2005. Tn5386, a novel Tn916-like mobile element in Enterococcus faecium D344R that interacts with Tn916 to yield a large genomic deletion. J. Bacteriol. 187, 6668-6677.

Rice, L.B., Carias, L.L., Marshall, S.H., Hutton-Thomas, R., Rudin, S., 2007. Characterization of Tn5386, a Tn916-related mobile element. Plasmid 58, 61-67.

Rice, L.B., Carias, L.L., Rudin, S., Hutton, R., Marshall, S., Hassan, M., Josseaume, N., Dubost, L., Marie, A., Arthur, M., 2009. Role of class A penicillin-binding proteins in the expression of beta-lactam resistance in Enterococcus faecium. J. Bacteriol. 191, 3649-3656.

Rice, L.B., Carias, L.L., Rudin, S., Hutton, R.A., Marshall, S., 2010. Multiple copies of functional, Tet(M)-encoding Tn916-like elements in a clinical Enterococcus faecium isolate. Plasmid

Rice, L.B., Bellais, S., Carias, L.L., Hutton-Thomas, R., Bonomo, R.A., Caspers, P., Page, M.G.P., Gutmann, L., 2004. Impact of specific pbp5 mutations on expression of {beta}-lactam resistance in Enterococcus faecium. Antimicrob. Agents Chemother. 48, 3028-3032.

Roberts, A.P., Johanesen, P.A., Lyras, D., Mullany, P., Rood, J.I., 2001. Comparison of Tn5397 from Clostridium difficile, Tn916 from Enterococcus faecalis and the CW459tet(M) element from Clostridium perfringens shows that they have similar conjugation regions but different insertion and excision modules. Microbiology 147, 1243-1251.

Roberts, A.P., Mullany, P., 2009. A modular master on the move: the Tn916 family of mobile genetic elements. Trends Microbiol. 17, 251-258.

Roberts, A.P., Mullany, P., 2011. Tn916-like genetic elements: a diverse group of modular mobile elements conferring antibiotic resistance. FEMS Microbiol. Rev.

Roberts, M.C., 2005. Update on acquired tetracycline resistance genes. FEMS Microbiol. Lett. 245, 195-203.

Roberts, M.C., Sutcliffe, J., Courvalin, P., Jensen, L.B., Rood, J., Seppala, H., 1999. Nomenclature for macrolide and macrolide-lincosamide-streptogramin B resistance determinants. Antimicrob. Agents Chemother. 43, 2823-2830.

Rodriguez-Martinez, J.M., Velasco, C., Briales, A., Garcia, I., Conejo, M.C., Pascual, A., 2008. Qnr-like pentapeptide repeat proteins in gram-positive bacteria. J. Antimicrob. Chemother. 61, 1240-1243.

Rosato, A., Pierre, J., Billot-Klein, D., Buu-Hoi, A., Gutmann, L., 1995. Inducible and constitutive expression of resistance to glycopeptides and vancomycin dependence in glycopeptide-resistant Enterococcus avium. Antimicrob. Agents Chemother. 39, 830-833.

Rosato, A., Vicarini, H., Leclercq, R., 1999. Inducible or constitutive expression of resistance in clinical isolates of streptococci and enterococci cross-resistant to erythromycin and lincomycin. J. Antimicrob. Chemother. 43, 559-562.

Rosvoll, T.C.S., Pedersen, T., Sletvold, H., Johnsen, P.J., Sollid, J.E., Simonsen, G.S., Jensen, L.B., Nielsen, K.M., Sundsfjord, A., 2009. PCR-based plasmid typing in Enterococcus faecium strains reveals widely distributed pRE25-, pRUM-, pIP501-

and pHTbeta-related replicons associated with glycopeptide resistance and stabilizing toxin-antitoxin systems. FEMS Immunology and Medical Microbiology 58, 254-268.

Ruggero, K.A., Schroeder, L.K., Schreckenberger, P.C., Mankin, A.S., Quinn, J.P., 2003. Nosocomial superinfections due to linezolid-resistant Enterococcus faecalis: evidence for a gene dosage effect on linezolid MICs. Diagn. Microbiol. Infect. Dis. 47, 511-513.

Ruiz-Garbajosa, P., Bonten, M.J., Robinson, D.A., Top, J., Nallapareddy, S.R., Torres, C., Coque, T.M., Canton, R., Baquero, F., Murray, B.E., Del, C.R., Willems, R.J., 2006. Multilocus sequence typing scheme for Enterococcus faecalis reveals hospital-adapted genetic complexes in a background of high rates of recombination. J. Clin. Microbiol. 44, 2220-2228.

Sader, H.S., Moet, G.J., Jones, R.N., 2009. Antimicrobial resistance among Gram-positive bacteria isolated in Latin American hospitals. J. Chemother. 21, 611-620.

Saeedi, B., Hallgren, A., Isaksson, B., Jonasson, J., Nilsson, L.E., Hanberger, H., 2004. Genetic relatedness of Enterococcus faecalis isolates with high-level gentamicin resistance from patients with bacteraemia in the south east of Sweden 1994-2001. Scand. J. Infect. Dis. 36, 405-409.

Sahlstrom, L., Rehbinder, V., Albihn, A., Aspan, A., Bengtsson, B., 2009. Vancomycin resistant enterococci (VRE) in Swedish sewage sludge. Acta Vet. Scand. 51, 24-

Sahm, D.F., Kissinger, J., Gilmore, M.S., Murray, P.R., Mulder, R., Solliday, J., Clarke, B., 1989. In vitro susceptibility studies of vancomycin-resistant Enterococcus faecalis. Antimicrob. Agents Chemother. 33, 1588-1591.

San Millan, A., Depardieu, F., Godreuil, S., Courvalin, P., 2009a. VanB-type Enterococcus faecium clinical isolate successively inducibly resistant to, dependent on, and constitutively resistant to vancomycin. Antimicrob. Agents Chemother. 53, 1974-1982.

San Millan, A., Depardieu, F., Godreuil, S., Courvalin, P., 2009b. VanB-type Enterococcus faecium clinical isolate successively inducibly resistant to, dependent on, and constitutively resistant to vancomycin. Antimicrob. Agents Chemother. 53, 1974-1982.

Schmitz, F.J., Witte, W., Werner, G., Petridou, J., Fluit, A.C., Schwarz, S., 2001. Characterization of the translational attenuator of 20 methicillin-resistant, quinupristin/dalfopristin-resistant Staphylococcus aureus isolates with reduced susceptibility to glycopeptides. J. Antimicrob. Chemother. 48, 939-941.

Schouten, M.A., Voss, A., Hoogkamp-Korstanje, J.A., 1997. VRE and meat. Lancet 349, 1258-

Schwarz, F.V., Perreten, V., Teuber, M., 2001. Sequence of the 50-kb conjugative multiresistance plasmid pRE25 from Enterococcus faecalis RE25. Plasmid 46, 170-187.

Sebaihia, M., Wren, B.W., Mullany, P., Fairweather, N.F., Minton, N., Stabler, R., Thomson, N.R., Roberts, A.P., Cerdeno-Tarraga, A.M., Wang, H., Holden, M.T., Wright, A., Churcher, C., Quail, M.A., Baker, S., Bason, N., Brooks, K., Chillingworth, T., Cronin, A., Davis, P., Dowd, L., Fraser, A., Feltwell, T., Hance, Z., Holroyd, S., Jagels, K., Moule, S., Mungall, K., Price, C., Rabbinowitsch, E., Sharp, S., Simmonds, M., Stevens, K., Unwin, L., Whitehead, S., Dupuy, B., Dougan, G., Barrell, B., Parkhill, J., 2006. The multidrug-resistant human pathogen Clostridium difficile has a highly mobile, mosaic genome. Nat. Genet. 38, 779-786.

Seedat, J., Zick, G., Klare, I., Konstabel, C., Weiler, N., Sahly, H., 2006. Rapid emergence of resistance to linezolid during linezolid therapy of an Enterococcus faecium infection. Antimicrob. Agents Chemother. 50, 4217-4219.

Shaw, J.H., Clewell, D.B., 1985. Complete nucleotide sequence of macrolide-lincosamide-streptogramin B-resistance transposon Tn917 in Streptococcus faecalis. J. Bacteriol. 164, 782-796.

Shin, E., Hong, H., Ike, Y., Lee, K., Park, Y.H., Cho, D.T., Lee, Y., 2006. VanB-vanA incongruent VRE isolated from animals and humans in 1999. J. Microbiol. 44, 453-456.

Shirano, M., Takakura, S., Yamamoto, M., Matsumura, Y., Matsushima, A., Nagao, M., Fujihara, N., Saito, T., Ito, Y., Iinuma, Y., Shimizu, T., Fujita, N., Ichiyama, S., 2010. Regional spread of vanA- or vanB-positive Enterococcus gallinarum in hospitals and long-term care facilities in Kyoto prefecture, Japan. Epidemiol. Infect. 1-7.

Sievert, D.M., Rudrik, J.T., Patel, J.B., McDonald, L.C., Wilkins, M.J., Hageman, J.C., 2008. Vancomycin-resistant Staphylococcus aureus in the United States, 2002-2006. Clin. Infect. Dis. 46, 668-674.

Sifaoui, F., Gutmann, L., 1997. Vancomycin dependence in a vanA-producing Enterococcus avium strain with a nonsense mutation in the natural D-Ala-D-Ala ligase gene. Antimicrob. Agents Chemother. 41, 1409-

Sillanpaa, J., Nallapareddy, S.R., Prakash, V.P., Qin, X., Hook, M., Weinstock, G.M., Murray, B.E., 2008. Identification and phenotypic characterization of a second collagen adhesin, Scm, and genome-based identification and analysis of 13 other predicted MSCRAMMs, including four distinct pilus loci, in Enterococcus faecium. Microbiology 154, 3199-3211.

Simjee, S., White, D.G., Wagner, D.D., Meng, J., Qaiyumi, S., Zhao, S., McDermott, P.F., 2002. Identification of vat(E) in Enterococcus faecalis isolates from retail poultry and its transferability to Enterococcus faecium. Antimicrob. Agents Chemother. 46, 3823-3828.

Simonsen, G.S., Haaheim, H., Dahl, K.H., Kruse, H., Lovseth, A., Olsvik, O., Sundsfjord, A., 1998. Transmission of VanA-type vancomycin-resistant enterococci and vanA resistance elements between chicken and humans at avoparcin-exposed farms. Microb. Drug Resist. 4, 313-318.

Sinclair, A., Arnold, C., Woodford, N., 2003. Rapid detection and estimation by pyrosequencing of 23S rRNA genes with a single nucleotide polymorphism conferring linezolid resistance in Enterococci. Antimicrob. Agents Chemother. 47, 3620-3622.

Singh, K.V., Malathum, K., Murray, B.E., 2001. Disruption of an Enterococcus faecium species-specific gene, a homologue of acquired macrolide resistance genes of staphylococci, is associated with an increase in macrolide susceptibility. Antimicrob. Agents Chemother. 45, 263-266.

Singh, K.V., Murray, B.E., 2005. Differences in the Enterococcus faecalis lsa locus that influence susceptibility to quinupristin-dalfopristin and clindamycin. Antimicrob. Agents Chemother. 49, 32-39.

Singh, K.V., Weinstock, G.M., Murray, B.E., 2002. An Enterococcus faecalis ABC homologue (Lsa) is required for the resistance of this species to clindamycin and quinupristin-dalfopristin. Antimicrob. Agents Chemother. 46, 1845-1850.

Sivertsen, A., Lundblad, E.W., Wisell, K.T., Liljequist, B., Billström, H., Ullberg, M., Heimer, D., Sjögren, I., Aasnaes, B., Sundsfjord, A., Hegstad, K., 2011. The widespread VRE outbreak in Swedish hospitals 2007-2009 was associated with clonal E. faecium CC17 genogroup strains harbouring several virulence traits and transferable vanB pRUM-like repA plasmids. Final Programme of the 21st ECCMID, Milano, May 7-10, 2011 Poster P924, 113-

Sletvold, H., Johnsen, P.J., Hamre, I., Simonsen, G.S., Sundsfjord, A., Nielsen, K.M., 2008. Complete sequence of Enterococcus faecium pVEF3 and the detection of an omega-epsilon-zeta toxin-antitoxin module and an ABC transporter. Plasmid 60, 75-85.

Sletvold, H., Johnsen, P.J., Simonsen, G.S., Aasnaes, B., Sundsfjord, A., Nielsen, K.M., 2007. Comparative DNA analysis of two vanA plasmids from Enterococcus faecium strains isolated from poultry and a poultry farmer in Norway. Antimicrob. Agents Chemother. 51, 736-739.

Sletvold, H., Johnsen, P.J., Wikmark, O.G., Simonsen, G.S., Sundsfjord, A., Nielsen, K.M., 2010. Tn1546 is part of a larger plasmid-encoded genetic unit horizontally disseminated among clonal Enterococcus faecium lineages. J. Antimicrob. Chemother. 65, 1894-1906.

Sng, L.H., Cornish, N., Knapp, C.C., Ludwig, M.D., Hall, G.S., Washington, J.A., 1998a. Antimicrobial susceptibility testing of a clinical isolate of vancomycin-dependent enterococcus using D-alanine-D-alanine as a growth supplement. Am. J. Clin. Pathol. 109, 399-403.

Sng, L.H., Cornish, N., Knapp, C.C., Ludwig, M.D., Hall, G.S., Washington, J.A., 1998b. Antimicrobial susceptibility testing of a clinical isolate of vancomycin-dependent enterococcus using D-alanine-D-alanine as a growth supplement. Am. J. Clin. Pathol. 109, 399-403.

Soderblom, T., Aspevall, O., Erntell, M., Hedin, G., Heimer, D., Hokeberg, I., Kidd-Ljunggren, K., Melhus, A., Olsson-Liljequist, B., Sjogren, I., Smedjegard, J., Struwe, J., Sylvan, S., Tegmark-Wisell, K., Thore, M., 2010. Alarming spread of vancomycin resistant enterococci in Sweden since 2007. Euro. Surveill 15, pii: 19620.

Sorum, M., Johnsen, P.J., Aasnes, B., Rosvoll, T., Kruse, H., Sundsfjord, A., Simonsen, G.S., 2006. Prevalence, persistence, and molecular characterization of glycopeptide-resistant enterococci in Norwegian poultry and poultry farmers 3 to 8 years after the ban on avoparcin. Appl. Environ. Microbiol. 72, 516-521.

Stamper, P.D., Shulder, S., Bekalo, P., Manandhar, D., Ross, T.L., Speser, S., Kingery, J., Carroll, K.C., 2010. Evaluation of BBL CHROMagar VanRE for detection of vancomycin-resistant Enterococci in rectal swab specimens. J. Clin. Microbiol. 48, 4294-4297.

Stamper, P.D., Cai, M., Lema, C., Eskey, K., Carroll, K.C., 2007. Comparison of the BD GeneOhm VanR Assay to culture for identification of vancomycin-resistant enterococci in rectal and stool specimens. J. Clin. Microbiol. 45, 3360-3365.

Stinear, T.P., Olden, D.C., Johnson, P.D., Davies, J.K., Grayson, M.L., 2001. Enterococcal vanB resistance locus in anaerobic bacteria in human faeces. The Lancet 357, 855-856.

Stobberingh, E., van Den, B.A., London, N., Driessen, C., Top, J., Willems, R., 1999. Enterococci with glycopeptide resistance in turkeys, turkey farmers, turkey slaughterers, and (sub)urban residents in the south of The Netherlands: evidence for transmission of vancomycin resistance from animals to humans? Antimicrob. Agents Chemother. 43, 2215-2221.

Straus, S.K., Hancock, R.E., 2006a. Mode of action of the new antibiotic for Gram-positive pathogens daptomycin: comparison with cationic antimicrobial peptides and lipopeptides. Biochim. Biophys. Acta 1758, 1215-1223.

Straus, S.K., Hancock, R.E., 2006b. Mode of action of the new antibiotic for Gram-positive pathogens daptomycin: comparison with cationic antimicrobial peptides and lipopeptides. Biochim. Biophys. Acta 1758, 1215-1223.

Tanimoto, K., Nomura, T., Maruyama, H., Tomita, H., Shibata, N., Arakawa, Y., Ike, Y., 2006. First VanD-Type vancomycin-resistant Enterococcus raffinosus isolate. Antimicrob. Agents Chemother. 50, 3966-3967.

Tenover, F.C., McDonald, L.C., 2005. Vancomycin-resistant staphylococci and enterococci: epidemiology and control. Curr. Opin. Infect. Dis. 18, 300-305.

Teuber, M., Schwarz, F., Perreten, V., 2003. Molecular structure and evolution of the conjugative multiresistance plasmid pRE25 of Enterococcus faecalis isolated from a raw-fermented sausage. International Journal of Food Microbiology 88, 325-329.

Thal, L.A., Silverman, J., Donabedian, S., Zervos, M.J., 1997. The effect of Tn916 insertions on contour-clamped homogeneous electrophoresis patterns of Enterococcus faecalis. J. Clin. Microbiol. 35, 969-972.

Toh, S.M., Xiong, L., Arias, C.A., Villegas, M.V., Lolans, K., Quinn, J., Mankin, A.S., 2007. Acquisition of a natural resistance gene renders a clinical strain of methicillin-resistant Staphylococcus aureus resistant to the synthetic antibiotic linezolid. Molecular Microbiology 64, 1506-1514.

Top, J., Willems, R., Blok, H., de Regt, M., Jalink, K., Troelstra, A., Goorhuis, B., Bonten, M., 2007. Ecological replacement of Enterococcus faecalis by multiresistant clonal complex 17 Enterococcus faecium. Clinical Microbiology and Infection 13, 316-319.

Top, J., Willems, R., Bonten, M., 2008a. Emergence of CC17 Enterococcus faecium: from commensal to hospital-adapted pathogen. FEMS Immunol. Med. Microbiol. 52, 297-308.

Top, J., Willems, R., van, d., V, Asbroek, M., Bonten, M., 2008b. Emergence of clonal complex 17 Enterococcus faecium in The Netherlands. J. Clin. Microbiol. 46, 214-219.

Torres, C., Reguera, J.A., Sanmartin, M.J., Perez-Diaz, J.C., Baquero, F., 1994. vanA-mediated vancomycin-resistant Enterococcus spp. in sewage. J. Antimicrob. Chemother. 33, 553-561.

Tsvetkova, K., Marvaud, J.C., Lambert, T., 2010. Analysis of the mobilization functions of the vancomycin resistance transposon Tn1549, a member of a new family of conjugative elements. J. Bacteriol. 192, 702-713.

Usacheva, E.A., Ginocchio, C.C., Morgan, M., Maglanoc, G., Mehta, M.S., Tremblay, S., Karchmer, T.B., Peterson, L.R., 2010. Prospective, multicenter evaluation of the BD GeneOhm VanR assay for direct, rapid detection of vancomycin-resistant Enterococcus species in perianal and rectal specimens. Am. J. Clin. Pathol. 134, 219-226.

Valdezate, S., Labayru, C., Navarro, A., Mantecon, M.A., Ortega, M., Coque, T.M., Garcia, M., Saez-Nieto, J.A., 2009. Large clonal outbreak of multidrug-resistant CC17 ST17 Enterococcus faecium containing Tn5382 in a Spanish hospital. J. Antimicrob. Chemother. 63, 17-20.

Van Caeseele, P., Giercke, S., Wylie, J., Boyd, D., Mulvey, M., Amin, S., Ofner-Agostini, M., 2001. Identification of the first vancomycin-resistant Enterococcus faecalis harbouring vanE in Canada. Can. Commun. Dis. Rep. 27, 101-104.

Van Den Bogaard, A.E., Mertens, P., London, N.H., Stobberingh, E.E., 1997. High prevalence of colonization with vancomycin- and pristinamycin-resistant enterococci in healthy humans and pigs in The Netherlands: is the addition of antibiotics to animal feeds to blame? J. Antimicrob. Chemother. 40, 454-456.

van den Braak, N., van Belkum, A., van Keulen, M., Vliegenthart, J., Verbrugh, H.A., Endtz, H.P., 1998. Molecular characterization of vancomycin-resistant enterococci from hospitalized patients and poultry products in The Netherlands. J. Clin. Microbiol. 36, 1927-1932.

van Schaik, W., Top, J., Riley, D.R., Boekhorst, J., Vrijenhoek, J.E.P.V., Schapendonk, C.M.E., Hendrickx, A.P.A., Nijman, I.J., Bonten, M.J.M., Tettelin, H., Willems, R.J.L., 2010. Pyrosequencing-based comparative genome analysis of the nosocomial pathogen Enterococcus faecium and identification of a large transferable pathogenicity island. BMC Genomics 11, 239-

van Schaik, W., Willems, R.J., 2010. Genome-based insights into the evolution of enterococci. Clin. Microbiol. Infect.

Weaver, K.E., Kwong, S.M., Firth, N., Francia, M.V., 2009. The RepA_N replicons of Gram-positive bacteria: a family of broadly distributed but narrow host range plasmids. Plasmid 61, 94-109.

Weber, P., Meziane-Cherif, D., Haouz, A., Saul, F.A., Courvalin, P., 2009. Crystallization and preliminary X-ray analysis of a D-Ala:D-Ser ligase associated with VanG-type vancomycin resistance. Acta Crystallogr. Sect. F. Struct. Biol. Cryst. Commun. 65, 1024-1026.

Weigel, L.M., Clewell, D.B., Gill, S.R., Clark, N.C., McDougal, L.K., Flannagan, S.E., Kolonay, J.F., Shetty, J., Killgore, G.E., Tenover, F.C., 2003. Genetic analysis of a high-level vancomycin-resistant isolate of Staphylococcus aureus. Science 302, 1569-1571.

Werckenthin, C., Schwarz, S., 2000. Molecular analysis of the translational attenuator of a constitutively expressed erm(A) gene from Staphylococcus intermedius. J. Antimicrob. Chemother. 46, 785-788.

Werckenthin, C., Schwarz, S., Westh, H., 1999. Structural alterations in the translational attenuator of constitutively expressed ermC genes. Antimicrob. Agents Chemother. 43, 1681-1685.

Werner, G., 2011. Surveillance of antimicrobial resistance among Enterococcus faecium and Enterococcus faecalis isolated from human (clinical/commensal), food animal, meat and environmental samples. In: Semedo-Lemsaddek, T., Barreto-Crespo, M.T., Tenreiro, R. (Eds), Enterococcus and safety. Nova Science Publishers Inc., Hauppage, N.Y., pp. [in press]-.

Werner, G., Bartel, M., Wellinghausen, N., Essig, A., Klare, I., Witte, W., Poppert, S., 2007a. Detection of mutations conferring resistance to linezolid in Enterococcus spp. by fluorescence in situ hybridization. J. Clin. Microbiol. 45, 3421-3423.

Werner, G., Coque, T.M., Hammerum, A.M., Hope, R., Hryniewicz, W., Johnson, A., Klare, I., Kristinsson, K.G., Leclercq, R., Lester, C.H., Lillie, M., Novais, C., Olsson-Liljequist, B., Peixe, L.V., Sadowy, E., Simonsen, G.S., Top, J., Vuopio-Varkila, J., Willems, R.J., Witte, W., Woodford, N., 2008a. Emergence and spread of vancomycin resistance among enterococci in Europe. Euro. Surveill 13, pii: 19046-

Werner, G., Dahl, K.H., Willems, R.J., 2006. Composite elements encoding antibiotic resistance in Enterococcus faecium and Enterococcus faecalis. In: Kobayashi, N. (Eds), Drug Resistance in Enterococci: Epidemiology and Molecular Markers. Research Signpost, Fort P.O., Trivandrum, Kerala, pp. 157-208.

Werner, G., Fleige, C., Ewert, B., Laverde-Gomez, J.A., Klare, I., Witte, W., 2010a. High-level ciprofloxacin resistance among hospital-adapted Enterococcus faecium (CC17). Int. J. Antimicrob. Agents 35, 119-125.

Werner, G., Fleige, C., Geringer, U., van, S.W., Klare, I., Witte, W., 2011a. IS element IS16 as a molecular screening tool to identify hospital-associated strains of Enterococcus faecium. BMC. Infect. Dis. 11, 80-

Werner, G., Freitas, A.R., Coque, T.M., Sollid, J.E., Lester, C., Hammerum, A.M., Garcia-Migura, L., Jensen, L.B., Francia, M.V., Witte, W., Willems, R.J., Sundsfjord, A., 2010b. Host range of enterococcal vanA plasmids among Gram-positive intestinal bacteria. J. Antimicrob. Chemother.

Werner, G., Freitas, A.R., Coque, T.M., Sollid, J.E., Lester, C., Hammerum, A.M., Garcia-Migura, L., Jensen, L.B., Francia, M.V., Witte, W., Willems, R.J., Sundsfjord, A., 2011b. Host range of enterococcal vanA plasmids among Gram-positive intestinal bacteria. J. Antimicrob. Chemother. 66, 273-282.

Werner, G., Gfrörer, S., Fleige, C., Witte, W., Klare, I., 2008b. Tigecycline-resistant Enterococcus faecalis strain isolated from a German ICU patient. J. Antimicrob. Chemother. 61, 1182-1183.

Werner, G., Hildebrandt, B., Witte, W., 2001a. Aminoglycoside-streptothricin resistance gene cluster aadE-sat4-aphA-3 disseminated among multiresistant isolates of Enterococcus faecium. Antimicrob. Agents Chemother. 45, 3267-3269.

Werner, G., Hildebrandt, B., Witte, W., 2001b. The newly described msrC gene is not equally distributed among all isolates of Enterococcus faecium. Antimicrob. Agents Chemother. 45, 3672-3673.

Werner, G., Hildebrandt, B., Witte, W., 2003a. Linkage of erm(B) and aadE-sat4-aphA-3 in multiple-resistant Enterococcus faecium isolates of different ecological origins. Microb. Drug Resist. 9 Suppl 1, S9-16.

Werner, G., Klare, I., Heier, H., Hinz, K.H., Bohme, G., Wendt, M., Witte, W., 2000. Quinupristin/dalfopristin-resistant enterococci of the satA (vatD) and satG (vatE) genotypes from different ecological origins in Germany. Microb. Drug Resist. 6, 37-47.

Werner, G., Klare, I., Konstabel, C., Witte, W., 2007b. The current MLVA typing scheme for Enterococcus faecium does not discriminate enough to resolve epidemic-virulent, hospital-adapted clonal types. BMC Microbiology 7, 28-

Werner, G., Klare, I., Spencker, F.B., Witte, W., 2003b. Intra-hospital dissemination of quinupristin/dalfopristin- and vancomycin-resistant Enterococcus faecium in a paediatric ward of a German hospital. J. Antimicrob. Chemother. 52, 113-115.

Werner, G., Klare, I., Witte, W., 1997. Arrangement of the vanA gene cluster in enterococci of different ecological origin. FEMS Microbiol. Lett. 155, 55-61.

Werner, G., Klare, I., Witte, W., 2002. Molecular analysis of streptogramin resistance in enterococci. Int. J. Med. Microbiol. 292, 81-94.

Werner, G., Serr, A., Schütt, S., Schneider, C., Klare, I., Witte, W., Wendt, C., 2011c. Comparison of direct cultivation on a selective solid medium, polymerase chain reaction from an enrichment broth, and the BD GeneOhm™ VanR Assay for identification of vancomycin-resistant enterococci in screening specimens. Diagnostic Microbiology and Infectious Diseases 70, 512-521.

Werner, G., Strommenger, B., Witte, W., 2008c. Acquired vancomycin resistance in clinically relevant pathogens. Future Microbiology 3, 547-562.

Werner, G., Klare, I., Fleige, C., Witte, W., 2007c. Increasing rates of vancomycin resistance among Enterococcus faecium isolated from German hospitals between 2004 and 2006 are due to wide clonal dissemination of vancomycin-resistant enterococci and horizontal spread of vanA clusters. International Journal of Medical Microbiology 298, 515-527.

Werner, G., Strommenger, B., Klare, I., Witte, W., 2004. Molecular detection of linezolid resistance in Enterococcus faecium and Enterococcus faecalis by use of 5' nuclease real-time PCR compared to a modified classical approach. J. Clin. Microbiol. 42, 5327-5331.

Willems, R.J., Hanage, W.P., Bessen, D.E., Feil, E.J., 2011. Population biology of Gram-positive pathogens: high-risk clones for dissemination of antibiotic resistance. FEMS Microbiol. Rev.

Willems, R.J., Homan, W., Top, J., van Santen-Verheuvel, M., Tribe, D., Manzioros, X., Gaillard, C., Vandenbroucke-Grauls, C.M., Mascini, E.M., van, K.E., Van Embden, J.D., Bonten, M.J., 2001. Variant esp gene as a marker of a distinct genetic lineage of vancomycin-resistant Enterococcus faecium spreading in hospitals. Lancet 357, 853-855.

Willems, R.J., Top, J., van Den, B.N., van, B.A., Mevius, D.J., Hendriks, G., van Santen-Verheuvel, M., Van Embden, J.D., 1999. Molecular diversity and evolutionary relationships of Tn1546-like elements in enterococci from humans and animals. Antimicrob. Agents Chemother. 43, 483-491.

Willems, R.J., van Schaik W., 2009. Transition of Enterococcus faecium from commensal organism to nosocomial pathogen. Future. Microbiol. 4, 1125-1135.

Willems, R.J., Top, J., Smith, D.J., Roper, D.I., North, S.E., Woodford, N., 2003. Mutations in the DNA mismatch repair proteins MutS and MutL of oxazolidinone-resistant or -susceptible Enterococcus faecium. Antimicrob. Agents Chemother. 47, 3061-3066.

Willems, R.J., Bonten, M.J., 2007. Glycopeptide-resistant enterococci: deciphering virulence, resistance and epidemicity. Current Opinion in Infectious Diseases 20, 384-390.

Woodford, N., Adebiyi, A.M., Palepou, M.F., Cookson, B.D., 1998. Diversity of VanA glycopeptide resistance elements in enterococci from humans and nonhuman sources. Antimicrob. Agents Chemother. 42, 502-508.

Woodford, N., Johnson, A.P., Morrison, D., Hastings, J.G., Elliott, T.S., Worthington, A., Stephenson, J.R., Chin, A.T., Tolley, J.L., 1994. Vancomycin-dependent enterococci in the United Kingdom. J. Antimicrob. Chemother. 33, 1066-

Woodford, N., Reynolds, R., Turton, J., Scott, F., Sinclair, A., Williams, A., Livermore, D., 2003. Two widely disseminated strains of Enterococcus faecalis highly resistant to gentamicin and ciprofloxacin from bacteraemias in the UK and Ireland. J Antimicrob. Chemother. 52, 711-714.

Worth, L.J., Slavin, M.A., Vankerckhoven, V., Goossens, H., Grabsch, E.A., Thursky, K.A., 2008. Virulence determinants in vancomycin-resistant Enterococcus faecium vanB: clonal distribution, prevalence and significance of esp and hyl in Australian patients with haematological disorders. J. Hosp. Infect. 68, 137-144.

Xu, X., Lin, D., Yan, G., Ye, X., Wu, S., Guo, Y., Zhu, D., Hu, F., Zhang, Y., Wang, F., Jacoby, G.A., Wang, M., 2010. vanM, a new glycopeptide resistance gene cluster found in Enterococcus faecium. Antimicrob. Agents Chemother. 54, 4643-4647.

Yoo, S.J., Sung, H., Cho, Y.U., Kim, M.N., Pai, C.H., Kim, Y.S., 2006. Role of horizontal transfer of the transposon Tn1546 in the nosocomial spread of vanA vancomycin-resistant enterococci at a tertiary care hospital in Korea. Infect. Control Hosp. Epidemiol. 27, 1081-1087.

Yoshimura, H., Ishimaru, M., Endoh, Y.S., Suginaka, M., Yamatani, S., 1998. Isolation of glycopeptide-resistant enterococci from chicken in Japan. Antimicrob. Agents Chemother. 42, 3333-

Young, H.L., Ballard, S.A., Roffey, P., Grayson, M.L., 2007. Direct detection of vanB2 using the Roche LightCycler vanA/B detection assay to indicate vancomycin-resistant enterococcal carriage - sensitive but not specific. J. Antimicrob. Chemother. 59, 809-810.

Zarrilli, R., Tripodi, M.F., Di, P.A., Fortunato, R., Bagattini, M., Crispino, M., Florio, A., Triassi, M., Utili, R., 2005. Molecular epidemiology of high-level aminoglycoside-resistant enterococci isolated from patients in a university hospital in southern Italy. J. Antimicrob. Chemother. 56, 827-835.

Zhanel, G.G., Calic, D., Schweizer, F., Zelenitsky, S., Adam, H., Lagace-Wiens, P.R., Rubinstein, E., Gin, A.S., Hoban, D.J., Karlowsky, J.A., 2010a. New lipoglycopeptides: a comparative review of dalbavancin, oritavancin and telavancin. Drugs 70, 859-886.

Zhanel, G.G., DeCorby, M., Adam, H., Mulvey, M.R., McCracken, M., Lagace-Wiens, P., Nichol, K.A., Wierzbowski, A., Baudry, P.J., Tailor, F., Karlowsky, J.A., Walkty, A., Schweizer, F., Johnson, J., Hoban, D.J., 2010b. Prevalence of antimicrobial-resistant pathogens in Canadian hospitals: results of the Canadian Ward Surveillance Study (CANWARD 2008). Antimicrob. Agents Chemother. 54, 4684-4693.

Zhanel, G.G., DeCorby, M., Laing, N., Weshnoweski, B., Vashisht, R., Tailor, F., Nichol, K.A., Wierzbowski, A., Baudry, P.J., Karlowsky, J.A., Lagace-Wiens, P., Walkty, A., McCracken, M., Mulvey, M.R., Johnson, J., Hoban, D.J., 2008a. Antimicrobial-resistant pathogens in intensive care units in Canada: results of the Canadian National Intensive Care Unit (CAN-ICU) study, 2005-2006. Antimicrob. Agents Chemother. 52, 1430-1437.

Zhanel, G.G., DeCorby, M., Nichol, K.A., Baudry, P.J., Karlowsky, J.A., Lagace-Wiens, P.R., McCracken, M., Mulvey, M.R., Hoban, D.J., 2008b. Characterization of methicillin-resistant Staphylococcus aureus, vancomycin-resistant enterococci and extended-spectrum beta-lactamase-producing Escherichia coli in intensive care units in Canada: Results of the Canadian National Intensive Care Unit (CAN-ICU) study (2005-2006). Can. J. Infect. Dis. Med. Microbiol. 19, 243-249.

Zhanel, G.G., Harding, G.K., Rosser, S., Hoban, D.J., Karlowsky, J.A., Alfa, M., Kabani, A., Embil, J., Gin, A., Williams, T., Nicolle, L.E., 2000. Low prevalence of VRE gastrointestinal colonization of hospitalized patients in Manitoba tertiary care and community hospitals. Can. J. Infect. Dis. 11, 38-41.

Zheng, B., Tomita, H., Inoue, T., Ike, Y., 2009. Isolation of VanB-type Enterococcus faecalis strains from nosocomial infections: first report of the isolation and identification of the pheromone-responsive plasmids pMG2200, Encoding VanB-type vancomycin resistance and a Bac41-type bacteriocin, and pMG2201, encoding erythromycin resistance and cytolysin (Hly/Bac). Antimicrob. Agents Chemother. 53, 735-747.

Zheng, B., Tomita, H., Xiao, Y.H., Ike, Y., 2007a. The first molecular analysis of clinical isolates of VanA-type vancomycin-resistant Enterococcus faecium strains in mainland China. Lett. Appl. Microbiol. 45, 307-312.

Zheng, B., Tomita, H., Xiao, Y.H., Wang, S., Li, Y., Ike, Y., 2007b. Molecular characterization of vancomycin-resistant Enterococcus faecium isolates from mainland China. J. Clin. Microbiol. 45, 2813-2818.

Zhu, W., Clark, N.C., McDougal, L.K., Hageman, J., McDonald, L.C., Patel, J.B., 2008. Vancomycin-resistant Staphylococcus aureus isolates associated with inc18-like vanA plasmids in Michigan. Antimicrob. Agents Chemother. 52, 452-457.

Zhu, W., Murray, P.R., Huskins, W.C., Jernigan, J.A., McDonald, L.C., Clark, N.C., Anderson, K.F., McDougal, L.K., Hageman, J.C., Olsen-Rasmussen, M., Frace, M., Alangaden, G.J., Chenoweth, C., Zervos, M.J., Robinson-Dunn, B., Schreckenberger, P.C., Reller, L.B., Rudrik, J.T., Patel, J.B., 2010. Dissemination of an Enterococcus Inc18-like vanA plasmid, associated with vancomycin-resistant Staphylococcus aureus. Antimicrob. Agents Chemother.

Zhu, X., Zheng, B., Wang, S., Willems, R.J., Xue, F., Cao, X., Li, Y., Bo, S., Liu, J., 2009. Molecular characterisation of outbreak-related strains of vancomycin-resistant Enterococcus faecium from an intensive care unit in Beijing, China. J. Hosp. Infect. 72, 147-154.

Zirakzadeh, A., Patel, R., 2006. Vancomycin-resistant enterococci: colonization, infection, detection, and treatment. Mayo Clin. Proc. 81, 529-536.

Zirakzadeh, A., Patel, R., 2005. Epidemiology and mechanisms of glycopeptide reistance in enterococci. Current Opinion in Infectious Diseases 18, 507-512.

Clinically Relevant Antibiotic Resistance Mechanisms Can Enhance the *In Vivo* Fitness of *Neisseria gonorrhoeae*

Elizabeth A. Ohneck[1], Jonathan A. D'Ambrozio[2],
Anjali N. Kunz[2], Ann E. Jerse[2] and William M. Shafer[3,4]
[1]*Emory University Laney Graduate School;*
[2]*Uniformed Services University of the Health Sciences;*
[3]*Emory University School of Medicine;*
[4]*Laboratories of Bacterial Pathogenesis, VA Medical Center (Atlanta, GA)*
USA

1. Introduction

In 2007 the Centers for Disease Control and Prevention placed *Neisseria gonorrhoeae* on the infamous "Super Bugs" list to highlight the high prevalence of strains resistant to relatively inexpensive antibiotics, such as penicillin, tetracycline and fluoroquinolones, previously used in therapy to treat gonorrhea (Shafer et al., 2010). This event was significant because the gonococcus, a strict human pathogen, causes > 95 million infections worldwide each year and since the mid-1940s mankind has relied on effective antibiotic therapy to treat infections and stop local spread of disease. Today, such therapy is threatened by antibiotic resistance. Specifically, the third generation cephalosporins, especially ceftriaxone, may be losing their effectiveness since some (albeit still rare) isolates in the Far East, most recently Japan, and Europe have displayed clinical resistance to currently used levels of ceftriaxone, and treatment failures have been reported (Ohnishi et al., 2011; Unemo et al., 2010). Concern has been raised that the spectrum of resistance expressed by some gonococcal strains may make standard antibiotic treatment for gonorrhea ineffective in the not too distant future (Dionne-Odom et al., 2011). Without new, effective antibiotics or novel combination therapies of existing antibiotics, the reproductive health of the world's sexually active population may be placed at risk due to such antibiotic resistant gonococci.

An important question regarding antibiotic resistance is whether a particular resistance mechanism has a fitness cost for the bacterium (Andersson & Levin, 1999; Andersson & Hughes, 2010), especially in the community where it competes with its antibiotic sensitive brethren. A fitness cost is typically experimentally measured as a deleterious change in bacterial growth rate in laboratory media or survival in experimental infection in the absence of antibiotic pressure. Fitness costs (or benefits) are best viewed during co-cultivation of isogenic strains that differ only in the resistance mechanism under study. For certain antibiotic resistance mechanisms, a significant fitness cost can be incurred. This general observation led to the idea that removal of the selective pressure imposed by the antibiotic in question would favor sensitive strains to predominate in the community and allow for the return of the antibiotic in question to treat the infection in question. By and large, this has proven not be the case (Andersson and Hughes, 2010). There are many reasons for this, including the unintentional selective pressure exerted by the widespread availability and use of antibiotics to treat bacterial infections in general, over-the-counter antimicrobials that confer selective pressure and provide cross-resistance (or decreased susceptibility) to the antibiotic in question, and host-derived antimicrobials that select for the particular resistance determinant. In addition to antimicrobial pressures, it has been repeatedly documented that compensatory, second site mutations can develop that reverse fitness costs while maintaining resistance (Schrag et al., 1997; Marcusson et al., 2009; Andersson and Hughes, 2010).

More recently, a new view has been taken regarding antibiotic resistance and fitness: some resistance systems actually provide the resistant strain with a fitness advantage over wild-type strains or can reverse a fitness burden imposed by a separate mutation that also participates in resistance to a particular antibiotic. Evidence for enhanced fitness of bacterial pathogens, in laboratory media or in experimental infection models, due to mutations or gene acquisition events that increase resistance to antibiotics has been provided for *Campylobacter jejuni* (Luo et al., 2005) and *Neisseria gonorrhoeae* (Warner et al., 2007, 2008). The idea that an antibiotic resistance mechanism could have negligible and even beneficial effects on fitness could help to explain, in part, why resistant strains persist in the community long after the antibiotic has been removed from the treatment regimen. For instance, gonococci expressing resistance to penicillin, tetracycline and/or fluoroquinolones have persisted in the community despite the removal of these antibiotics from the recommended gonorrhea treatment regimen for several years. Against this background, we herein review data and provide models as to how two mechanisms of antibiotic resistance expressed by *N. gonorrhoeae* can enhance fitness *in vivo*. The *in vivo* system employed in these studies is a female mouse model of lower genital tract infection that recapitulates many features of infection in human females, most notably the development of inflammation that occurs during cervicitis (Jerse, 1999; Packiam et al., 2010; Song et al., 2008). The two resistance mechanisms discussed below are multi-drug efflux by the MtrC-MtrD-MtrE pump (Hagman et al., 1995; Jerse et al., 2003) and quinolone resistance that develops due to point mutations in *gyrA* and *parC*. We discuss concepts regarding the evolution of antibiotic resistance expressed by gonococci in the context of how these resistance mechanisms may have endowed this strict human pathogen with a fitness advantage during infection.

2. Antimicrobial efflux and gonococcal fitness

The MtrC-MtrD-MtrE efflux pump of *N. gonorrhoeae* is a resistance-nodulation-division (RND) efflux pump family member that recognizes a diverse array of hydrophobic antimicrobial agents and exports these toxic compounds out of the gonococcal cell (Hagman et al., 1995). The *mtrCDE* operon is composed of three structural genes that encode the core proteins of the efflux pump: *mtrC*, which encodes a periplasmic membrane fusion protein; *mtrD*, encoding an energy-dependent inner membrane transporter; and *mtrE*, which encodes a TolC-like outer membrane channel protein (Delahay et al., 1997; Hagman et al., 1995; Hagman et al., 1997). In addition to these core efflux proteins, an accessory protein termed MtrF is required for high-level resistance to substrates of the pump and its gene (*mtrF*) is also located within the *mtr* locus (Figure 1) (Veal & Shafer, 2003).

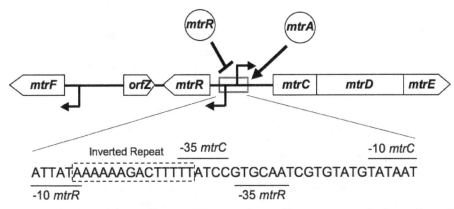

Fig. 1. **Organization of the *mtr* locus of *N. gonorrhoeae*.** Bent arrows mark the *mtrR*, *mtrF*, and *mtrCDE* promoters. *mtrR* and *mtrCDE* are divergently transcribed on opposite strands. Circles represent the transcriptional regulatory proteins MtrR and MtrA. The box represents the location of the expanded sequence. The *mtrR* and *mtrCDE* promoter elements are indicated in the expanded sequence; the dashed box marks the inverted repeat element of the *mtrR* promoter.

Transcription of the *mtrCDE* operon is negatively regulated by the TetR family transcriptional regulator, MtrR, which represses *mtrCDE* expression by the binding of two homodimers to pseudo-direct repeats within the *mtrCDE* promoter (Hoffman et al., 2005; Lucas et al., 1997). The *mtrR* gene is located 250 base pairs upstream of and is transcribed divergently from *mtrCDE* (Pan & Spratt, 1994). Additionally, transcription of *mtrCDE* may be induced in the presence of sub-lethal concentrations of nonionic, membrane-acting detergents through the action of an AraC/XylS family transcriptional activator, MtrA (Rouquette et al., 1999). Expression of *mtrF* is negatively regulated by both MtrR and the AraC family regulator MpeR (Folster and Shafer, 2005), as well as the availability of free iron (Mercante et al., 2012).

The MtrC-MtrD-MtrE efflux pump mediates resistance to structurally diverse hydrophobic antimicrobial agents, including ß-lactam antibiotics such as penicillin, macrolide antibiotics including erythromycin and azithromycin, dyes such as crystal violet, and detergents such as Triton X-100 and nonoxynol-9 (Hagman et al., 1995; Rouquette et al., 1999). Additionally, MtrC-MtrD-MtrE confers resistance to host antimicrobial compounds, including fatty acids, bile salts, progesterone, and the antimicrobial peptide LL-37 (Jerse et al., 2003; Morse et al., 1982; Shafer et al., 1995; Shafer et al., 1998). MtrC-MtrD-MtrE efflux pump-deficient mutants are highly attenuated in a female BALB/c mouse model of lower genital tract infection, even in the absence of pump substrate antibiotic treatment (Jerse et al., 2003). This attenuation is likely due to an increased susceptibility to host antimicrobial compounds, highlighting the importance of the *mtr* system in establishing gonococcal infection.

The production of efflux pumps is an energy-expensive process, and it might be hypothesized that high levels of MtrC-MtrD-MtrE production could stress the gonococcus, resulting in slower or defective growth, thereby conferring a fitness cost on strains with increased *mtrCDE* expression. In this respect, Eisenstein and Sparling noted that a mutant strain displaying the Mtr phenotype, now known to be due to a single base pair deletion in the inverted repeat in the *mtrR* promoter (Figure 1) that results in high-level antibiotic resistance through increased transcription of *mtrCDE* (Hagman & Shafer, 1995), had a slower growth rate *in vitro* (Eisenstein & Sparling, 1978). However, this same mutation confers a fitness advantage during competitive infection against wild-type strain FA19 in the female mouse model of infection in the absence of antibiotics (Warner et al., 2008) and is frequently found in clinical isolates (Shafer et al., 1995; Zarantonelli et al., 1999), particularly from men who have sex with men (Shafer et al., 1995; Xia et al., 2000). Additional mutations in the *mtrR* coding region and the *mtrR* promoter have been identified in clinical isolates that increase resistance to MtrC-MtrD-MtrE pump substrates as well as confer a survival advantage in the female mouse infection model (Table 1) (summarized in Warner et al., 2008). Mutations in the *mtrR* coding region, particularly those resulting in radical amino acid changes in the MtrR helix-turn-helix DNA binding domain, lead to low or intermediate levels of antimicrobial resistance that corresponds to a low to intermediate survival advantage during competitive infection in female mice (Warner et al., 2008). The single nucleotide deletion in the inverted repeat of the *mtrR* promoter and a recently identified mutation 120 base pairs upstream of the *mtrC* start codon (*mtr*$_{120}$) confer high-level resistance to pump substrates as well as a greater fitness advantage *in vivo* (Warner et al., 2008). These changes in fitness require an active efflux pump, as the effects were reversed in the regulatory mutant strains when the efflux pump system was genetically inactivated. Thus, it appears that the level of antibiotic resistance due to increased *mtrCDE* expression corresponds positively to the strength of the fitness advantage observed *in vivo*.

Genotype	CI at day 3
Single bp deletion in *mtrR* promoter	1000
mtr$_{120}$ point mutation	1000
A39T change in DNA binding domain of MtrR	100
mtrA::Km^R	0.005
mtrA::Km^R *mtrR*$_{1-53}$	100
mtrA::Km^R *mtrR*$_{E202G}$	10
mpeR::Km^R	1

Table 1. Fitness of *mtr* regulatory mutants in mice compared to wild-type. CI: competitive index. Ratio of mutant to wild-type CFU (vaginal isolates) divided by mutant to wild-type CFU (inoculum).

Induction of *mtrCDE* expression by the activator MtrA is also important for gonococcal survival *in vivo*. Strains carrying a disrupted *mtrA* gene display a significant fitness disadvantage during competitive infection with wild-type strain FA19 in the female mouse model of infection (Warner et al., 2007). MtrA induction of *mtrCDE* expression occurs in the presence of nonionic detergents such as Triton X-100 (Rouquette et al., 1999). The presence of host antimicrobial factors that are pump substrates, such as fatty acids or CRAMP-38, the mouse homologue of the human cathelicidin LL-37, may have a similar effect. The decreased fitness of the *mtrA* mutants *in vivo* would therefore be attributed to failure of the gonococcus to respond to host defense factors due to inability to upregulate expression of the pump.

Interestingly, in a study by Warner et al., 2007, some $mtrA$-deficient strains developed mutations in the $mtrR$ gene ($mtrR_{1-53}$ and $mtrR_{E202G}$) after inoculation into mice in the absence of antibiotics; these strains were recovered in high numbers and displayed increased antibiotic resistance as well as a fitness advantage during subsequent competitive infection against wild-type FA19 (Table 1). The development of compensatory mutations to overcome the cost of $mtrA$ disruption highlights the importance of the MtrC-MtrD-MtrE efflux pump to gonococcal fitness $in\ vivo$.

The importance of the MtrC-MtrD-MtrE efflux pump $in\ vivo$, even in the absence of antibiotic treatment, suggests that this pump originally evolved as a mechanism to aid the gonococcus in escaping host defense mechanisms, rather than in response to the introduction of antibiotics to treat gonococcal infection. Increasing antibiotic use and the availability of the over-the-counter spermicide nonoxynol-9 may then have selected for pump mutants, such as those containing $mtrR$ mutations frequently isolated from patients with gonococcal infection. These strains are not only able to resist antibiotic treatment, but also better able to resist host antimicrobial compounds, giving them a survival advantage $in\ vivo$ and in the community (Xia et al., 2000). Thus, increased production of the MtrC-MtrD-MtrE efflux pump represents a mechanism of antibiotic resistance that imparts a fitness advantage upon the gonococcus, rather than a fitness cost. It is important to note that homologues of both the pump and its regulatory proteins exist in other Gram-negative bacteria. For example, the AcrA-AcrB-TolC efflux system of $Salmonella\ enterica$ enhances the capacity of this pathogen to cause experimental infection in chickens (Webber et al., 2009). Lessons learned with the gonococcus regarding drug efflux and fitness may therefore have broader implications for how bacterial pathogens escape both classical antibiotics and host defense compounds.

3. Quinolone resistance and gonococcal fitness

The limited use of quinolones in the treatment of bacterial infections began after the 1962 discovery of nalidixic acid as a product of chloroquine synthesis. Subsequent development of fluoroquinolone derivatives amassed broad-spectrum appeal due to their effective targeting of many Gram-positive and Gram-negative pathogens (Emmerson, 2003). Continued development of this class of antibiotics was fueled by the concurrent progression of bacterial resistance to penicillin and tetracycline, including $N.\ gonorrhoeae$ (Covino et al., 1990). By 1993, fluoroquinolones were recommended by the CDC as the first-line treatment option for uncomplicated gonococcal infections; however, within 10 years, over 80% of gonococcal isolates in the western Pacific region were ciprofloxacin resistant (Cip[R]) (Tapsall, 2005; Trees et al., 2001). The eventual spread of quinolone resistant $N.\ gonorrhoeae$ (QRNG) in the United States led to the removal of fluoroquinolones from the list of recommended first-line antibiotics for treatment of gonorrhea and related conditions by the CDC in 2007 (CDC, 2007).

Quinolones induce bacterial cell death by inhibiting the activity of the bacterial type IIA DNA topoisomerases DNA gyrase and topoisomerase IV (Emmerson, 2003; Hooper 1999). These enzymes are responsible for managing the topological state of genomic DNA and are necessary for resolving regions of topological stress that occur during critical cell processes such as DNA replication and the regulation of gene expression. DNA gyrase and topoisomerase IV are heterotetramers that bind to DNA and generate a double-stranded break in one region of the bound DNA duplex, which results results in a complex referred to as the G-segment. A second region of distant DNA duplex, referred to as the T-segment, passes through the G-segment and the cleaved substrate held in the G-segment is subsequently religated to complete a single round of topological adjustment (Bates et al., 2011; Chen and Lo 2003; Morais Cabral et al., 1997). Quinolones specifically target the G-segment of the enzyme-DNA complex. Presently, there is no universally accepted mechanism of how quinolones kill bacteria; however, mounting evidence suggests that two quinolone molecules stabilize the cleaved DNA duplex, resulting in the accumulation of lethal lesions within the genome of the cell (Laponogov et al., 2009).

Quinolone resistance in *N. gonorrhoeae* is due to point mutations in the quinolone resistance determining region (QRDR) of the A subunits of DNA gyrase (*gyrA*) and topoisomerase IV (*parC*) (Tanaka et al., 2000; Trees et al., 2001). Belland and colleagues were the first to delineate the genetic basis of quinolone resistance in *N. gonorrhoeae* in 1994. By analyzing ciprofloxacin resistant (Cip[R]) mutants selected *in vitro*, these investigators showed Cip[R] in *N. gonorrhoeae* is a two step process in which intermediate level ciprofloxacin resistance (Cip[I]) occurs via point mutations in *gyrA* that encode amino acid substitutions at positions Ser91 and Asp95. Cip[I] *gyrA* mutants then become Cip[R] when point mutations occur in *parC* (Belland et al., 1994). This sequence of events is consistent with data from numerous molecular epidemiologic studies (Kam et al., 2003; Morris et al., 2009; Starnino et al., 2010; Tanaka, 1992; Trees et al., 2001; Vereshchagin et al., 2004). Analyses of clinical isolates have also provided insights into the nature of mutations directly associated with fluoroquinolone resistance in *N. gonorrhoeae*. Commonly isolated substitutions in the Ser91 position of the GyrA subunit include amino acids with bulky side chains (phenylalanine and tyrosine) and the hydrophobic leucine, while arginine is the most common substitution at position Asp95 (Kam et al., 2003; Morris et al., 2009; Ruiz et al., 2001; Starnino et al., 2010; Tanaka et al., 2000; Trees et al., 2001; Vereshchagin et al., 2004; Vernel-Paulillac et al., 2009). Double point mutations in *gyrA* that result in these amino acid substitutions are sufficient and also largely responsible for sterically hindering the intercalation of quinolone molecules (Xiong et al., 2011). The location specificity of *parC* mutations that lead to high level Cip[R] appears to be less stringent than mutations in *gyrA*, with alterations at position 91 (the most common), 86, 87, or 88 identified among Cip[R] isolates (Dewi et al., 2004; Morris et al., 2009; Tanaka et al., 2000; Trees et al., 2001) (Figure 2).

The impact of quinolone resistance mutations on microbial fitness has been studied in several bacterial species. Topoisomerase mutations often are associated with an *in vitro* fitness cost, although not all *gyrA* mutations or combinations of *gyrA* mutations or *gyrA*, *parC* mutations result in decreased growth *in vitro* (Bagel et al., 1999; Marcusson et al., 2009, Pope et al., 2008; Luo et al., 2005). Interestingly, in 2005 Zhang and colleagues showed *gyrA* mutations confer a fitness benefit to *C. jejuni in vivo* using a chicken intestinal colonization model (Luo et al., 2005). Based on this report and the wide prevalence of QRNG strains, we hypothesized that fluoroquinolone resistance mutations in *N. gonorrhoeae* may be accompanied by a transmission or survival advantage. To address the possibility that QRNG may be more fit *in vivo*, we constructed Cip[I] and Cip[R] mutants in *N. gonorrhoeae* strain FA19 that carry the commonly isolated *gyrA* (Ser91Phe and Asp95Asn) or *gyrA* (Ser91Phe and Asp95Asn) and *parC* (Asp86Asn) mutations, respectively, and measured their fitness relative to the Cip[S] parent strain in the murine genital tract infection model. No *in vitro*

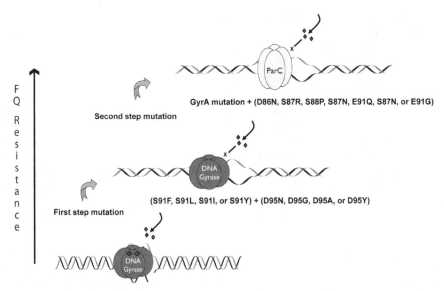

Fig. 2. **Evolution of quinolone resistance in *N. gonorrhoeae*.** Quinolone resistance in *N. gonorrhoeae* is a two-step process, beginning with point mutations in the QRDR of *gyrA*, which increase resistance to intermediate levels. Positions 91 and 95 are most often altered, with Ser91Phe and Asp95Asn the most common substitutions. Other substitutions have also been reported. High level resistance occurs upon mutation of the QRDR of *parC* mutation. *parC* mutations carried by Cip^R gonococci most often cause amino acid substations at position 91, 86, 87 or 88 (Kam et al., 2003; Ghanem et al., 2005; Morris et al., 2009; Ruiz 2001; Starnino et al., 2010; Tanaka et al., 2000; Trees et al., 2001; Vereshchagin et al., 2004; Vernel-Paulillac 2009).

fitness cost was associated with acquisition of the *gyrA*$_{91/95}$ mutations based on comparing the growth rates of the *gyrA*$_{91/95}$ mutant and the Cip^S wild-type strain, although a slight reduction (3-fold) in the recovery of the mutant was observed when co-cultured with the Cip^S wild-type strain (Table 2). Interestingly, however, the Cip^I *gyrA*$_{91/95}$ mutant exhibited a clear fitness advantage *in vivo* as evidenced by high competitive indices (CIs) over time and the isolation of only Cip^I bacteria from some mice on days 5 and 7 post-inoculation. In contrast, the Cip^R *gyrA*$_{91/95}$, *parC*$_{86}$ mutant grew significantly more slowly *in vitro* and exhibited reduced fitness *in vivo* relative to the wild-type Cip^S strain (Table 2) (Kunz et al., In Press).

Genotype	CI at day 3
gyrA$_{91/95}$	5-fold increase; 30-fold increase on day 5 compared to Cip^S wild-type strain
gyrA$_{91/95}$, *parC*$_{86}$	2-fold decrease compared to Cip^S wild-type strain
gyrA$_{91/95}$, *mtrR-79*	40-fold increase compared to Cip^S *mtr-56* mutant parent strain
gyrA$_{91/95}$, *parC*$_{86}$, *mtrR-79*	50-fold decrease compared to Cip^S *mtr-56* mutant parent strain

Table 2. Fitness of FQ-R mutations in mice compared to wild-type or *mtr* mutant Gc. CI: competitive index. Ratio of mutant to wild-type CFU (vaginal isolates) divided by mutant to wild-type CFU (inoculum).

As discussed, it is well established that mtr locus mutations increase gonococcal fitness in the mouse model, and we therefore wondered whether the fitness benefit conferred by $gyrA_{91/95}$ mutations would enhance the fitness advantage afforded by increased efflux of host substrates through the MtrC-MtrD-MtrE active efflux pump. Our alternative hypothesis was that increasing numbers of resistance mutations would impair growth to such an extent as to abrogate the fitness benefits associated with either resistance mutation. To test this hypothesis, we constructed $gyrA_{91/95}$ and $gyrA_{91/95}$, $parC_{86}$ mutants in an mtr mutant of strain FA19 that carries a commonly isolated $mtrR$ promoter mutation (the single base pair deletion in the $mtrR$ promoter termed hereafter as $mtrR$-79). The $gyrA_{91/95}$, $mtrR$-79 mutant (Cip^I) showed no fitness difference compared to the $mtrR$-79 mutant parent strain in $vitro$, but significantly out-competed the $mtrR$-79 mutant during experimental murine infection. In contrast, the highly Cip^R $gyrA_{91/95}$, $parC_{86}$, $mtrR$-79 mutant was severely attenuated both in $vitro$ and in $vivo$ relative to the $mtrR_{-56}$ mutant, with only $mtrR_{-56}$ mutant gonococci recovered from a majority of mice 5 days after inoculation (Table 2) (Kunz et al., In Press).

From these studies we conclude that the $gyrA_{91/95}$ mutation confers a fitness benefit to $N.$ $gonorrhoeae$ that is independent of the MtrC-MtrD-MtrE efflux pump system, but that an additional $parC_{86}$ mutation results in a net fitness cost. These data are intriguing and may help to explain the frequent isolation of Cip^R gonococci that also carry $mtrR$ promoter or $mtrR$ structural gene mutations, which has been interpreted by others as evidence that active efflux through the MtrC-MtrD-MtrE pump is another mechanism of fluoroquinolone resistance in $N.$ $gonorrhoeae$ (Dewi et al., 2004; Vereshchagin et al., 2004). The fact that we found no difference in the Cip MICs of the $gyrA_{91/95}$ versus $gyrA_{91/95}$, $MtrR$-79 mutants or of $gyrA_{91/95}$, $parC_{86}$ versus $gyrA_{91/95}$, $parC_{86}$, $mtrR$-79 mutants (Kunz et al., submitted), is strong genetic evidence that mtr mutations do not contribute to Cip^R in $N.$ $gonorrhoeae$. Instead, the prevalence of Cip^R mtr strains may reflect increased microbial fitness conferred by these mutations.

It is important to remember that while mutations in both $gyrA$ and $parC$ led to reduced fitness in the mouse model, compensatory mutations may occur in nature that restore fitness while maintaining high level Cip^R. There is much evidence that fitness compensation can occur in bacteria without loss of antibiotic resistance (Balsalobre et al., 2011; Bjorkholm et al., 2001; Bjorkman et al., 1998; Giraud et al., 1999; Komp Lindgren et al., 2005; Marcussen et al., 2009; Nagaev et al., 2001). In support of this possibility for QRNG, we have observed that while Cip^R gonococci were outcompeted by Cip^S (wild-type) or Cip^I bacteria in a majority of mice tested, only Cip^R gonococci were recovered from some mice (10-17%) as infection progressed in each of several experiments (Figure 3). To further investigate this observation, we analyzed Cip^R bacteria isolated on day 5 in pure culture from a mouse inoculated with a mixture of Cip^I ($gyrA_{91/95}$, $mtrR$-79) and Cip^R ($gyrA_{91/95}$, $parC_{86}$, $mtrR$-79) mutants. Interestingly, these Cip^R bacteria grew better than the Cip ^{I} and Cip^R strains used to inoculate the mouse and the Cip^S mtr parent of the Cip^I and Cip^R strains. Unlike either of these strains, the in $vivo$-selected Cip^R mutant had a wild-type mtr locus and a $gyrA$ allele that was predicted to encode a leucine instead of phenylalanine residue at position 91 (Phe91Leu) (Kunz et al., In Press). We conclude that one or more compensatory mutations occurred during infection that allowed highly Cip^R gonococci to out-compete Cip^I bacteria in $vivo$.

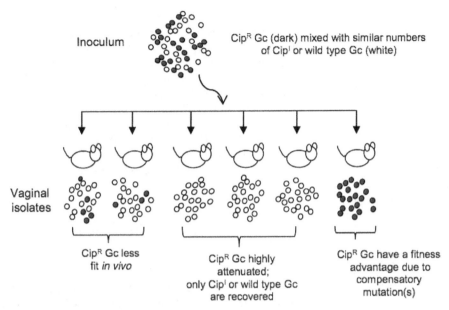

Fig. 3. **The fitness disadvantage of Cip^R gonococci can be overcome by selection for compensatory mutations**. Vaginal inoculation of estradiol-treated BALB/c mice with populations of Cip^S or Cip^I gonococci (white) mixed with similar numbers of Cip^R gonococci (black) results in the recovery of a higher proportion of Cip^S or Cip^I CFU, with some mice clearing the Cip^R bacteria. However, in 10-17% of mice tested, high numbers of only Cip^R CFU were recovered as infection progressed, most likely due to compensatory mutations (Kunz et al, In Press).

The basis for the reported *in vivo* fitness benefit shown by *gyrA* mutants in *N. gonorrhoeae* or *C. jejuni* (Luo et al., 2005) is not known. As topoisomerase mutations are accompanied by alterations in supercoiling (Bagel et al., 1999; Luo et al., 2005), changes in the expression of genes important for colonization, growth on mucosal surfaces, or evasion of host defenses are one possible explanation (Luo et al., 2005; Zhang et al., 2006). It is also possible that the *in vivo* fitness benefit exhibited by *gyrA*$_{91/95}$ mutants in *N. gonorrhoeae* is due to secondary mutations that were selected to compensate for alterations in GyrA as proposed by Marcusson *et al.* to explain the increased fitness of *gyrA* mutants of *E. coli* in a urinary tract infection model (Marcusson et al., 2009). The *E. coli* mutants tested in this study showed various degrees of fitness costs *in vitro*, however, and thus it is reasonable to assume that one or more compensatory mutations would be needed to promote fitness *in vivo*. In contrast, while *gyrA* mutations are associated with increased *in vivo* fitness in *C. jejuni* (Luo et al., 2005) and *N. gonorrhoeae* (Kunz et al., In Press), these mutations do not confer a significant growth cost *in vitro*; therefore, secondary mutations that restore growth may not be required for full fitness *in vivo*. Additionally, while not definitive evidence that *gyrA* mutations alone are responsible for the fitness we observe in the mouse model, we recently demonstrated that *gyrA*$_{91/95}$ mutations are accompanied by a pronounced fitness benefit in two other *N. gonorrhoeae* strains, and that this benefit was detected within one day of infection (Jonathan A. D'Ambrozio & Ann E. Jerse, unpublished observation).

Identification of the mechanism by which *gyrA* mutations enhance gonococcal fitness during experimental murine infection is important as it may reveal new and interesting facets of gonococcal pathogenesis. Additionally, our data suggest Cip^I strains may serve as a reservoir for Cip^R in *N. gonorrhoeae* since a single step mutation in *parC* is all that is then required for high-level resistance. We postulate the following scenario by which this may occur. First, low-levels of antibiotic pressure due to fluoroquinolone treatment for other infections or self-medication selects for Cip^I strains. Cip^I strains are then maintained within sexual networks, or even flourish, due to the fitness benefit conferred by the *gyrA*$_{91/95}$ mutations. Highly Cip^R strains would not flourish, possibly due to the more severe growth defect construed by mutation in *parC*$_{86}$ or the possibility that the *parC*$_{86}$ mutation or the combination of the *parC*$_{86}$, *gyrA*$_{91/95}$ mutations may have a negative impact on the expression of genes important for survival *in vivo*. However, some Cip^R gonococci will be selected due to compensatory mutations that restore fitness while maintaining high level Cip^R. Continued study of the frequency and nature of compensatory mutations that allow maintenance of high level Cip^R is important for understanding the spread of QRNG.

4. Conclusion

Antibiotic resistance expressed by many of the bacterial pathogens that infect humans represents one of the most important public health challenges for clinical medicine in the 21st century. During the early years of the antibiotic era of medicine (circa. 1945-1950) it became clear to physicians that antibiotic treatment failures were frequently the result of the infecting bacteria being resistant to the antibiotic being used; indeed, penicillinase-producing strains of *Staphylococcus aureus* were recognized and became wide-spread soon after penicillin was introduced as a therapeutic agent in 1943 (Bud, 2007). As the antibiotic era progressed and more antibiotics became available, disturbing reports of treatment failures became more prevalent. Fortunately, researchers trained in microbial physiology and bacterial genetics undertook studies to learn the mechanisms used by bacteria to resist a given antibiotic. These early investigators soon learned that while an antibiotic resistant strain had an advantage over a susceptible strain in the presence of the antibiotic in question, the resistance mechanism frequently came at a cost in the absence of the antibiotic. Thus, in the absence of the selective pressure brought by the antibiotic, the resistant strain frequently grew slower *in vitro* and in model systems of infection (cell culture or animals). However, for some resistance mechanisms, there was little if any cost when compared to a sensitive, but otherwise isogenic strain. The resulting dogma from this work was that antibiotic resistance in the absence of selective pressures could be costly for bacteria. In this case, removing the selective pressure would result in the evolution of more susceptible strains that would have an advantage in the community. By and large, this has not been the case (Anderson & Hughes, 2010).

Less clear, however, was whether in the absence of selective pressure, a resistant strain would have a fitness benefit during an infection over a sensitive counterpart. In this respect, the report of Luo *et al.* (2005) dealing with the increased fitness of a ciprofloxacin resistant strain of *C. jejuni* over a sensitive parent strain *in vivo* was a "game-changer" for antibiotic resistance researchers. Briefly, it forced us to consider the rather scary possibility that a mechanism of antibiotic resistance can actually enhance the ability of a pathogen to survive in the community. This possibility has a number of important implications for our understanding of bacterial pathogenesis and bacterial infections that should be considered. First, are there "antibiotic substitutes" *in vivo* that the resistance mechanism recognizes, allowing the resistant strain to out-compete the sensitive strain? Might these "host antibiotics" provide the selective pressure in the community? This is certainly likely for the fitness benefit imparted to those *N. gonorrhoeae* strains that over-express the Mtr efflux pump system. This pump, along with similar pumps produced by other Gram-negatives (Shafer et al., 2010), recognizes host antimicrobials (e.g., antimicrobial peptides) in addition to antibiotics such as beta-lactams and macrolides. In this context, efflux pump inhibitors (Lomovskaya & Bostian, 2006) may have clinical use as they would increase bacterial susceptibility to classical antibiotics as well as host antimicrobials. A second issue that requires further investigation is whether a resistance mechanism has secondary effects on the physiology of the resistant strain that results in an advantage during infection. This hypothesis may help to explain why $gyrA_{91/95}$ mutations can enhance the fitness of Cip^I strains of *N. gonorrhoeae*. Hopefully, ongoing transcriptional profiling studies that compare isogenic Cip^I and Cip^S strains will provide insights that will help us to understand fitness differences. A third point merits consideration: stable mutations that decrease bacterial susceptibility to a given antibiotic, but not to an extent that it pushes them across the MIC breakpoint, may be more advantageous for the bacteria than previously thought. In this respect, as emphasized throughout this text, mutations in *mtrR* or *gyrA* provide gonococci with a fitness advantage *in vivo*, but do not push them across the MIC breakpoint for either beta-lactams or quinolones, respectively. Importantly, both are necessary for clinically significant levels of resistance imparted by other mutations. Accordingly, strains bearing *mtrR* and/or *gyrA* mutations may not only be more fit during infection, but also more likely to subsequently develop clinical resistance to beta-lactams and quinolones than fully sensitive strains. This issue is of greater urgency now because the gonococcal strain that caused a ceftriaxone-resistant infection in Japan is an *mtrR* mutant (Ohnishi et al., 2011) even though the mutation by itself has little impact on the level of beta-lactam resistance (Veal & Shafer, 2003). Finally, if a resistance mutation enhances fitness and is stably maintained in a bacterial pathogen for years, it may be yet another reason why antibiotic re-cycling after extended absence from the treatment regimen may not be a viable option to combat the emergence and spread of antibiotic resistant bacteria.

We have used *N. gonorrhoeae* as a model human pathogen for studies on how bacterial fitness can be impacted by mechanisms of antibiotic resistance. Having been intimately associated with humans for thousands of years, it is of no surprise that the gonococcus has evolved novel ways to evade or resist the multitude of toxic agents that it encounters during infection. The continued emergence of strains expressing decreased susceptibility or even clinical resistance to frontline antibiotics used today (e.g., ceftriaxone) in therapy emphasizes the remarkable adaptive ability of this pathogen. The examples provided herein with the gonococcus emphasize that mechanisms of antibiotic resistance can enhance bacterial virulence, as defined by increased *in vivo* fitness. Understanding the processes that lead to increased fitness of the gonococcus (or any other pathogen) due to antibiotic resistance may result in novel strategies that could be used to inhibit bacterial replication *in vivo* directly or indirectly by enhancing the efficacy of the defensive systems of the host that operate locally.

5. Acknowledgments

This work was supported by the National Institute of Allergy and Infectious Diseases at the National Institute of Health [RO1 AI42053 and U19 AI31496 to A.E.J.; R37 AI21150 to

W.M.S.], and a USUHS training grant [C073-RT to A.N.K.]. W.M.S. was supported in part by a Senior Research Career Scientist Award from the VA Medical Research Service.

6. References

Andersson, D. & Levin, B. (1999) The Biological Cost of Antibiotic Resistance. *Current Opinion in Microbiology*, Vol. 2, No. 5, pp. 489 – 493, ISSN 1369-5274

Andersson, D. & Hughes, D. (2010) Antibiotic Resistance and Its Cost: Is It Possible to Reverse Resistance? *Nature Reviews Microbiology*, Vol. 8, No. 4, pp. 260 – 271, ISSN 1740 - 1526

Bagel, S., Hullen, V., Wiedemann, B. & Heisig, P. (1999) Impact of *gyrA* and *parC* Mutations on Quinolone Resistance, Doubling Time, and Supercoiling Degree in *Escherichia coli*. *Antimicrobial Agents and Chemotherapy*, Vol. 43, No. 4, pp. 868-875, ISSN 0066-4804

Balsalobre, L., Ferrandiz, J., de Alba, G. & de la Campa, A. (2011) Nonoptimal DNA Topoisomerases Allow Maintenance of Supercoiling Levels and Improve Fitness of *Streptococcus pneumoniae*. *Antimicrobial Agents and Chemotherapy*, Vol. 55, No. 3, pp. 1097-1105, ISSN 0066-4804

Bates, A., Berger, J. & Maxwell, A. (2011) The Ancestral Role of ATP Hydrolysis in Type II Topoisomerases: Prevention of DNA Double-Strand Breaks. *Nucleic Acids Research*, Vol. 39, No. 15, pp. 6327 – 6339, ISSN 0305-1048

Belland, R., Morrison, S., Ison, C. & Huang, W. (1994) *Neisseria gonorrhoeae* Acquires Mutations in Analogous Regions of *gyrA* and *parC* in Fluoroquinolone-Resistant Isolates. *Molecular Microbiology*, Vol. 14, No. 2, pp. 371-380, ISSN 0950-382X

Bjorkman J., Hughes, D. & Andersson, D. (1998) Virulence of Antibiotic-Resistant *Salmonella typhimurium*. *Proceedings of the National Acadamy of Science, USA*, Vol. 95, No. 7, pp. 3949-3953, ISSN 0027-8424

Bjorkholm, B., Sjolund, M., Falk, P., Berg, O., Engstrand, L. & Andersson, D. (2001) Mutation Frequency and Biological Cost of Antibiotic Resistance in *Helicobacter pylori*. *Proceedings of the National Acadamy of Science, USA*, Vol. 98, No. 25, pp. 146077-14612, ISSN 0027-8424

Bud, R. (2007) Fighting Resistance with Technology. In: *Penicillin: Triumph and Tragedy*, pp. 116 – 139, Oxford University Press, ISBN 978-0-19-925406-4, Oxford, UK

Centers for Disease Control and Prevention (CDC). (2007) Update to CDC's Sexually Transmitted Diseases Treatment Guidelines, 2006: Fluoroquinolones No Longer Recommended for Treatment of Gonococcal Infections. *Morbidity and Mortality Weekly Report*, Vol. 56, pp. 332-336

Chen, F.-J. & Lo, H.-J. (2003) Molecular Mechanisms of Fluoroquinolone Resistance. *Journal of Microbiology, Immunology, and Infection*, Vol. 36, No. 1, pp. 1-9, ISSN 1684-1182

Covino, J., Cummings, M., Smith, B., Benes, S., Draft, K. & McCormack, W. (1990) Comparison of Ofloxacin and Ceftriaxone in the Treatment of Uncomplicated Gonorrhea Caused by Penicillinase-Producing and Non-Penicillinase-Producing Strains. *Antimicrobial Agents and Chemotherapy*, Vol. 34, No. 1, pp. 148–149, ISSN 0066-4804

Delahay, R., Robertson, B., Balthazar, J., Shafer, W. & Ison, C. (1997) Involvement of the Gonococcal MtrE Protein in the Resistance of *Neisseria gonorrhoeae* to Toxic Hydrophobic Agents. *Microbiology*, Vol. 143, No. 7, pp. 2127 – 2133, ISSN 0002-1485

Dewi, B., Akira, S., Hayashi, H. & Ba-Thein, W. (2004) High Occurrence of Simultaneous Mutations in Target Enzymes and MtrRCDE Efflux System in Quinolone-Resistant

Neisseria gonorrhoeae. *Sexually Transmitted Diseases*, Vol. 31, No. 6, pp. 353-359, ISSN 0148-5717

Dionne-Odom, J., Tambe, P., Yee, E., Weinstock, H. & del Rio, C. (2011) Antimicrobial Resistant Gonorrhea in Atlanta: 1988 – 2006. *Sexually Transmitted Diseases*, Vol. 38, No. 12, pp. 780 – 782, ISNN 0148-5717

Eisenstein, B. & Sparling, P. (1978) Mutations to Increased Antibiotic Susceptibility in Naturally-Occurring Gonococci. *Nature*, Vol. 271, No. 5642, pp. 242 – 244, ISSN 0028-0836

Emmerson, A. M. (2003) The Quinolones: Decades of Development and Use. U.S. Patent 90001. *Journal of Antimicrobial Chemotherapy*, Vol. 51, Suppl1, pp. 13–20

Folster, J. & Shafer, W. (2005) Regulation of *mtrF* Expression in *Neisseria gonorrhoeae* and Its Role in High-Level Antimicrobial Resistance. *Journal of Bacteriology*, Vol. 187, N. 11, pp. 3713 – 3720, ISSN 0021-9193

Ghanem, K., Giles, J. & Zenilman, J. (2005) Fluoroquinolone-Resistant *Neisseria gonorrhoeae*: the Inevitable Epidemic. *Infectious Disease Clinics of North America*, Vol. 19, No. 2, pp. 351–365, ISSN 0891-5520

Giraud, E., Brisabois, A., Martel, J.-L. & Chaslus-Danclai, E. (1999) Comparative Studies of Mutations in Animal Isolates and Experimental *in vitro-* and *in vivo*-Selected Mutants of *Salmonella* spp. Suggest a Counterselection of Highly Fluoroquinolone-Resistant Strains in the Field. *Antimicrobial Agents and Chemotherapy*, Vol. 43, No. 9, pp. 2131-2137, ISSN 0066-4804

Hagman, K. & Shafer, W. (1995) Transcriptional Control of the *mtr* Efflux System of *Neisseria gonorrhoeae*. *Journal of Bacteriology*, Vol. 177, No. 14, pp. 4162 – 4165, ISSN 0021-9193

Hagman, K., Pan, W., Spratt, B., Balthazar, J., Judd, R. & Shafer, W. (1995) Resistance of *Neisseria gonorrhoeae* to Antimicrobial Hydrophobic Agents is Modulated by the *mtrRCDE* Efflux System. *Microbiology*, Vol. 141, No. 3, pp. 611 – 622, ISSN 0001-9400

Hagman, K., Lucas, C., Balthazar, J., Snyder, L., Nilles, M., Judd, R. & Shafer, W. (1997) The MtrD Protein of *Neisseria gonorrhoeae* is a Member of the Resistance/Nodulation/Division Protein Family Constituting Part of an Efflux System. *Microbiology*, Vol. 143, No. 7, pp. 2117 – 2125, ISSN 0002-1486

Hoffmann, K., Williams, D., Shafer, W. & Brennan, R. (2005) Characterization of the Multiple Transferable Resistance Repressor, MtrR from *Neisseria gonorrhoeae*. *Journal of Bacteriology*, Vol. 187, No 14, pp. 5008 – 5012, ISSN 0021-9193

Hooper, D. (1999) Mode of Action of Fluoroquinolones. *Drugs*, Vol. 58, Suppl 2, pp. 6–10, ISSN 0012-6667

Jerse, A. (1999) Experimental Gonococcal Genital Tract Infection and Opacity Protein Expression in Estradiol-Treated Mice. *Infection and Immunity* Vol. 67, No 11, pp. 5699-5708, ISSN 0019-9567

Jerse, A., Sharma, N., Simms, A., Crow, E., Snyder, L. & Shafer, W. (2003) A Gonococcal Efflux Pump System Enhances Bacterial Survival in a Female Mouse Model of Genital Tract Infection. *Infection and Immunity*, Vol. 71, No. 10, pp. 4476 – 5582, ISSN 0019-9567

Kam, K., Kam, S., Cheung, D., Tung, V., Au, W. & Cheung, M. (2003) Molecular Characterization of Quinolone-Resistant *Neisseria gonorrhoeae* in Hong Kong. *Antimicrobial Agents and Chemotherapy*, Vol 47, No. 1, pp. 436–439, ISSN 0066-4804

Komp Lindgren P., Marcusson, L., Sandvang, D., Frimodt-Moller, N. & Hughes, D. (2005) Biological Cost of Single and Multiple Norfloxacin Resistance Mutations in

Escherichia coli Implicated in Urinary Tract Infections. *Antimicrobial Agents and Chemotherapy*, Vol. 49, No. 6, pp. 2343-2351, ISSN 0066-4804

Kunz A., Begum, A., Wu, H., D'Ambrozio, J., Robinson, J., Shafer, W., Bash, M. & Jerse, A. (2012), Impact of Fluoroquinolone Resistance Mutations on Gonococcal Fitness and *in vivo* Selection for Compensatory Mutations. *Journal of Infectious Diseases* (In Press)

Laponogov, I., Sohi, M., Veselkov, D., Pan, X.-S., Sawhney, R., Thompson, A., McAuley, K., Fisher, L. & Sanderson, M. (2009) Structural Insight into the Quinolone–DNA Cleavage Complex of Type IIA Topoisomerases. *Nature Structural and Molecular Biology*, Vol. 16, No. 6, pp. 667–669, ISSN 1545-9993

Lomovskaya, O. & Bostian, K. (2006) Practical Applications and Feasibility of Efflux Pump Inhibitors in the Clinic — A Vision for Applied Use. *Biochemical Pharmacology*, Vol. 71, No. 7, pp. 910 – 918, ISSN 0006-2952

Lucas, C., Balthazar, J., Hagman, K. & Shafer, W. (1997) The MtrR Repressor Binds the DNA Sequence between the *mtrR* and *mtrC* Genes of *Neisseria gonorrhoeae*. *Journal of Bacteriology*, Vol. 179, No. 13, pp. 4123 – 4128, ISSN 0021-9193

Luo, N., Pereira, S., Sahin, O., Lin, J., Huang, S., Michel, L. & Zhang, Q. (2005) Enhanced *in vivo* Fitness of Fluoroquinolone-Resistant *Campylobacter jejuni* in the Absence of Antibiotic Selection Pressure. *Proceedings of the National Acadamy of Science, USA*, Vol. 102, No. 3, pp. 541-546, ISSN 0027-8424

Marcusson L., Frimodt-Moller, N. & Hughes, D. (2009) Interplay in the Selection of Fluoroquinolone Resistance and Bacterial Fitness. *PLoS Pathogens*, Vol. 5, No. 8, pp. e1000541, ISSN 1553-7366

Morais Cabral, J., Jackson, A., Smith, C., Shikotra, N., Maxwell, A. & Liddington, R. (1997) Crystal Structure of the Breakage-Reunion Domain of DNA Gyrase. *Nature*, Vol. 388, No. 6645, pp. 903–906, ISSN 0028-0836

Morris S., Moore, D., Hannah, P., Wang, S., Wolfe, J., Trees, D., Bolan, G. & Bauer, H. (2009) Strain Typing and Antimicrobial Resistance of Fluoroquinolone-Resistant *Neisseria gonorrhoeae* Causing a California Infection Outbreak. *Journal of Clinical Microbiology*, Vol. 47, No. 9, pp. 2944-2949, ISSN 0095-1137

Morse, S., Lysko, P., McFarland, L., Knapp, J., Sandstrom, E., Critchlow, C. & Holmes, K. (1982) Gonococcal Strains from Homosexual Men have Outer Membranes with Reduced Permeability to Hydrophobic Molecules. *Infection and Immunity*, Vol. 37, No. 2, pp. 432 – 438, ISSN 0019-9567

Mercante, A.D., Jackson, L., Johnson, P. J. T., Stringer, V. A., Dyer, D. W., & Shafer, W. M. (2012) MpeR Regulates the mtr Efflux Locus in *Neisseria gonorrhoeae* and Modulates Antimicrobial Resistance by an Iron-Responsive Mechanism. *Antimicrobial Agents and Chemotherapy*, Vol. 56, No. 3, pp. 1491 - 1501, ISSN 0066-4804.

Nagaev, I, Bjorkman, J., Andersson, D., & Hughes, D. (2001) Biological Cost and Compensatory Evolution in Fusidic Acid Resistant *Staphylococcus aureus*. *Molecular Microbiology*, Vol. 40, No. 2, pp. 443-449, ISSN 0950-382X

Ohnishi, M., Golparian, D., Shimuta, K., Saika, T., Hoshina, S., Iwasaku, K., Nakayama, S., Kitawaki, J. & Unemo, M. (2011) Is *Neisseria gonorrhoeae* Initiating a Future Era of Untreatable Gonorrhea?: Detailed Characterization of the First Strain with High-Level Resistance to Ceftriaxone. *Antimicrobial Agents and Chemotherapy*, Vol. 55, No. 7, pp. 3538 – 3545, ISSN 0066-4804

Packiam, M., Veit, S., Anderson, D., Ingalls, R. & Jerse, A. (2010) Mouse Strain-Dependent Differences in Susceptibility to *Neisseria gonorrhoeae* Infection and Induction of Innate Immune Responses. *Infection and Immunity*, Vol. 78, No. 1, pp. 433-440, ISSN 0019-9567

Pan, W. & Spratt, B. (1994) Regulation of the Permeability of the Gonococcal Cell Envelope by the *mtr* System. *Molecular Microbiology*, Vol. 11, No. 4, pp. 769 – 775, ISSN 0950-382X

Pope, C., Gillespie, S., Pratten, J. & McHugh, T. (2008) Fluoroquinolone-Resistant Mutants of *Burkholderia cepacia*. *Antimicrobial Agents and Chemotherapy*, Vol. 52, No. 3, pp. 1201-1203, ISSN 0066-4804

Rouquette, C., Harmon, J. & Shafer, W. (1999) Induction of the *mtrCDE*-Encoded Efflux Pump system of *Neisseria gonorrhoeae* Requires MtrA, an AraC-Like Protein. *Molecular Microbiology*, Vol. 33, No. 3, pp. 651 – 658, ISSN 1365-2958

Ruiz J., Jurado, A., Garcia-Méndez, E., Marco, F., Aguilar, L., Jiménez de Anta, M. & Vila, J. (2001) Frequency of Selection of Fluoroquinolone-Resistant Mutants of *Neisseria gonorrhoeae* Exposed to Gemifloxacin and Four Other Quinolones. *Journal of Antimicrobial Chemotherapy*, Vol. 48, No. 4, pp. 545-548, ISSN 0305-7453

Schrag, S., Perrot, V. & Levin, B. (1997) Adaptation to the Fitness Costs of Antibiotic Resistance in *Escherichia coli*. Proceedings of the Royal Society of Biological Sciences, Vol. 264, No. 1386, pp. 1287 – 1291, ISSN 0962-8452

Shafer, W., Balthazar, J., Hagman, K. & Morse, S. (1995) Missense Mutations that Alter the DNA-Binding Domain of the MtrR Protein Occur Frequently in Rectal Isolates of *Neisseria gonorrhoeae* that are Resistant to Fecal Lipids. *Microbiology*, Vol. 141, No. 4, pp. 907 – 911, ISSN 0001-9525

Shafer, W., Qu, X., Waring, A. & Lehrer, R. (1998) Modulation of *Neisseria gonorrhoeae* Susceptibility to Vertebrate Antibacterial Peptides due to a Member of the Resistance/Nodulation/Division Efflux Pump Family. *Proceedings of the National Academy of Science*, Vol. 95, No. 4, pp. 1829 – 1833, ISSN 0027-8424

Shafer, W., Folster, J. & Nicholas, R. (2010) Molecular Mechanisms of Antibiotic Resistance Expressed by the Pathogenic *Neisseria*. In: *Neisseria: Molecular Mechanisms of Pathogenesis*, Genco, C. & Wetzler, L. (Ed.), pp. 245 – 267, Caister Academic Press, ISBN 978-1-904455-51-6, Norfolk, UK

Song, W., Condron, S., Mocca, B., Veit, S., Hill, D., Abbas, A. & Jerse, A. (2008) Local and Humoral Immune Responses Against Primary and Repeat *Neisseria gonorrhoeae* Genital Tract Infections of 17ß-Estradiol-Treated Mice. *Vaccine*, Vol. 26, pp. 5741-5751, ISSN 0264-410X

Starnino, S., Conte, I., Matteelli, A., Galluppi, E., Cusini, M., Carlo, A., Delmonte, S. & Stefanelli, P. (2010) Trend of Ciprofloxacin Resistance in *Neisseria gonorrhoeae* Strains Isolated in Italy and Analysis of the Molecular Determinants. *Diagnostic Microbiology and Infectious Disease*, Vol. 67, No. 4, pp. 350–354, ISSN 0732-8893

Tanaka, M., Nakayama, H., Haraoka, M., Saika, T., Kobayashi, I., & Naito, S. (2000) Antimicrobial Resistance of *Neisseria gonorrhoeae* and High Prevalence of Ciprofloxacin-Resistant Isolates in Japan, 1993-1998. *Journal of Clinical Microbiology*, Vol. 38, No. 2, pp. 521-525, ISSN 0095-1137

Tapsall, J. W. (2005) Antibiotic Resistance in *Neisseria gonorrhoeae*. *Clinical Infectious Diseases*, Vol. 41, Suppl 4, pp. S263-8

Trees, D., Sandul, A., Neal, S., Higa, H., & Knapp, J. (2001) Molecular Epidemiology of *Neisseria gonorrhoeae* Exhibiting Decreased Susceptibility and Resistance to Ciprofloxacin in Hawaii, 1991-1999. *Sexually Transmitted Diseases*, Vol. 28, No. 6, pp. 309-14, ISSN 0148-5717

Unemo, M., Golparian, D., Syversen, G., Vestrheim, D. & Moi, H. (2010) Two Cases of Verified Clinical Failures Using Internationally Recommended First-Line Cefixime for Gonorrhoea Treatment, Norway, 2010. *Euro Surveillance*, Vol. 15, No. 47, ISSN 1025-496X

Veal, W. & Shafer, W. (2003) Identification of a Cell Envelope Protein (MtrF) Involved in Hydrophobic Antimicrobial Resistance in *Neisseria gonorrhoeae*. *Journal of Antimicrobial Chemotherapy*, Vol. 51, No. 1, pp. 27 – 37, ISSN 0305-7453

Vereshchagin V., Ilina, E., Malakhova, M., Zubkov, M., Sidorenko, S., Kuhanova, A. & Govorun, V. (2004) Fluoroquinolone-Resistant *Neisseria gonorrhoeae* Isolates from Russia: Molecular Mechanisms Implicated. *Journal of Antimicrobial Chemotherapy*, Vol. 53, No. 4, pp. 653-656, ISSN 0305-7453

Vernel-Pauillac F., Hogan, T., Tapsall, J. & Goarant, C. (2009) Quinolone Resistance in *Neisseria gonorrhoeae*: Rapid Genotyping of Quinolone Resistance-Determining Regions in *gyrA* and *parC* Gene by Melting Curve Analysis Predicts Susceptibility. *Antimicrobial Agents and Chemotherapy*, Vol. 53, No. 3, pp. 1264-1267, ISSN 0066-4804

Warner, D., Folster, J., Shafer, W. & Jerse, A. (2007) Regulation of the MtrC-MtrD-MtrE Efflux-Pump System Modulations the *in vivo* Fitness of *Neisseria gonorrhoeae*. *Journal of Infectious Diseases*, Vol. 196, No. 12, pp. 1804 – 1812, ISSN 0022-1899

Warner, D., Shafer, W. & Jerse, A. (2008) Clinically Relevant Mutations that Cause Derepression of the *Neisseria gonorrhoeae* MtrC-MtrD-MtrE Efflux Pump System Confer Different Levels of Antimicrobial Resistance and *in vivo* Fitness. *Molecular Microbiology*, Vol. 70, No. 2, pp. 462 – 478, ISSN 1365-2958

Webber, M., Baily, A., Blair, J., Morgan, E., Stevents, M., Hinton, J., Ivens, A., Wain, J. & Piddock, L. (2009) The Global Consequence of Disruption of the AcrAB-TolC Efflux Pump in *Salmonella enterica* Includes Reduced Expression of SPI-1 and Other Attributes Required to Infect the Host. *Journal of Bacteriology*, Vol. 191, No. 13, pp. 4276 – 4285, ISSN 0021-9193

Xia, M., Whittington, W., Shafer, W. & Holmes, K. (2000) Gonorrhea Among Men Who Have Sex with Men: Outbreak Caused by a Single Genotype of Erythromycin-Resistant *Neisseria gonorrhoeae* with a Single Base Pair Deletion in the *mtrR* Promoter Region. *Journal of Infectious Diseases*, Vol. 181, No. 6, pp. 2080 – 2082, ISSN 0022-1899

Xiong, X., Bromley, E., Oelschlaeger, P., Woolfson, D. & Spencer, J. (2011) Structural Insights into Quinolone AntibioticRresistance Mediated by Pentapeptide Repeat Proteins: Conserved Surface Loops Direct the Activity of a Qnr Protein from a Gram-Negative Bacterium. *Nucleic Acids Research*, Vol. 39, No. 9, pp. 3917–3927, ISSN 0305-1048

Zhang, Q., Sahin, O., McDermott, P. & Payot, S. (2006) Fitness of Antimicrobial-Resistant *Campylobacter* and *Salmonella*. *Microbes and Infection*, Vol. 8, No. 7, pp. 1972-1978, ISSN 1286-4579

Zarantonelli, L., Borthagaray, G., Lee, E. & Shafer, W. (1999) Decreased Azithromycin Susceptibility of *Neisseria gonorrhoeae* Due to *mtrR* Mutations. *Antimicrobial Agents and Chemotherapy*, Vol. 43, No. 10, pp. 2468 – 2472, ISSN 0066-4804

3

Single Cell Level Survey on Heterogenic Glycopeptide and β-Lactams Resistance

Tomasz Jarzembowski, Agnieszka Jóźwik,
Katarzyna Wiśniewska and Jacek Witkowski
Medical University of Gdańsk,
Poland

1. Introduction

Traditional microbiological methods, which involve the study of populations rather than individual cells, obscure heterogeneity of microorganisms. Now this phenomenon is widely reported and study of individual cells rather than populations seems to be highly reasonable. Differences between cells can be observed, especially in bacterial biofilm structure. In the case of wide variety of cells in the mixture, flow cytometry has proved to be a successful method in investigating varied populations of cells. This technique operates essentially by monitoring bacteria in suspension flowing, so that only one cell at a time passes by a sensor. The information acquired based on size and inner complexity of particles as well as fluorescence emission following previous staining can deliver great amount of information. This process also provides an immediate assessment of cells populations.

Although more than three decades ago flow cytometry has been applied to measure bacteria (Paau et al. 1977, Bailey et al. 1977), its use in microbiology is still underestimated and far from fully utilized. One of the reasons for that is that bacteria in comparison to mammalian cells are so much more difficult to work with in terms of their size and cell structure. Nevertheless with increasingly sensitive equipment, flow cytometry is finding its utility in dealing with highly heterogeneous bacterial populations.

The best known example of heterogeneity of bacteria is antibiotic resistance (Davey et al., 2003; Falagas et al., 2008). It is defined as resistance to antibiotics expressed by a subpopulation of cells within strains susceptible to antibiotics according to traditional in-vitro susceptibility testing. The heteroresistance has been observed in a range of microbes, including Staphylococcus aureus, coagulase-negative staphylococci, Acinetobacter baumannii , Mycobacterium tuberculosis, Streptococcus pneumoniae , Enterococcus faecium and Cryptococcus neoformans (Alvarez-Barrientos et al., 2000). Most observations on heteroresistance reported in the literature concern staphylococci resistant to methicillin, vancomycin, and/or inhibitors of teichoic acid synthesis (Finan at all., 2002). Recently, β-lactams heteroresistance of S. pneumoniae and vancomycin heteroresistance of enterococci have been also reported (Hasman et al., 2006; Nottasorn et al., 2005). The mechanism of β-lactams resistance is a change in the affinity of penicillin-binding proteins or overproduction of specific penicillin-binding proteins. Williamson et al. showed that at least five PBPs had been found in E. faecalis. Vancomycin resistance is usually determined by one of the two related gene clusters, vanA and vanB, that encode a dehydrogenase (VanH or VanHB) and ligase (VanA or VanB). Expression of VanA- and VanB-type resistance is regulated by the VanRS and VanRBSB two-component regulatory systems, respectively (Arthur et al., 1992; Evers and Courvalin, 1996).

As flow cytometry involves the study of single cells, it is an excellent method for studying heterogeneous populations. While analyzing many more cells than by conventional cytometry, rare cell types are more likely to be detected and the results are accessible to statistical analysis. The multiparametric nature of flow cytometric measurements is also an advantage. These include differences in cell size, DNA content or antigenic properties. Additionally, many supplementary modifications of flow cytometry are used. An example is the study of heterogenic vancomycin resistance with the use of reporter system for single-cell analysis of van gene expression. In the study, plasmid containing gene coding a green fluorescent protein was constructed for fluorescence-activated cell sorter (FACS) analysis (Cormack et al., 1996).

So far flow cytometry has been found useful in general microbiology with some clinical uses, as well as in its more specific branches such as environmental (Troussellier et al., 1999) or industrial microbiology (Gunasekera et al., 2000). First attempts to use flow cytometry for bacterial detection in body fluids are dated for the 80's when a test was developed enabling E. coli detection in blood samples (Mansour et al., 1985). The approach using flow cytometry has been continued and was reported later to be successful in bile, pleural fluid, ascites and cerebrospinal fluid (Takashi et al., 2000). Lately new tools based on flow cytometry have been developed, providing detection of significant bacteriuria as well as enumeration of bacterial particles, appearing to be an effective screening method (Hiroshi et al., 2006).

The emergence of multi-drug resistant microbial strains has emphasised the need for rapid detection method of antibiotic resistance and in this case as well flow cytometry appeared to be an extremely attractive tool.

Population analysis, among others, is the golden standard for the identification of hetero resistant vancomycin intermediate Staphylococcus aureus (hVISA) due to the fact that a proportion of MRSA found to harbor hVISA can be up to 8.3%. Moreover, for as yet unknown reasons, virtually all clinical E. faecalis isolates are tolerant to β-lactams and glycopeptides. Minimal inhibitory concentrations (MICs) of antimicrobials remain the same but the minimal bactericidal concentrations (MBCs) increase in tolerance.

Enterococcus faecalis usually plays a role in commensal flora in the human gastrointestinal tract. However, it can become a pathogen involved in various infections such as endocarditis, urinary tract infections, meningitis, sepsis and intraabdominal infections. It is also a leading cause of nosocomial infections, and the emergence of vancomycin- and multidrug-resistant E. faecalis in the clinical setting is of particular concern (Bizzini et al., 2009).

Here, the authors will present the analysis of heterogeneity of resistance studied by flow cytometry with use of fluorescent antibiotics binding bacterial cells and fluorescent probes targeting resistance genes. The proposal of vancomycin and methicilin heteroresistant strain model will be presented. With use of the model, results obtained for clinical E.faecalis and S.aureus strain are discussed.

2. Material and methods

The study was performed on reference and clinical strains listed in Tab 1. Fourteen MRSA strains were isolated from patients of various wards of the University Clinical Centre in Gdańsk and 12 Enterococcus faecalis from patients of Kościerzyna Medical Centre. The staphylococcal strains were isolated in the hospital laboratory during the period March 2008 to March 2009 and were sent to the Microbiology Department of the Medical University of Gdańsk for epidemiological typing. One isolate per patient was included in the study. Bacteria were cultured from swabs: wound (4 isolates), nose (2 isolates) and fluids: tracheostomy tube fluid (3 isolates), blood (1 isolate), abscess fluid (1 isolate), pus (1 isolate), bronchial fluid (1 isolate), urine (1 isolate). The data about clinical recognitions were not available. The isolates were cultured on sheep blood agar and were identified as *S.aureus* by colony morphology, a positive plasma coagulase reaction and by biochemical tests (API, bioMerieux, France). Resistance to methicillin was primary tested using disc diffusion method with cefoxitin disc (Clinical and Laboratory Standards Institute,2006) and then was confirmed by detection of *mec A* gene by the Polymerase Chain Reaction (PCR) as described previously (Barski et al., 1996). DNA of bacterial isolates was extracted according to the previous report (Barski et al., 1996). For further analyses, the isolates were subcultured on nutrient broth and stored with glycerol at - 70°C.

Spa typing and BURP analyses. The polymorphic X region of the protein A gene (*spa*) was amplified from the isolates by PCR with primers and according to procedure described by Kobayashi (1999). *Spa* types were determined by using Ridom Staph Type software, according to Harmsen et al (2003). The *spa* types were clustered into *spa*–CCs (clonal complexes) using the algorithm BURP - based upon repeat pattern (Rupptisch et al., 2006).

Phage typing was performed according to Blair and Williams (1961). Two sets of phages were used as follows: a basic set of 23 phages with additional phages 88,89,187 and an additional set of phages MR8, MR12, MR25, 30, 33, 38, M3, M5, 622, 56B supplied by the Central Public Health Laboratory in London for use on MRSA strains (Richardson et al., 1999). The phages were used in concentrations at routine test dilution (RTD) and 100xRTD. Reactions for phages were noted as described by Blair and Williams (1961). The phage type was defined by all the phages with strong reaction.

The susceptibility of the MRSA isolates to antimicrobial agents other than cefoxitin was determined by the disc diffusion method according to the guidelines (Clinical and Laboratory Standards Institute. 2006). The following drugs were used for test: erythromycin, clindamycin, ciprofloxacin, co–trimoxazole, tetracycline, gentamycin, vancomycin, teicoplanin, fusidic acid, rifampicin, linezolid, synercid, chloramphenicol. For isolates identified as resistant to erythromycin, but susceptible to clindamycin, D-test was performed to detect inducible clindamycin resistance. For vancomycin, additionally, the minimal inhibitory concentration (MIC) was determined by E-tests as described by the manufacturer (AB Biodisc, Sweden).

Enterococci were identified by esculin hydrolysis on Coccosel agar (bioMerieux). Species-level identification was based on rapid Strep ID (bioMerieux). Susceptibility testing was performed by following the current guidelines of the National Committee for Clinical Laboratory Standards (2002). Isolates were additionally tested for resistance to nitrofurantoin, gentamycin, amikacin, tobramycin, kanamycin, streptomycin ,neomycin, penicilin, meropenem, ampicillin, piperacilin and differentiated by antibiotic resistance pattern.

No.	Clinical source	Antibiotic resistance pattern	Phage group	Phage type	Spa type
SA1	Urine	Te C	III	42E/53/75/83A	010
SA1	Nose	E Cc Cip	III	54/75/83A	003
SA3	Nose	Sensitive	I/V	55/94/96	018
SA4	Tracheostomy tube fluid	E Cc Cip	III	47/54/75/83A	003
SA5	Blood	Cip Te C/	NT	-	008
SA6	Wound	Cip Te C/	III	53/83A	2065
SA7	Pus	E Cc Cip Sxt Te Rf C/Ge	NT	-	037
SA8	Bronchial fluid	E Cc Cip Te Ge	NT	-	008
SA9	Tracheostomy tube fluid	E Cc Cip Te Ge	III	47/54/75/83A	008
SA10	Tracheostomy tube fluid	E Cc Cip C	III	47/54/75/83A	151
SA11	Wound	E Cc Cip	II	55/71	003
SA1	Abscess	E Cc Cip	III	75/83A	003
SA2	Wound	E Cc Cip	III	83A	003
SA12	Wound	E Cc Cip	NT	-	002
SA	ATCC 25923		-	-	
SA	ATCC 29213		-	-	
E.F	wound	Te,FM, Rf, E,CC,An,NN,K,S	-	-	
E.F	Bronchial fluid	Te,Rf,E,CC,NN,K,N,Me,Am	-	-	
E.F	urine	FM,C,E,CC,Ge,An,NN,K,S,N	-	-	
E.F	urine	CC,An,NN,K,S,N,	-	-	
E.F	wound	FM,Cip,Ra,C,CC,An,NN,K,S,N	-	-	
E.F	wound	Te,FM,CC,Ge,NN,K,S,N	-	-	
E.F	faeces	Te,FM,C,CC,An,NN,K,S	-	-	
E.F	wound	Te,Rf,C,CC,An,NN,K,N,P,	-	-	
E.F	faeces	Te,Cip,Ra,C,CC,NN,K,	-	-	
E.F	faeces	Te,Ra,CC,NN,	-	-	
E.F	faeces	Cip,Ra,C,CC,An,NN,K,S,N	-	-	
E.F	faeces	FM,Cip,Rf,C,CC,An,NN,K,N,P, Mem,Am,PIP	-	-	
E.F	ATTC 51299	Van-R	-	-	
E.F	ATTC 29212	Van-S	-	-	

S.A Staphylococcus aureus, E.F. Enterococcus faecalis, ICU- intensive care unit; DVA - dermatology, venerology, alergology department; E - erytromycin; Cc – clindamycin (/ -inducible resistance to macrolides); Cip -ciprofloxacin; Te - tetracycline; C - chloramphenicol; Rf – rifampicin; Sxt trimetoprim/ sulfamethoxazole; Ge – gentamicin NT - non- typable; ° - inhibition reaction with phages; Cc – clonal complex; MIC – minimal inhibitory concentration; Va –vancomycin; FM- Nitrofurantoin, , Ge- gentamycin, AN- Amikacin, NN –Tobramycin, K- Kanamycin, S-streptomycin , N- Neomycin, P- penicilin, MeM- Meropenem, AM- Ampicilin, PIP piperacilin

Table 1. List of strains used in the study.

For flow cytometry analysis, the isolates were grown overnight on Tryptic Soy Broth (TSB) at 37°C and standardized to OD 1 (600 nm). The cells were then centrifuged 5 min at 2500 rpm, washed and suspended in 200 µl PBS buffer. The binding assay was carried out by adding solution of Bocillin @fl or vancomycin @fl respecitivelly to the cell suspension of each strain. The reaction mixtures were incubated for 30 min at 37°C and centrifuged. The pellets were collected and washed three times in 1 ml of PBS. Fluorescence of particles was determined by a FACS Scan flow cytometer (Becton Dickinson, San Jose, CA, USA).

2.1 Optymalisation of bocillin@fl and vancomycin@fl binding

In the previous study the relation between fluorescence and amount of used bocillin@fl was described by equation below;

$$y = 4.469\ln(x) + 3.427, \quad R^2 = 0.944 \tag{1}$$

Following these results (Jarzembowski et al., 2008) and similar results obtained during study of vancomycin @fl binding (Jarzembowski et al., 2009) we stained cells by addition of 1µg/ml vancomycin@fl. Because of inductive mechanism of vancomycin resistance , before staining strain was cultured in presence of 2ug/ml vancomycin (Sigma). The reaction mixtures were incubated for 45 min at 37°C and again centrifuged. The pellets were collected and washed three times in 1 ml of PBS. Fluorescence of particles was determined with the use of FACS Scan flow cytometer (Becton Dickinson, San Jose, CA, USA). Results of induction of reference resistant strain are shown on Fig 1.

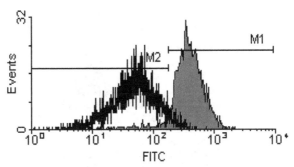

Fig. 1. Fluorescence (FL1) inducted (red) and uninducted (black) vancomycin resistant reference strain after staining with vancomycin@fl

To ensure cell nature of analysed particles we have excluded from procedure particles sized below 1µm based on value for size standard (Polysciences. Inc) and particles with low PI (propidium iodide) binding (Fig2).

2.2 Modeling of vancomycin heteroresistant strain

Mixture of the reference strains in proportion staring from 1.25 up to 50 % of resistant cells were composed to create model of heteroresistant strain. Cells binding and not binding vancomycin @fl were differentiated by markers consisting of 99.69 % of susceptible (M1) and 94% of resistant (M2) cells (Fig 3)

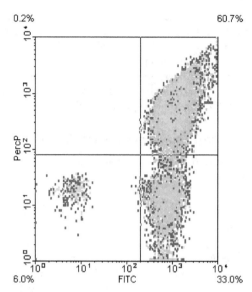

Fig. 2. Green (x axis) vancomycin@fl fluorescence and red (y axis) PI fluorescence reference susceptible strain. Only upper regions were included into further analysis.

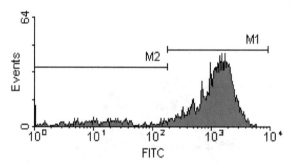

Fig. 3. Fluorescence (FL1) of mixed culture consisting of 25% resistant cells

2.3 Design and testing of DNA probes

Oligonucleotide probes were designed with the software package (Biosoft: Beacon Designer) and rRNA sequences were obtained from the Ribosomal Database Project (RDP) supplemented with newly deposited rRNA sequences from GenBank. As a positive control, Enfl84 probe (3'-ACGTGAGTTAACCTTTCTCC, Waar et al. 2005) targeting 16sRNA gene was used. Fluorescein-labelled oligonucleotides against selected specific target sequences (van genes) of *E. faecalis* were synthesized commercially (Metabion) and tested for specificity against the set of reference organisms. For hybridization, procedure described by Waar et al (2005) was adopted. Briefly, cell membrane was permeabilizated by incubation for 30 min at 37 °C in permeabilization buffer consisting of 1 mg lysozyme ml^{-1} (DNA Gdańsk). The cells were then centrifuged 5 min at 2500 rpm, washed and suspended in 200µl PBS buffer.

Subsequently, 200μl hybridization buffer containing FITC- labelled probe (1ng) was added. The probes were hybridizated at 50°C for 45 min.

3. Results and discussion

Heteroresistance, defined as a presence of subpopulations of resistant cells within susceptible majority was observed against β-lactams and glycopeptides. However, mechanism of actions of these groups of antibiotics is different.

The emergence of community acquired methicillin resistant Staphylococcus aureus (cMRSA) has renewed interest in the mechanisms of methicillin resistance (Okuma et al., 2002; Nunes et al., 2007). In contrast to vancomycin resistance, resistance to β-lactams (methicillin resistance) is constitutively mediated by a affinity change in penicillin-binding proteins (enzymes involved in cell wall synthesis). Because many genes are involved in cell wall biosynthesis, explanation of the nature of heterogeneous expression of methicillin resistance is very difficult (Markova et al., 2008). Since 2001, an increase in the number of MRSA strains with heteroresistance to oxacillin has been observed in the Netherlands. These strains can spread unnoticed, as their phenotypic heterogeneous resistance to beta-lactams affects the results of susceptibility testing (Wannet 2002). Coexistence of two subpopulations (susceptible and resistant) within a clinical isolate and expression of resistance only in a small number of cells leads to diagnostic problems in clinical laboratories (Markova et al., 2008). In methicillin-resistant Staphylococcus strain degree of heterogeneity is quite low: only 1 CFU of 10^4–10^7 CFU are phenotypically resistant (De Lencastre et al., 1993).

Invention of Bocillin@fl, commercially avaible fluorescent penicillin, significantly increased possibility of studying heteroresistance (Jarzembowski et al., 2010). Results of flow cytometry were found to be correlated with reference heteroresistant strain properties. Furthermore, use of fluorescent antibiotics in flow cytometry proved linear nature of heteroresistance (Fig.4.).

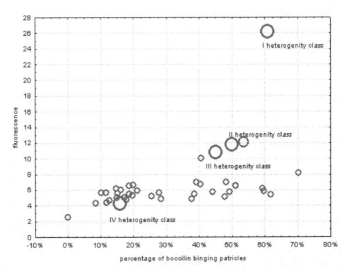

Fig. 4. Variance of bocillin @fl binding by medical isolates of S.aureus in relation to reference value

However, even in susceptible cell culture we always detect at least 1.47% antibiotic unbinding particles so it seems that the number of resistant cells in this method is overestimated.

Results of Markova et al study (2008) showed that also changes of cell structure can be involved in mechanism of heteroresistance. Both heteroresistant and methicillin susceptible strains (MSSA) may transform into cell wall-deficient form after exposure to sub tolerant conditions. The finding that methicillin sensitive strain and heteroresistant strain give rise to L-form colonial growth both on oxacillin-free and oxacillin-containing media appeared to be remarkable. It is known that the heterogeneous resistance phenotype of *mecA*-positive MRSA strains progresses to homogeneous resistance upon incubation with methicillin (Sakoulas et al., 2001). Study results of resistance demonstrate that differences reduction of antibiotic binding after preincubation can be proved with the use of flow cytometry (Fig.5).

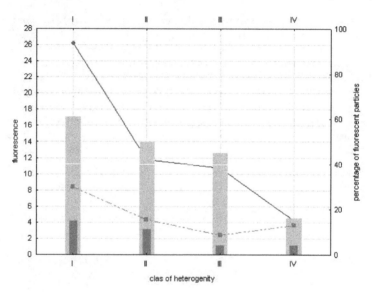

Fig. 5. Influence of incubation of heteroresistant strain with methicillin on Bocillin@fl binding

In contrast to MSSA and heteroresistant strains, homogenic MRSA strains did not convert to the cell wall-deficient forms (Markova et al., 2008).

Vancomycin resistance is an example of inductive reaction on presence of antibiotic. In presence of vancomycin high amount of cell wall precursor with low affinity to vancomycin (d-ala-d alla) is synthesized while native precursors are removed (Hasman et al., 2006). Because we aimed to detect resistant cells between susceptible majorities, the induction condition should be set to prevent inhibition of growth of susceptible strain. Thus, we set up inductive concentration below breakpoint value, at 0.016µg 0.8 µg, 2µg and 4µg/ml. The results showed optimal induction with final vancomycin concentration of 2µg/ml (data not shown). While there are no reference strains of different degree of vancomycin heteroresistance, model obtained by combination of resistant and susceptible strain was prepared. Vancomycin@fl binding by cells in this model is presented on fig 6. The high correlation between percentage of fluorescent particles and percentage of resistant cells can be seen. (Fig. 6)

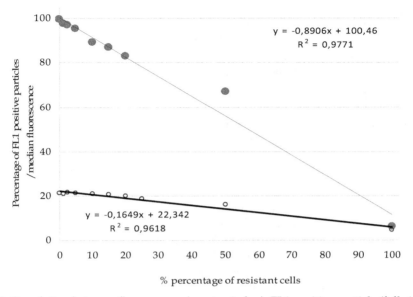

Fig. 6. Correlation between fluorescence (empty circles), FL1 positive particle (full circles) and percentage of resistant cells

The obtained model of vancomycin heteroresistance was then used for analysis of clinical strains. The percentage of stained particles ranged from 6.07% in resistant up to 99.66% in susceptible reference strains. Percentage in resistant unindicted strains was similar to the susceptible one (94.62 %). Reference strains showed also differences in fluorescence but they were not so significant (Tab. 3.) Similar, constant divergence was observed in the study of methicillin heteroresistance (Jarzembowski et al., 2010). Despite satisfactory differentiation of heteroresistance, the results showed some limitations of the method. Even in resistant strains some particles bind vancomycin@fl according to the chosen criteria. Among clinical strains, the percentage of unstained particles varies from 46.32 to 98.53 while median fluorescence varied from 547 to 1980.96. (Tab 2.). Generally, fluorescence of staphylococci was higher than fluorescence of enterococci

	percentage of FL1 positive particles	Median fluorescence	Mean fluorescence per particle
max in staphylococci	97.77	1980.96	37.01
max in enterococci	98.53	1684.85	27.26
Min in staphylococci	46.32	572.55	10.87
Min in enterococci	90.47	547.37	9.01
resistant reference strain	6.07	239.28	4.6
Susceptible reference strain	99.69	10009.04	21.2
Resistant uninducted strains	94.62	403.15	11.5

Table 2. Comparison of estimator values in groups of strains

In contrast to results of MIC based screening of vancomycin resistance, the results obtained in flow cytometry suggest heteroresistance of some strains (Fig. 7). It is obvious if we consider that presence of heteroresistant strains in US and Europe is quite high. Nunes et al. (2007) found a prevalence of 8.5 % (9/106) of glycopeptides-heteroresistant staphylococci isolated from bacteremia while others 7.4% (Frebourg et al., 1998).

None of the tested strains had a MIC value below 4µg/ml, so all of them should be considered as vancomycin susceptible. On the other hand, determination of MICs have shown good accuracy only to detect vancomycin intermediate Staphylococcus aureus (VISA) and fail in the detection of glycopeptides heteroresistant strains (Nunes et al., 2007). Heterogeneous phenotypes of clinical strains of *S. aureus* and CNS present MIC value below 4µg/ml (Nunes et al., 2007). That is why heteroresistance of the strains could be missed out in routine diagnostic.

The heteroresistance has been considered responsible for failure in the treatment. Unfortunately, there is no widely accepted method to detect heteroresistant strains. The lack of a standardized method makes it difficult to determine the clinical significance in the treatment of an infection with vancomycin. In the presence of vancomycin not only van genes change expression. There is some evidence that vancomycin influences biofilm formation, at least in S. epidermidis culture. Changes of cell surface structure and size seen in flow cytometry as SSC and FSC values were explained by the studied effect of the glycopeptide antibiotic on cell envelope properties and biofilm formation. SEM examination of cells grown in the presence of vancomycin revealed the presence of polymorphic form. Such changes in cell morphology could be the reason of extremely high fluorescence of some strains after staining with vancomycin@fl.

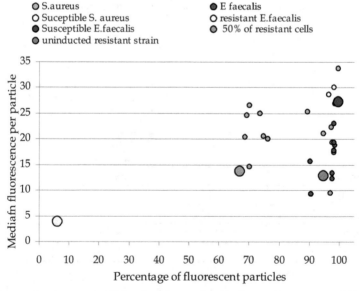

Fig. 7. Variance of vancomycin@fl binding by medical isolates of S.aureus and E. faecalis in relation to reference value

Both in study of vancomycin heteroresistance and study of methicillin resistance, median fluorescence per particle seems to be a very effective estimator (Fig. 1, 7). It is interesting to compare FCM results of "native 'methicillin heteroresistance (Fig. 4) and "artificial' model of vancomycin heteroresistance. Despite different resistance mechanism, changes of estimators are very similar. Both fluorescence and percentage of fluorescent particle decrease with amount of resistant cells (Fig. 7).

Detailed information about mechanism of heteroresistance can be explained by the study of resistance gene expression. At the first stage of our ongoing study we adopt protocol described by Warr (2005) to detect 16sRNA gene. In fact, Fig. 8 demonstrates successful detection of E. faecalis cells in flow cytometry. Furthermore, the protocol used determines the amount of cells in mixed culture.

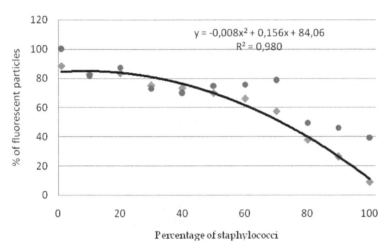

Fig. 8. Correlation between percentages of detectable particles in FLOW-FISH and proportion of E. faecalis cells in mixed culture stained by fluorescent 16sRNA probe

Detection of 16s RNA gene, which appeared to be successful in single cells, ranged between 10^4 and 10^5 ribosomes and, consequently, as many copies of 5S and 16Sand 23S-like rRNAs (Amman et al., 1990) making it was quite easy to get satisfactory signal. Despite the proven usefulness, serious limitations of FLOW- FISH technique in its sensitivity and resolution constitute an obstacle. It is believed that probes containing nucleic acid analogs with higher affinity for DNA and RNA may have the potential to reduce these problems (Kelly et al., 2009). An example of such probe is peptide nucleic acid (PNA), which binds to DNA and RNA with high affinity.

For our study, we decided to use another class of nucleic acid analogs in which the ribose sugar is constrained by a methylene bridge between 20-oxygen and 40-carbon, resulting in an N-type (3-endo) conformation , so called locked nucleic acids (LNAs) (Kelly et al., 2009).

LNA is able to hybridize with DNA and RNA according to Watson–Crick base-pairing rules and does so with unprecedented high affinity. As a result, LNAs have been shown to significantly improve the sensitivity and specificity.

This technique is expected to be particularly useful for the detection of lower mRNA transcript levels. In fact, preliminary results (Fig. 9) are promising. On the other hand, further studies are needed for validation of chosen approach.

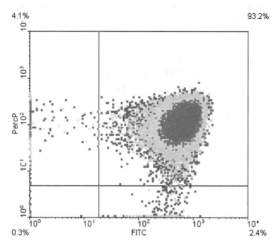

Fig. 9. Results of regulatory vancomycin gene detection with LNA probe (x axe- binding of probe, Y axe PI staining)

3. Conclusion

According to obtained results, fluorescent antibiotics are excellent tools both, for detection of resistance and studies of heteroresistance in flow cytometry. Model of vancomycin heteroresistance was successfully prepared and used in studies of clinical strains. Because it is believed that heteroresistance mechanism involves changes of cell structure, it is especially profitable in terms of antibiotic binding and changes in cell structure can be observed. However, overestimation of resistant cells in culture remain unsolved.

Preliminary results of FLOW-FISH are also promising. It seems, that use of LNA probes allows to express detection in single cells in culture. On the other hand, it is obvious that further studies are needed to evaluate the specifity ad sensitivity of this approach.

4. Acknowledgment

We thank Dr Agnieszka Daca and prof Ewa Bryl (Department of Physiopathology, Medical Unversity of Gdańsk) for their support of flow cytometry analysis of this study.

This study was supported by grants from: National Science CentreNN 401 597540

5. References

Amann, R., I.; Binder, B.; Olson, R., J.; Chisholm, S., W.; Devereux, R.; Stahl, D.,A.(1990)[1] Combination of 16S rRNA-Targeted Oligonucleotide Probes with Flow Cytometry for Analyzing Mixed Microbial Populations. Applied And Environmental Microbiology, 56, pp. 1919-1925

Alvarez-Barrientos, A.; Arroyo, J.; Canton, R.; Nombela, C.; Sanchez- Perez, M.(2000). Application of flow cytometry to clinical microbiology. Clin Microbiol Rev , 13, pp.167–195

Baptista, M.; Rodrigues, P.; Depardieu, F.; Courvalin, P.; Arthur, M.(1999) Single-cell analysis of glycopeptide resistance gene expression in teicoplanin-resistant mutants of a VanB-type Enterococcus faecalis. Molecular Microbiology , 32(1), pp.17±28

Barski, P.; Piechowicz, L.; Galiński, J.; Kur, J. (1996). Rapid assay for detection of methicillin-resistant *Staphylococcus aureus* using multiplex PCR. Molec. Cellul. Probs., 10, pp. 471–475

Bizzini, A.; Zhao, H.; Auffray, H., Hartke, A. The Enterococcus faecalis superoxide dismutase is essential for its tolerance to vancomycin and penicillin. Journal of Antimicrobial Chemotherapy, 64, pp. 1196–1202

Blair, J.E.; Williams, R.,E.,O. (1961). Phage typing of Staphylococci. Bull. World Health Organ, 24, pp. 771–784.

Cargill, S.; Upton, L. (2003). Low concentrations of vancomycin stimulate biofilm formation in some clinical isolates of Staphylococcus epidermidis. Curr. Issues Mol. Biol., 5, pp. 9-15.

Clinical and Laboratory Standards Institute. 2006. Performance standards for antimicrobial susceptibility testing; sixteenth informational supplement., Vol. 26, No. 3.

Davey, H.; Winson, M. (2003). Using Flow Cytometry to Quantify Microbial Heterogeneity Curr. Issues Mol. Biol., 5, pp. 9-15

De Lencastre, H.; Figueiredo, A.; Tomasz,. A. (1993). Genetic control of population structure in heterogeneous strains of methicillin resistant Staphylococcus aureus. Eur J Clin Microbiol Infect Dis , 12, pp. 13–18

Device , O.; Toshiro, S.; Akinobu, Gotoh.; Yutaka, K.; Satoru , Muto.; Hisamitsu, I.; Yukio, H.; Horie, S.(2006). Enumeration of Bacterial Cell Numbers and Detection of Significant Bacteriuria by Use of a New Flow Cytometry-Based Journal of Clinical Microbiology, pp. 3596–3599

Falagas, M., E.,; Makris, C., G., ; Dimopoulos, G.,; Matthaiou, D., K. (2008). Heteroresistance: a concern of increasing clinical significance? Clin Microbiol Infect , 14, pp 101–104

Fiebelkorn, K.,R.; Crawford, S.,A.; Mc Elmeel, M.,L.; Jorgensen, J.,H. et al. (2003). Practical disc diffusion method for detection of inducible clindamycin resistance in *Staphylococcus aureus* and coagulase- negative staphylococci. J. Clin. Microbiol., 41, pp. 4740-4744.

Finan, J., E.; Rosato, A.,E.; Dickinson, T.,M.; Ko, D.; Archer, G.,L. (2002). Conversion of oxacillin-resistant staphylococci from heterotypic to homotypic resistance expression. Antimicrob Agents Chemother, 46, pp. 24–30

Frebourg, N., B.; Nouet, D.; Lemée, L.; Martin , E; Lemeland, J.,F.(1998). Comparison of ATB staph, rapid ATB staph, Vitek, and E-test methods for detection of oxacillin heteroresistance in staphylococci possessing mecA. Clin Microbiol. , (Jan 1998) 36, (1) pp. 52-7..

Gazzola, S.; Cocconcelli, P., S. (2008). Vancomycin heteroresistance and biofilm formation in Staphylococcus epidermidis from food. Microbiology, 154, pp. 3224-3231

Gunasekera, T., S.; Attfield, P.,V.; Veal, D.,A.(2000). A flow cytometry method for rapid detection and enumeration of total bacteria in milk. Applied and Environmental Microbiology, 66, pp.1228-1232.

Hartman, B., J.; Tomasz, A. (1986). Expression of methicillin resistance in heterogeneous strains of Staphylococcus aureus. Antimicrob Agents Chemother, 29, pp. 85–92

Harmsen, D.; Claus, H.; Witte, W.; Rothganger, J.; Turnwald, D. et al., (2003). Typing of methicillin-resistant *Staphylococcus aureus* in a university hospital setting by using novel software for *spa* repeat determination and database management. J. Clin. Microbiol., 41, pp. 5442-5448.

Hasman, H.; Aarestrup, FM.; Dalsgaard, A.;Guardabassi, L. (2006) Heterologous expression of glycopeptide resistance vanHAX gene clusters from soil bacteria in Enterococcus faecalis Journal of Antimicrobial Chemotherapy 57, 648–653

Jarzembowski, T.; Wiśniewska, K.; Jóź wik, A.; Bryl, E.; Witkowski ,J. (2008). Flow cytometry as a rapid test for detection of penicillin resistance directly in bacterial cells in Enterococcus faecalis and Staphylococcus aureus. Curr Microbiol, 57, pp. 167–169

Jarzembowski, T.; Wiśniewska, K.; Jóź wik, A.; Witkowski ,J. (2009). Heterogeneity of Methicillin-Resistant Staphylococcus aureus Strains (MRSA) Characterized by Flow Cytometry, Curr Microbiol, 59, pp. 78–80

Jarzembowski, T.; Wiśniewska, K.; Jóź wik, A.; Witkowski ,J. (2010). Flow Cytometry Approach Study of Enterococcus faecalis Vancomycin Resistance by Detection of Vancomycin@FL Binding to the Bacterial Cells. Curr Microbiol , 61, pp. 407–410

Kelly, L.; Robertson, A.; Dzung, C., Thach, C.(2009). LNA flow–FISH: A flow cytometry–fluorescence in situ hybridization method to detect messenger RNA using locked nucleic acid probesAnalytical Biochemistry. 390, pp. 109–114

Kobayashi, N.; Urasawa, S.; Uehara, N.; Watanabe, N.(1999). Analysis of genomic diversity within the Xr-region of the protein A gene in clinical isolates of *Staphylococcus aureus*. Epidemiol. Infect., 122, pp. 241-249.

Mansour JD, Robson JA, Arndt CW, Schulte Detection of *Escherichia coli* in Blood Using Flow Cytometry. Cytometry, 6, pp. 186-190

Markova, N.; Haydoushka, I.; Michailova, L.; Ivanova, R.; Valcheva, V.; Jourdanova, M.; Popova, T.; Radoucheva, T. (2008). Cell wall deficiency and its effect on methicillin heteroresistance in *Staphylococcus aureus*.International Journal of Antimicrobial Agents , 31, pp. 255–260

National Committee for Clinical Laboratory Standards (2002). Methods for dilution antimicrobial susceptibility tests for bacteria that grow aerobically. 5th edn. Approved standard M7-A5. National Committee for Clinical Laboratory Standards, Wayne,PA

Nunes, A., P., F.; Schuenck, R., P.; Bastos, C., C.; Magnanini, M., M., F.; Long, J., B.; Iorio, N.; Netto dos Santos, K., R.(2007). Heterogeneous resistance to vancomycin and teicoplanin among *Staphylococcus* spp. isolated from bacteremia. Brazilian Journal of Infectious Diseases ,vol.11, no.3 (June 2007).

Nottasorn, P.; Gilat, L.; Heidi, B.; Thomson, R. (2005). Unstable vancomycin heteroresistance is common among clinical isolates of methiciliin-resistant Staphylococcus aureus Journal of clinical microbiology, Vol. 43, No. 5,(May 2005), pp. 2494–2496

Okuma, K.; Iwakawa , K.; Turnidge, J., D. et al (2002). Dissemination of new methicillin-resistant Staphylococcus aureus clones in the community. J Clin Microbiol, 40, pp. 4289–4294

Pe'richon, B., Courvalin, P.(2006). Synergism between _-Lactams and Glycopeptides against VanA-Type Methicillin-Resistant Staphylococcus aureus and Heterologousn Expression of the vanA Operon. Antimicrobial agents and chemotherapy, Vol. 50, No. 11 (Nov. 2006), pp. 3622–3630

Richardson, J.,F.; Rosdahl, V.,T.; van Leeuwen, W.,J.; Vickery, A.,M.; Vindel, A. et al. (1999).Phages for methicillin-resistant *Staphylococcus aureus*: an international trial. Epidemiol. Infect., 122, pp. 227-233.

Rupptisch, W.; Indra, A.; Stoger, A. et al. (2006). Classifying *spa* types in complexes improves interpretation of typing results for methicillin-resistant *Staphylococcus aureus*.J. Clin. Microbiol., 44, pp. 2442-2448.

Sakoulas, G.; Gold, H.,S.;Venkataraman, L.; Degirolami, P., C.; Eliopoulos, G., M. Qian, Q. (2001). Methicillin-Resistant *Staphylococcus Aureus*: Comparison Of Susceptibility Testing Methods And Analysis Of *Meca*-Positive Susceptible Strains. Journal Of Clinical Microbiology, 39, vol 11, pp. 3946–3951.

Saribas, S; Bagdatli, Y.(2004). Vancomycin tolerance in enterococci. Chemotherapy, 50, pp. 250–4.

Takashi, S.; Yoshitsugu, I.; Shunji, T.; Naoko, F.; Junya, I.; Yukio, H.; Satoshi, I.(2005). Feasibility of flow cytometry for the detection of bacteria from body fluid samples. J Infect Chemother, 11, pp. 220–225

Trousscllier, M.; Courties, P.; Servais, P. (1999).Flow cytometric discrimination of bacterial populations in seawater based on SYTO 13 staining of nucleic acids. FEMS Microbiology Ecology, 29, pp. 319-330

Wannet, W., J. Spread of an MRSA clone with heteroresistance to oxacillin in the Netherlands. Euro Surveill. 2002;7(5):pii=367. Available online: http://www.eurosurveillance.org/ViewArticle.aspx?ArticleId=367

Wong, S.,S.,Y.; Ho, P.,L.; Woo, P.,C.,Y.; Yuen, K.,Y. (1999)Bacteremia caused by staphylococci with inducible vancomycin heteroresistance. Clin Infect Dis ,29, pp. 760-7.

Waar, K.; Degener, J.,E.; van Luyn, M., J.; Harmsen, H.,J.(2005) Fluorescent in situ hybridization with specific DNA probes offers adequate detection of Enterococcus faecalis and Enterococcus faecium in clinical samples. J Med Microbiol., 54, pp. 937-44.

Zhao, G.; Meier, T., I.; Kahl, S., D.; Gee, K., R.; Blaszczak, L.,C. (1999). Bocillin fl, a sensitive and commercially available reagent for detection of penicillin-binding proteins. Antimicrob Agents Chemother, 43, pp. 1124–1128

Zwirglmaier, K.; Ludwig, W.; Schleifer, K.,H.(2004). Recognition of *in* dividual *g* enes in a
        single bacterial cell by fluorescence *in situ* hybridization – RING-FISH Molecular
        Microbiology , 51, vol 1, pp. 89–96

4

Mechanisms of Antibiotic Resistance in *Corynebacterium* spp. Causing Infections in People

Alina Olender
Department of Medical Microbiology, Medical University of Lublin
Poland

1. Introduction

In recent years we can observe an increasing number of publications describing different incidents of infections, where species of *Corynebacterium* are isolated as the etiological factor of infection (Anderson et al., 2008; Campanile et al., 2009; Chiner et al., 1999; Dela et al., 2008; Fernandez-Roblas et al., 2009; Funke et al., 1997a; Funke et al., 1997b; Lagrou et al., 1998; Otsuka et al., 2005; Ostuka et al., 2006; Williams et al., 1993). It is a large and very diverse group of microorganisms, in which *Corynebacterium diphtheriae* is the most important species, with the most important human-pathogenic significance (Gomes et al., 2009; Wagner et al., 2011; Wilson, 1995). Strains of this species produce a strong exotoxine and are responsible for causing diphtheria. Well-developed procedures for diagnosis of diphtheria and conducted large-scale vaccinations resulted in erradication of diphtheria in most countries. Beside the typical human-pathogenic *C. diphtheriae*, the genus *Corynebacterium* comprises more than 85 different species of pathogenic significance. This type includes species pathogenic for animals, e.g. *C. pseudotuberculosis* (Baird & Fontanie, 2007; Nieto et al., 2009), *C. kutscheri* (Amao et al., 2008; Suzuki et al., 1988), *C. canis* (Funke et al., 2009) and a very large group of species colonizing the skin and mucous membranes of man, which in favorable circumstances, may become the cause of serious infections in humans. These opportunistic organisms, e.g. *C. jeikeium* (Ifantidou et al., 2010; Pitcher et al., 1990; Rosato et al., 2001), *C. urealyticum* (Funke et al., 1997b; Garcia-Bravo et al. 1996; López-Medrano et al., 2008), *C. amycolatum* (Anderson et al., 2008; Dela et al., 2008; Funke et al., 1997b), *C. striatum* (Campanile et al., 2009; Funke et al., 1997b; Martinem-Martinez et al., 1995; Ostuka et al., 2006; Roberts et al., 1992), *C. pseudodiphtehriticum* (Chiner et al., 1999; Dorello et al., 2006; Freman et al., 1994; Olender & Niemcewicz, 2010), may cause infections of various course: mild, chronic and acute, as well as of invasive nature, life-threatening to a patient. The genus *Corynebacterium* includes also species unrelated to the human organism, e.g. *C. glutamicum*, producing L-glutamic acid and lysine, used in biotechnological processes on the industrial scale and in genetic studies (Katsumata et al., 1984; Serwold-Davis et al., 1987; Tauch et al., 1998; Wendisch et al., 2006; Valbuena et al., 2007, Yague Guirao et al., 2005).

Application of modern molecular biology techniques in genetic studies of unknown strains isolated from infections resulted in the detection and description of new species such as: *C. singulare* (Riegel etal., 1997), *C. auriscanis* (Collins et al., 1999), *C. resistens* (Otsuka et al. 2005),

C. imitans (Funke at al., 1997a), *C. sputi* (Yassin & Siering, 2008) and the reclassification of previously inaccurately determined ones, e.g.: *C. cystitidis*, *C. pilosum* (Takahashi et al., 1995).

In view of a widely conducted taxonomic research of species belonging to the genus *Corynebacterium*, the term "dyphteroids" has also been changed, which was used commonly for the opportunistic species, suggesting a direct relationship with *C. diphtheriae*. Nowadays taxonomists more and more replace it by a more universal name for this group of bacteria "coryneform" (Anderson et al., 2008; Balci et al., 2002; Funke et al., 1996; Funke et al., 1997b; Gomez-Garces et al., 2007; Lagrou et al., 1998; Ostuka et al., 2005), which seems fully justified.

Many opportunistic strains of the genus *Corynebacterium*, isolated from clinical materials, belong to species whose characteristics determining the pathogenic effect on the human body have not been thoroughly recognised and characterized yet. Therefore, the assessment of their role as pathogens is often very difficult. Undoubtedly, the common occurrence of coryneform on mucous membranes and the skin may cause doubts in interpretation of their contribution to infections, especially when the material is sampled from places non-sterile physiologically and there might be a suspicion of its contamination.

An increasing number of recognized and described incidents of infections and the observed increase in the number of publications on this topic is probably connected with the microbiological diagnostics currently carried out at a higher level and development of quick commercial tests for identification of species based on their biochemical properties. In reference to strains difficult to identify or requiring verification of uncertain biochemical determination, oftener methods of molecular biology are used, which has resulted in detection of new species and the reclassification of ones previously poorly assayed.

Infections caused by opportunistic *Corynebacterium spp.* generally refer to a group of people, who experience symptoms of immunodeficiency. The group of patients with a particular risk of infection includes primarily people with immunodeficiency due to disorders of bone marrow activity, the ongoing processes of cancer, post surgery or urological surgery, invasive diagnostic procedures and patients with AIDS. The risk of infection is increased by long-term hospitalization, antibiotic therapy, radiotherapy, treatment with cytostatics or steroids. A disturbing fact is occurrence of such infections in a group of people called "immunocompetent", in whom no symptoms of immunodeficiency were reported before (Chiner et al., 1999; Frejman et al., 1994).

The basis for treatment of infections caused by *Corynebacterium spp.* is taking up of an effective antibiotic therapy. For this group of microorganisms, until recently an obstacle in the evaluation of drug resistance was use of different criteria of interpretation that were recommended for other groups of microorganisms and determination of drug resistance with various methods, yet results presented by different authors have become the basis for information about   occurrence of strains with high resistance to antibiotics among opportunistic *Corynebacterium spp.*, which indicate existence of different mechanisms of resistance in these strains.

The described multidrug-resistant strains of *C. jeikeium* (Rosato et al., 2001; Yagye Guirao et al., 2005) *C. amycolatum* (Yagye Guirao et al., 2005; Yoon et al., 2011), *C. striatum* (Campanile et al., 2009; Martinem-Martinez et al., 1995; Otsuka et al., 2006; Roberts et al., 1992) i *C. resistens* (Otsuka et al., 2005) confirm presence in *Corynebacterium spp.* of different mechanisms of resistance and genes, which may be differently located. Phenotypic tests of resistance to antibiotics have become the basis for search of the genes responsible for them and their transmission paths. They have also contributed to analyses and study of similarity in occurrence of resistance genes in other groups of microorganisms, often unrelated to the genus *Corynebacterium*, such as *Staphylococcus spp.* (Roberts et al., 1999), *Enterococcus* spp.(Power et al., 1995), *E. coli* (Deb & Noth,1999; Serwold-Davis et al., 1990; Serwold-Davis et al., 1987).

2. Mechanisms of resistance to antibiotics most commonly occurring in *Corynebacterium* spp.

The conducted study characterizing resistance to antibiotics isolated from clinical material of different species of the genus *Corynebacterium* (Anderson et al., 2008; Fernandez-Roblas et al., 2009; Funke et al., 1997a; Funke et al., 1997b; Garcia-Bravo et al., 1996; Gomez-Garceset al., 2007; Martinem-Martinez et al., 1995; Otsuka et al., 2006; Roberts et al., 1992, Troxler R et al., 2001, Weiss et al., 1996) draw attention to the most frequently occuring mechanisms of resistance to antibiotics in this group of microorganisms. The results show participation of extrachromosomal genetic elements in transmission of resistance genes in both pathogenic and potentially pathogenic - opportunistic and typically nonpathogenic ones, e.g. present in the soil or strains of *Corynebacterium spp.* (Kono et al., 1983; Vertes et al., 2005).

Antibiotic resistance genes in species of *Corynebacterium spp.* are often located on large plasmids, e.g. resistance to tetracycline, chloramphenicol, erythromycin and streptomycin on plasmid pTP10 in *C. xerosis* (Deb & Nath, 1999; Hodgson et al., 1990), but also on trensposons (Delal et al., 2008).

2.1 Resistance to macrolides, lincosamides and streptogramins B

The occurrence of simultaneous resistance to three groups of antibiotics: macrolides, lincosamides and streptogramins B, determined in short as MLSB, is characteristic mainly of staphylococci and streptococci. It is connected with occurrence of three different mechanisms of the effects of activity: modification of the ribosome binding site associated with methylation or mutation, the mechanism of active efflux of antibiotic from the cell and the least significant - enzymatic inactivation of the antibiotic. The first two MLSB resistance mechanisms are of the highest importance.

Methylation of the binding site causes conformational changes of the subunit 23S rRNA, which prevents binding of the antibiotic molecules in the peptidyltransferase center within the 50S ribosome subunit and leads to the blockade of the mRNA translation and inhibition of bacterial protein synthesis. In species of the genus *Corynebacterium* it is connected with presence of genes belonging to class *erm* (erythromycin ribosome methylation), encoding the rRNA methylase enzyme, which causes dimethylation of adenine present in the 23S rRNA (Arthur et al., 1990). The gene *erm* occurring in *Corynebacterium spp*, responsible for this mechanism of resistance has been classified as class X of genes *erm* (Roberts et al., 1999). Despite a high degree of homology between genes *ermX* isolated from different species of *Corynebacterium* (*C. diphtheriae, C. jeikeium and C. xerosis*), it has been found that they exhibit different locations. The gene *ermX* in *C. diphtheriae* was found within the 14.5-kbp plasmid pNG2 (Coyle et al., 1979), while the gene *ermX* in *C. xerosis* turned out to be located on transposon Tn5432, whose carrier is the 50-kbp plasmid pTP10 (Delal et al., 2008). In the strain *C. jeikeium* (Pitcher et al., 1990) and *C. striatum* (Roberts et al., 1992), the gene *ermX* was found on the chromosome, which has been confirmed also in other analysed strains of *C. jeikeium* (Rosato et al., 2001). Despite detection of different locations of genes *ermX* in certain strains of *C. jeikeium* and *C. xerosis*, it is assumed that its most typical location is primarily the transposon Tn5432. At the same time in other examined *Corynebacterium spp.*, in which the MLSB mechanism is not related to the location of genes *ermX* on transposon Tn5432, interesting results of research were obtained, indicating the possibility of reorganization of fragments of the transposon Tn5432 and presence of all its components in the strain genome (Hall et al., 1999).

It is possible that mobile transpositional elements IS1249 containing *ermX* may create new composite transposons containing other multidrug- resistant genes. This phenomenon is particularly disturbing since transposition of the insertional sequence IS1249 is known for its capabilities to insert and transfer Tn5432 from genomes of unrelated bacteria (Rosato et al., 2001).

Different results of studies suggesting different locations of the detected genes *ermX* referred to the species of *Corynebacterium*, which were isolated from strains coming from different geographical regions, which may explain such diversified locations in the genome. The strain of *C. diphthariae*, containing pNG2 and *C. striatum* came from patients from the north-western USA (Coyle et al., 1979; Hodgson et al., 1990; Roberts et al., 1992), *C. xerosis* from pTP10 from Japan (Tauch et al.1995), *C. jeikeium* from France (Rosato et al.2001) and *C. jeikeium* and *C. amycolatum* from Spain (Yague Guirao et al., 2005).

It is very likely that different locations of genes *ermX* may indicate the possibility of acquiring resistance genes by multidrug-resistant strains of *Corynebacterium spp.* from microorganisms colonizing the skin or mucous membranes. *ErmX* occurring in *C. diphtheriae* is contained in plasmid pNG2, similar to plasmids isolated from *Corynebacterium spp.* occurring on the skin (Serwold-Davis & Groman, 1986). The replicon 2.6-kb EcoRI-ClaI fragment (oriR) may be possessed by many microorganisms, including a popular commensal *E. coli* (Deb & Nath, 1999; Serwold-Davis et al., 1990; Serwold-Davis et al., 1987).

At the same time, as research indicates, the plasmid pNG2 seems an unlikely place of origin for genes *erm* occurring in *Corynebacterium spp.* More likely is transposon Tn5432 associated with the chromosome, which may be mobile (Trauch et al., 1995). Tn5432 was also found in the occuring on the skin strains of *Propionibacterium acnes*, *P. granulosum* and *P. avidum*, which suggests that multidrug –resistant strains of the genus *Corynebacterium* may be an important source in horizontal transfer of resistance genes to other human pathogens (Ross et al., 2002). Another source, from which strains may be derived or to which they may arrive, is bacterial flora occurring in animals. It may be confirmed by detection of gene *ermX* in the strain of *Corynebacterium spp.* isolated from pasteurized milk. It showed resistance to erythromycin and/or spiromycin (Perrin-Guyomard et al., 2005).

Beside gene *ermX*, in strains of *Corynebacterium* Group A with the MLSB mechanism of resistance, also gene *erm* class B has been found (Luna et al., 1999), which occurs in *Enterococcus spp.* and *Streptococcus spp.*, which may also suggest the participation of these microorganisms in spread of the MLSB mechanism in *Corynebacterium spp.*

The expression of the MLSB resistance may be constitutive or induced. In the case of the constitutive type of resistance, active mRNA, permitting synthesis of methylase, is created without an inducer, while the induced MLSB - inactive mRNA is synthesized, which is activated only under the influence of an inducer, which allows synthesis of the enzyme. Occurrence of the constitutive MLSB resistance mechanism is very popular in strains of *C. pseudodiphtheriticum*, present in mucous membranes of the upper respiratory tract in humans (Olender & Niemcewicz, 2010).

Formation of cross-resistance associated with the MLSB mechanism is also accompanied by the process of active efflux of antibiotic from the cell. In staphylococci they are transporters of the membrane protein nature (ETP - binding cassette), encoded by genes *msrA* (macrolide streptogramin resistance), carried on plasmids. These transporters act as a specific pump removing macrolides of 14 - and 15-membered lactone ring and streptogramins B from the bacterial cell. Macrolides of 16-membered lactose ring, lincosamides and telithromycin are not transported. In this case, this mechanism is referred to as MSB (Leclercq, 2002; Douthwaite &Champney, 2001)

It was found that presence of gene *msrA* is also associated with resistance to macrolides and streptogramins B in strains of *Corynebacterium spp.* (Ojo et al., 2006) and similarly with production of an active transport system of the antibiotic pumped out from the cell (macrolide efflux proteins). Gene *msrA* had been previously found only in *Staphylococcus spp.* (Roberts et al., 1999). It encodes the ATP relay needed by the cell to gain energy from hydrolysis ATP for active transport of erythromycin and streptogramin B, and enables synthesis of the ABC family of transporters, i.e. multiprotein systems to actively pump out the antibiotic from the cell.

In turn in reference to *S.pneumoniae*, *S. pyogenes*, *S. agalactiae* and other species of streptococci and enterococci, the efflux mechanism is associated with presence of the MCF transporters (macrolide-specific efflux) and refers only to macrolites with 14 - and 15-membered lactose rings. It does not apply to macrolites with a 16-membered lactose ring, ketolides, linkosamides and streptogramin B. It is associated with low levels of resistance to macrolides (Appelbaum, 2002).

Gene *mef*, causing active efflux of macrolides from the bacterial cell was also found in *Corynebacterium* group A, *C. jeikeium* and strains of *Corynebacterium spp.* (Luna et al., 1999).

2.2 Resistance to fluoroquinolones

In species of the genus *Corynebacterium*, resistance has been also observed to fluoroquinolones. It is associated with point mutations within the structural gene region of the gyrase subunit A, which is defined as the region determining resistance to quinolones (QRDR - quinolone resistance determining region).

Mutations are of the spontaneous nature, leading to changes in the amino acid sequences, on which depends the range of resistance to certain fluoroquinolones. The resulting level of resistance depends largely on the type of the amino acid that has been built-in as a result of mutation in place of the pre-existing one. Some of them cause a small loss of affinity and a slight decrease in sensitivity, other reduce potently the affinity and activity of fluoroquinolones. It is confirmed by studies of strains of *C. macginleyi*, in which resistance has been found to norfloxacin, ciprofloxacin and levofloxacin. By analyzing gene *gyraA* encoding the gyrase subunit A, a change of the amino acid in position 83 in the QRDR region was found (Serine to Arginine), which resulted in resistance in *C. macginleyi* to norfloxacin. A double mutation has been also found, leading to amino acid changes in positions 83 and 87, which conditioned resistance to all fluoroquinolones. It was observed that double mutations occurred in Ser-83 and Asp-87 in all strains of *C. macginleyi* with a high level of resistance (Eguchi et al., 2008).

Studies of the gene *gyr*A sequence were also conducted in strains of *C. striatum* and *C. amycolatum* (Sierra et al., 2005). A high resistance to quinolones in *C.amycolatum* resulted from a double mutation and amino acid changes in positions 87 and 97 or 87 and 88 (unusual location of mutation in *gyr*A). In the case of *C. striatum* mutations of amino acids in positions 87 and 91 occurred in *gyr*A, corresponding to resistance characterized by very high MIC values for ciprofloxacin and levofloxacin, while only moderately increased MIC values for moxifloxacin.

These studies showed various complex and intricate mechanisms of resistance to quinolones in the studied species of *Corynebacterium spp.* (Sierra et al., 2005), which depend on the number of mutations and the type of changed amino acids.

2.3 Resistance to tetracyclines

Phenotypic studies constituted the basis for detection of resistance to tetracycline in *Corynebacterium spp.* In the case of *C. striatum*, it was found in 97% of the tested strains (Martinem-Martinez, 1995). These observations were confirmed by detection of the gene *tet*M, responsible for resistance to all tetracyclines, which is due to the protective effect on the protein ribosome with the mass of about 72-72.5 kDa (Roberts et al., 1992).

In strains of *C. striatum* M82B resistance to tetracycline is associated with the region 50-kb R-plasmid pTP10. An analysis of the nucleotide sequence revealed two reading frames called *tet*A and *tet*B. For analysis of the *tet*AB genes function, their expression in *C. glutamicum* was used and thus it was confirmed that they are responsible for resistance to tetracycline, oxytetracycline, and at a low level to other derivatives, such as chlortetracycline, minocycline and doxycycline. At the same an increased MIC value for oxacycline was found in this strain. This effect is associated with participation of the *tet*AB genes that determine resistance of the transport nature. It creates a powerful mechanism of active transport (efflu) causing pumping out of drugs from the cell via specific transport protein localized in the cytoplasmic membrane (Tauch et al., 1999).

R-plasmid pTP10 found in *C. xerosis* also contains determinants of resistance to tetracycline with parallel resistance to other antibiotics, such as chloramphenicol, kanamycin and erythromycin (Kono et al., 1983; Tauch et al., 1995) whereas, in strains of *C. melassecola*, the species used to produce glutamate, the resistance gene to tetracycline was found on another mobile element - plasmid pAG1 (Deb & Nath, 1999).

2.4 Resistance to beta-lactam antibiotics

The common susceptibility to penicillin in toxic and nontoxic strains of *C. diphtheriae* made it one of the most frequently prescribed antibiotics in treatment of diphtheria (Wilson, 1995).

Despite this opinion, there have been cases observed in which it showed no efficacy. Phenotypic tests consisuted the basis (Von Hunostein et al., 2002), in which penicillin sensitivity of 24 nontoxic strains of C. diphtheriae biotype gravis was determined in the broth microdilution method and by Etests. The research conducted with two methods showed a high 98% consistency of results. MIC values for penicillin were in the range from 0.064 to 0.250 mg/l, with simultaneous very low values for erythromycin (MIC ≤ 0.016 mg/l), whereas MBC (Minimal Bactericidal Concentaration) - MBC50 and MBC90 for penicillin were respectively 2.0 and 8.0 mg/l and 17.0 and 24.0. In 71% of the tested strains the ratio MBC/MIC was ≥ 32. The results of the study indicated the insensitivity (tolerance) to penicillin, which was confirmed by a lack of a positive effect of treatment despite the MIC values indicating sensitivity of the tested strains to this antibiotic. Such an effect was also observed in the case of tolerance to amoxicillin in the strain C. diphtheriae isolated from the case of endocarditis (Dupon et al., 1995).

In other strains of Corynebacterium spp. a similar situation was found, i.e. creation of insensitivity to oxacillin with low MIC values. This effect was not associated with the existing mechanism of resistance to beta-lactam antibiotics, but with a very high phenotypic expression and activity of a pair of genes tetA and tetB present on the Tn3598-transposon Class II - 12kb, which determined resistance to tetracycline. The activity of these genes, which consists of powerful active pumping, resulted also in removal of a structurally different antibiotic, which was oxacillin (Tauch et al., 2000).

Based on the analysis of results of phenotypic and genotypic studies of different species of the genus Corynebacterium showing resistance to beta-laktam antibiotics, it can be concluded that both resistance mechanisms organisms occur in these microorganisms, i.e. production of beta-laktamases and modification of penicillin-binding proteins. It is confirmed by e.g. resistance to penicillin (MIC 90> 4 μg/ml) in strains of C. jeikeium and C. urealyticum, ampicillin (MIC90> 8 μg/ml) (Gomez-Garces et al., 2007), in C. resistens to penicillin, cefazolin, cefotiam, cefmetazol, cefepime (MIC> 64 μg/ml) and imipenem (MIC> 32 μg/ml) (Otsuka et al., 2005), in strains of C. striatum to penicillin, ampicillin (MIC90 = 16 μg/ml), cefazolin, cefotiam, cefotaxime, imipenem (MIC90> 32 μg/ml) (Otsuka et al., 2006). Just like in hospital strains of C. urealyticum, in which resistance to penicillin and cefotaxime was particularly high (MIC90> 512 μg/ml) (Garcia-Bravo et al., 1996).

It can be also confirmed by an analysis of the genome sequence of C. glutamicum, which showed presence of four genes encoding proteins PBP (Penicillin Binding Proteins) HMW (high-molecular-weight), i.e. PBP1a, PBP1b, PBP2a, PBP2b, two genes encoding PBP4, PBP4b (low-molecular-weight) and two probably encoding beta-laktamases (Valbuena et al., 2007).

2.5 Resistance to glycopeptides

An antibiotic recommended by many authors in the empirical treatment of invasive infections caused by species of the genus Corynebacterium is vancomycin. It is connected with the common sensitivity to this antibiotic of even multidug-resistant species, which pose the greatest problems in infections. It refers to such species as C. jeikeium, C. resistant, C. amycolatum and C. striatum (Wiliams et al., 1993). Unfortunately, still cases of isolated strains of C. aquaticum and C. group B1 resistant to vancomycin have been reported.

Only single cases are described, in treatment of which other alternative antibiotics give very good results. An example might be a case of infection in a 44-year-old patient with *endocarditis* 4 months after a prosthetic mitral valve (Barnas et al., 1991). The strain of *Corynebacterium spp.* isolated from the blood turned out resistant to vancomycin and penicillin G, erythromycin, gentamicin and rifampicin. The use of imipenem and ciprofloxacin resulted in an effective cure of the infection.

In related species of Coryneform *Oerskovia turbata 892* and *Arcanobacterium* (former *Corynebacterium*) *haemolyticum 872,* resistance to vancomycin and teicoplanin was found of the constitutive nature. Presence of the VanA gene was detected, found on plasmids of 15 and 20 kb. In strains of *A. haemolyticum 872* the VanA gene sequence turned out the same as in vancomycin-resistant *Enterococcus faecium BM4147.* In the case of *O. turbata 892* a change of sequence occurred in three points. Species *A. haemoliticum* and *O. turbata* show a natural sensitivity to vancomycin and teicoplanin, and resistance found in the tested strains resulted from presence of the VanA gene (Power et al., 1995). The resistance phenotype associated with presence of the VanA gene is characterized by a high degree of resistance to vancomycin and teicoplanin.

2.6 Resistance to chloramphenicol

Resistance genes to chloramphenicol were detected on plasmids - in the strain *Corynebacterium spp.* on the pXZ10145 plasmid - 5.3 kb and in *C. xerosis* on pTP10 - 45.0 kb (Deb & Nath, 1999). In *C. striatum* strain M82B (former *C. xerosis* M82B) (Tauch et al., 1998) chloramphenicol resistance gene cmx (chloramphenicol and exports) was detected as an integral part of the transposon Tn5564, which contains a complete copy of the insertion sequence IS1513. The *cmx* gene is responsible for encoding of a specific protein (transmembran chloramphenicol efflux protein), which inhibits the passage of the antibiotic into the cytoplasm, and gives the bacetrial cell resistance to chloramphenicol.

3. Problems with diagnostic of infection by coryneform

The increasing isolation of multidrug-resistant strains of the genus *Corynebacterium* from clinical materials draws attention to the emerging issues related to treatment of infections caused by this group of opportunistic bacteria. The problem is all the more important since the infections often concern diagnostically difficult cases, long-hospitalized patients, the chronically ill, often with an accompanying disease causing immunosuppression. The underrated contribution of coryneform in infections may lead to therapeutic errors. Their common occurrence on the mucous membranes and skin causes doubts about their recognition as the etiologic factor of the infection.

The next problem, that may determine the accuracy of microbiology result as well as confirmation of the presence of opportunistic *Corynebacterium spp.* in infection, is a choice of appropriate culture method – bacterial culture media, which composition supports the growth of different coryneforms species. It is applied mostly for lipophilic species, as *C. jeikeium, C. urealyticum.* It is very important to identify the isolated strains precisely, as this enables tracking multi drug-resistance in specific strains, their existence on specific areas and routes of transmission. These informations are specifically important for hospital areas, facilitating to make proper decision on limiting these types of infections.

Accurate microbiological diagnostics of infections caused by species of the genus *Corynebacterium*, identification of strains of the isolated species and determination of antibiotic susceptibility with methods enabling determination of the MIC values permit assessment of the existing and emerging mechanisms of drug resistance and result in making right decisions about the most appropriate antibiotic therapy for a given case. It is extremely important to apply correct interpretation criteria of the determined drug resistance for species of the genus *Corynebacterium*, specific for this group of microorganisms, based on the established and generally accepted recommendations (Clinical and Laboratory Standards Institute [CLSI], 2006; Łętowska & Olender, 2010). Application of methods of molecular biology and examination of resistance genes, their locations and transmission paths is a very important direction of research on monitoring of resistance mechanisms in coryneform and gives the ability to track and determine their role in transmission of genes also among other species.

4. Antibiotic therapy used in infections of *Corynebacterium spp.*

The basis for monitoring of the emerging multi-drug resistant strains for all bacteria, as well as species of the genus *Corynebacterium*, is conducting research characterizing their sensitivity to antibiotics, which is potentially useful in treating infections. Publication of such data is extremely important due to tips received about the most effective antibiotic therapy for a given group of microorganisms.

An analysis of sensistivity to antibiotics of a large group of strains of *C. urealyticum*, *C. amycolatum*, *C. jeikeium*, *C. coyleae*, *C. striatum*, *C. aurimucosum* and *C. afermentans* was conducted with assays using Etests (Fernandez-Roblas et al., 2009). The authors found that strains of all tested species were susceptible to glycopeptides, linezolid, chinupristin/dalphopristin and daptomycin, which was also confirmed in other studies (Funke et al., 1997a; Funke et al., 1997b).

The results obtained from research done in Italy, involving strains of *C. striatum* isolated from different infections, also indicated the need of analysis of drug resistance in *Corynebacterium*. Genetic studies of strains of *C. striatum* MDR (multidrug-resistant) revealed presence of a multidrug-resistant clone, whose strains isolated from cases of pneumonia, catheter related bacteremia and wound infections showed, despite resistance to other classes of antibiotics, susceptibility to glycopeptides, tigecyclin, chinupristyn/dalphopristin, daptomycin and linezolid (Campanile et al., 2009).

One of the most resistant species, which causes the biggest problems in hospitals and is frequently isolated from infections in hospitalized patients, is *C. jeikeium*. The study of 66 strains of *C. jeikeium* (Johnson et al. 2004) showed resistance to penicillin in all of them, in 94% resistance to erythromycin, and in 74% to tetracycline. Twenty-two strains of other examined species of the genus *Corynebacterium* had a significantly lower level of the resistant. But what is extremely important, all examined strains were susceptible to vancomycin (MIC = 0.5-4.0 mg/l), linezolid (MIC = 0.5-2.0 mg/l) and daptomycin (MIC ≤ 1mg/l) with the exception of two isolates of *C. auaticum*, whose MIC for daptomycin was 8 mg/l. At the same time effecacy of daptomycin was confirmed in the successfully applied combination with rifampicin in a patient with *endocarditis* caused by *C. amycolatum* (Dala et al., 2008) i *C. striatum* (Shah & Murillo, 2005).

Linezolid, as shown in published works, was also characterized by a very good action. High activity of linezolid was found in studies of 190 strains of coryneform (Gomez-Garces et al.,2007). It confirmed the possibility of equally successful application of this antibiotic in infections caused by Coryneform.

Diversity of antibiotic resistance in species of the genus *Corynebacterium* is strictly connected with the locations, in which the tested strains occur. As found in the conducted studies (Garcia-Bravo et al., 1996) strains of *C. urealyticum* coming from hospitalized patients show significantly higher resistance to antibiotics than those isolated from outpatients, from outside of the hospital environment. An analysis of frequency and duration of antibiotic therapy used in patients from both groups of respondents was conducted. It confirmed unequivocally that the hospital environment and more frequently used antibiotics in the hospitalized patients is conducive to occurence of multidrug-resistant strains, and the hospital environment in which such patients stay is the place from which strains of *C. urealyticum* came, causing infections in the hospitalized patients. At the same time considerably lower resistance to antibiotics of isolates coming from the outpatients indicates that the strains of *C.urealyticum* most likely are derived from microflora colonizing the skin of the examined outpatients.

A very disturbing fact is discovery of new multidrug-resistant species of the genus *Corynebacterium*, which suggests a progressive character of multidrug-resistance occurring in this group. It is confirmed by a description of a new multidrug-resistant species of *C. resistens* in 2005. It is lipophilic, with low fermentation properties (it ferments glucose), does not reduce nitrates, does not produce urease and pyrazinamidase. It is characterized by resistance to penicillin and cephalosporins (MIC > 64 µg/ml), imipenem (MIC > 32 µg/ml), aminoglycosides (MIC > 3 µg/ml 2), macrolides (MIC > 16 µg/ml), quinolones (MIC > 32 µg/ml) and sensitivity to teicoplanin (MIC ≤ 0.5 µg/ml) and vancomycin (MIC = 2 µg/ml) (Otsuka et al., 2005).

5. Conclusion

Presented by several authors results of their studies on antibiotics resistance show, that even though *Corynebacterium spp.* are the members of the normal flora, they are not universally susceptible to antibiotics, as could be expected. Opportunistic *Corynebacterium spp.*, until now considered as bacteria of low pathogenicity, may pose a diagnostic and therapeutic problems, as they are more and more commonly isolated from serious, life-threatening invasive infections. Observed in many cases multi drug-resistance may be connected with the possibility to acquire resistance genes by gene transfer within bacteria regarded as normal flora present in large number on a given body area (skin, mucous membranes). Drug resistance occurrence in opportunistic species is the result of antibiotics overuse. It is obvious that antibiotics used also influence on saprophytic bacteria. Resulting selection of resistant strains is commonly known and regarded as important process leading to multi drug-resistance. For these reasons, analysis of the process in opportunistic *Corynebacterium* is an important element in monitoring new multi drug-resistant strains derived from saprophytic flora, mostly in infections in patients from risk groups, under immunosuppression, hospitalized for long time. Studying mechanisms of drug resistance on the basis of phenotypic and genotypic expression is important for proper antibiotic therapies in infections caused by this group of microorganisms.

Studies on sensitivity to antibiotics of different multidrug-resistant species of the genus *Corynebacterium* indicate that the highest efficacy in treatment of infections is shown by glycopeptides, linezolid, daptomycin, tigecyclin and chinupristin/dalphopristin.

6. References

Adderson, E. E., Boudreaux, J. W. & Hayden, R. T. (2008). Infections caused by coryneform bacteria in pediatric oncology patients. *Pediatr Infect.* 27 (2): 136-141.

Amao, H., Moriguchi, N., Komukai, Y., Kawasami, H., Takahashi, S. & Sawada, T. (2008). Detection of *Corynebacterium kutscheri* in the feaces of subclinically infectied mice. *Lab Anim.* 42 (3): 376-382.

Appelbaum, P. C. (2002). Resistance among *Streptococcus pneumoniae*: Implications for drug selection. *Clin Infect Dis.* 34 (12): 1613-20.

Arthur, M., Nolinas, C., Mabilat, C. & Courvalin, P. (1990). Detection of erythromycin resistance by the Polymerase Chain Reaction using primers in conserved refion of *erm* rRNA methylase genes. *Antimicrob Agents Chemother.* 34 (10): 2024-26.

Baird, G. J., and Fontanie, M. C. (2007). *Corynebacterium pseudotuberculosis* and its role in ovine caseous lymphadenitis. *J Comp Pathol.* 137 (4): 179-210.

Balci, I., Esik, F., & Bayram, A. (2002). Coryneform bacteria isolated from blond cultures and their antibiotic susceptibilities. *J Intern Med Res.* 30 (4): 422-7.

Barnass, S., Holland, K. & Tabaqchali, S. K. (1991). Vancomycin-resistant *Corynebacterium species* causing prosthetic valve endocarditis successfully treated with imipenem and ciprofloxacin. *J Infect.* 22(2): 161-9.

Campanile, F., Carretto, E., Barbarini, D., Grigis, A., Falcone, M., Goglio, A., Venditti, M. & Stefani, S. E. (2009). Clonal multidrug - resistant *Corynebacterium striatum* strains, Italy. *Emerg Infect Dis.* 15(1): 75-78.

Chiner, E., Arriero, J. M., Signes-Costa, J., Marco, J., Corral, J., Gomez-Esparrago, A., Ortiz de la Tabla, V. & Martin, C. (1999). *Corynebacterium pseudodiphtheriticum* pneumonia in an immunocompetent patient. *Monaldi Arch Chest Dis.* 54 (4): 325-327.

Clinical and Laboratory Standards Institute. (2006). Method for antimicrobial dilution and disk susceptibility testing of infrequently isolated or fastidious bacteria. Approved standard M45-A. Wayne, PA. Clinical and Laboratory Standards Institute.

Collins, M. D., Hoyles, L., Lawson, P. A., Falsen, E., Robson, R. L. & Foster, G. (1999). Phenotypic and phylogenetic characterization of a new *Corynebacterium* species from dogs: description of *Corynebacterium auriscanis* sp.nov. *J Clin Microbiol.* 37(11): 3443-7.

Coyle, M. B., Minshew, B. H., Bland, J. A. & Hsu, P. C. (1979). Erythromycin and clindamycin resistance in *Corynebacterium diphtheriae* from skin lesion. *Antimicrob Agents Chemother.* 16 (4): 525-7.

Dalal, A., Urban, C. & Segal-Maurer, S. (2008). Endocarditis due *Corynebacterium amycolatum*. *J Med Microbiol.* 57 (10): 1299-1302.

Deb, J. K., and Nath, N. (1999). Plasmids of corynebacteria. *FEMS Microbiology Letters.* 175 (1): 11-20.

Dorella, F. A., Pacheco, L. G., Oliveira, S. C., Miyoshi, A. & Azevedo, V. (2006). *Corynebacterium pseudotuberculosis*: microbiology, biochemical properties, pathogenesis and molecular studies of virulence. *Vet Res.* 37 (2): 201-18.

Douthwaite, S., and Champney, W. S. (2001). Structures of ketolides and macrolides determine their mode of interaction with the ribosomal target site. *J Antimicrob Chemother.* 48 (Suppl T1): 1–8.

Dupon, C., Turner, L., Rouveix, E., Nicolas, M. H. & Dorra, M. (1995). Endocardite à *Corynebacterium diphtheriae* tolerant à l'amoxicillin. *Presse Med.* 24 (24): 1135.

Eguchi, H., Kuwahara, T., Miyamoto, T., Nakayama-Imaohji, H., Ichimura, M., Hayashi, T. & Shiota, H. (2008). High-level fluoroquinolone resistance in ophthalmic clinical isolates belonging to the species *Corynebacterium macginleyi*. *J Clin Microbiol.* 46 (2): 527-32.

Freeman, J. D., Smith, H. J., Haines, H. G. & Hellyar, A. G. (1994). Seven patients with respiratory infection due to *Corynebacterium pseudodiphtheriticum*. *Pathology.* 26 (3): 311-4.

Fernandez-Roblas, R., Adames, H., Martin-de-Hijas, N. Z., Garcia Almeida, D., Gadea, I. & Esteban, J. (2009). In vitro activity of tigecycline and 10 other antimicrobials against clinical isolates of the genus *Corynebacterium*. *Int J Antimicrob Agents.* 33 (5): 353-5.

Funke, G., Efstratiou, A., Kiklinska, D., Hutson, R., De Zoysa, A., Engler, K. H. & Collins, M. D. (1997a). *Corynebacterium imitans* sp.nov. isolated from patients with suspected diphtheria. *J Clin Microbiol.* 35 (8): 1978-83.

Funke, G., Englert, R., Frodl, R., Bernard, K. A. & Stenqer S. (2010). *Corynebacterium canis* sp. nov., isolated from a wound infection caused by a dog bite. *Int J Syst Evol Microbiol.* 60 (11): 2544-7.

Funke, G., Punter, V. & von Graevenitz, A. (1996). Antimicrobial susceptibility patterns of some recently established coryneform bacteria. *Antimicrob Agents Chemother.* 40 (12): 2874-8.

Funke, G., von Graevenitz, A., Clarridge III, J. E. & Bernard, K. A. (1997b). Clinical Microbiology of coryneform bacteria. *Clin Micrbiol Rev.*10 (1): 125-159.

Garcia-Bravo, M., Aguado, J. M., Morale, J. M. & Norwega, A. R. (1996). Influence of external factors in resistance of *Corynebacterium urealyticum* to antimicrobial agents. *Antimicrob. Agents Chemother.* 40 (2): 497-499

Gomes, D. L, Martins, C. A, Faria, L. M, Santos, L. S, Santos, C. S, Sabbadini, P. S, Souza, M. C, Alves, G. B, Rosa, A. C, Nagao, P. E, Pereira, G. A, Hirata, R. Jr, & Mattos-Guaraldi, A. L. (2009). *Corynebacterium diphtheriae* as an emerging pathogen in nephrostomy catheter-related infection: evaluation of traits associated with bacterial virulence. *J Med Microbiol.* 58 (11): 1419-27.

Gomez-Garces, J-L., Alos, J-I. & Tamayo, J. (2007). *In vitro* activity of linezolid and 12 other antimicrobials against coryneform bacteria, *Int J Antimicro Agents.* 29 (6): 688-692.

Hall, R. M., Collis, C. M., Kim, M. J., Partridge, S. R., Recchia, G. D. & Stokes, H. W. (1999). Mobile gene cassettes and integrons in evolution. *Ann N Y Acad Sci.* 18 (870): 68-80.

Hodgson, A.L., Krywult, J. & Radford, A. J. (1990). Nucleotide sequence of the erythromycin resistance gene from the *Corynebacterium* plasmid pNG2. *Nucleic Acods Res.* 18 (7): 1891.

Ifantidou, A. M, Diamantidis, M. D, Tseliki, G., Angelou, A. S., Christidou, P., Papa, A. & Pentilas, D. (2010). *Corynebacterium jeikeium* bacteremia in a hemodialyzed patient. *Int J Infect Dis.* 14 (3): 265-8.

Johnson, A. P., Mushtaq, S., Warner, M. & Livermore, D. M. (2004).Activity of daptomycin against multi-resistant Gram-positive bacteria including enterococci and *Staphylococcus aureus* resistant to linezolid. *Int J Antimicrob Agents*. 24 (4): 315-319.

Katsumata, R., Ozaki, A., Oka, T. & Furuya, A. (1984). Protoplast transformation of glutamate-producting bacteria with plazmid DNA. *J Bacteriol*. 159 (1): 306-311.

Kono, M., Sasatsu, M. & Aoki, T. (1983). R plasmids in *Corynebacterium xerosis* strains. *Antimicrob Agents Chemother*. 23 (3): 506-508.

Lagrou, J., Verhaegen, M., Janssens, G., Wauters, G. & Verbist, L. (1998). Prospective study of catalase-positive coryneform organisms in clinical specimens: identification, clinical relevance, and antibiotic susceptibility. *Diagn Microbiol Infect Dis*. 30 (1): 7-15.

Leclercq, R. (2002). Mechanisms of resistance to macrolides and lincosamides: nature of the resistance elements and their clinical implications. *Clin Infect Dis*. 34 (4): 482–92.

López-Medrano, F., García-Bravo, M., Morales, J. M., Andrés, A., San Juan, R., Lizasoain, M. & Aguado, J. M. (2008). Urinary tract infection due to *Corynebacterium urealyticum* in kidney transplant recipients: an underdiagnosed etiology for obstructive uropathy and graft dysfunction-results of a prospective cohort study. *Clin Infect Dis*. 46 (6): 825-30.

Luna, V.A., Coates, P., Eady, A., Cove, J. H., Nguyen, T. T. H. & Roberts, M. C. (1999). A variety of Gram-positive bacteria carry mobile mef genes. *J Antimicrob Chemother*. 44 (1): 19-25.

Łętowska, I. and Olender, A. (2010). Rekomendacje doboru testów do oznaczania wrażliwości bakterii na antybiotyki i chemioterapeutyki 2010. Oznaczanie wrażliwości pałeczek Gram-dodatnich z rodzaju *Corynebacterium* spp. Krajowy Ośrodek ds. Lekowrażliwości KORLD. www.korld.edu.pl

Martinez-Martinez, L., Suarez, A. I., Winstanley, J., Ortega, M. C. & Bernard, K. (1995). Phenotypic characteristics of 31 strains of *Corynebacterium striatum* isolated from clinical sample. *J Clin Microbiol*. 33 (9): 2458-2461.

Nieto, N. C, Foley, J. E, MacLachlan, N. J, Yuan, T. & Spier, S. J. (2009). Evaluation of hepatic disease in mice following intradermal inoculation with *Corynebacterium pseudotuberculosis*. *Am J Vet Res*. 70 (2): 257-62.

Ojo, K. K., Striplin, M. J., Ulep, C. C., Close, N. S., Zittle, J., Luis, H., Bernardo, M., Leitao, J. & Roberts, M. C. (2006). *Staphylococcus* efflux *msr*(A) gene characterized in *Streptococcus, Enterococcus, Corynebacterium,* and *Pseudomonas* isolates. *Antimicrob Agents Chemother*. 50 (3): 1089-1091.

Olender, A. and Niemcewicz, M. (2010). Macrolide, lincosamide, and streptogramin B-constitutive tract resistance in *Corynebacterium pseudodiphtheriticum* isolated from upper respiratory tract specimens. *Microb Drug Resist*. 16 (2): 119-22.

Otsuka, Y., Kawamura, Y., Koyama, T., Iihara, H., Ohkusu, K. & Azeki, T. (2005). *Corynebacterium resistens* sp.nov., a new multi-resistant coryneform bacterium isolated from human infection. *J Clin Microbiol*. 43 (8): 3713- 17.

Otsuka, Y., Ohkusu, K.,Kawamura, Y., Baba, S., Azeki, T. & Kiura, S. (2006). Emergence of multidrug-resistant *Corynebacterium striatum* as a nosocomial pathogen in long-term hospitalized patients with underlying diseases. *Diagn Microbiol Infect Dis*. 54 (2): 109-14.

Perrin-Guyomard, A., Soumet, C., Leclercq, R., Doucet-Populair, R. & Sanders, P. (2005). Antibiotic susceptibility of bacteria isolated from pasteurized milk and characterization of macrolide-lincosamide-streptogramin resistance genes. *J Food Prot*. 68 (2): 347-352.

Pitcher, D., Johnson, A., Allerberger, F., Woodford, N. & George, R. (1990). An investigation of nosocomial infection with *Corynebacterium jeikeium* in surgical patients using a ribosomal RNA gene probe. *Eur J Clin Microbiol Infect Dis*. 9 (9): 643-648.

Power, E. G., Abdullah, Y. H., Talsania, H. G., Spice, W., Aathithan, S. & French, G. L. (1995) VanA genes in vancomycin-resistant clinical isolates of *Oerskovia turbata* and *Arcanobacterium (Corynebacterium) haemolyticum*. *J Antimicrob Chemother*. 36 (4): 595-606.

Riegel, P., Ruimy, R., Renard, F. N. R., Freney, J., Prevost, G., Jehl, F., Christen, R. & Monteil, H. (1997). *Corynebacterium singulare* sp. nov., new species for urease-positive strains related to *Corynebacterium minutissimum*. *Int J Syst Bacteriol*. 36 (4): 1092-1096.

Roberts, M. C., Leonard, R. B., Briselden, A., Schoenknecht, F. D., & Coyle, M. B. (1992). Characterization of antibiotic-resistant *Corynebacterium striatum* strains. *J Antimicrob Chemother*. 30 (4): 463-474.

Roberts, M. C., Sutcliffe, J., Courvalin, P., Jensen, L. B., Rood, J. & Seppala, H. (1999). Nomenclature for macrolide and macrolide-lincosamide-streptogramin B resitance determinants. *Antimicrob Agents Chemother*. 43 (12): 2823-30.

Rosato, A. E., Lee, B. S. & Nash, K. A. (2001). Inducible macrolide resistance in *Corunebacterium jeikeium*. *Antimicrob Agents Chemother*. 45 (7): 1982-89.

Ross, J. I., Eady, A. A., Carnegle, E. & Cove, J. H. (2002). Detection of transposon Tn5432 - mediated macrolide- lincosamide-streptogramin B (MLSB) resistance in cutaneus propionibacterie from six European cities. *J Antimicrob Chemiother*. 49 (1): 165-168.

Serwold-Davis, T. M. and Groman, N. B. (1986). Mapping and cloning of *Corynebacterium diphtheriae* plasmid pNG2 and characterization of ist relatedness to plasmids from skin corynefrms. *Antimicrob Agents Chemother*. 30 (1): 69-72.

Serwold-Davis, T. M., Groman, N. B. & Kao, C. C. (1990). Localization of an orgin of replication in *Corynebacterium diphtheriae* broad host range plasmid pNG2 that also functions in Escherichia coli. *FEMS Microbiol Lett*. 54 (1-3): 119-23.

Serwold-Davis, T. M., Groman, N. & Rabin M. (1987). Transformaction of *Corynebacterium diphtheriae*, *Corynebacterium ulcerans*, *Corynebacterium glutamicum* and *Escherichia coli* with the *C.diphtheriae* plasmid pNG2. *Poc Natl Acad Sci USA*. 84 (14): 4964-68.

Shah, M. and Murillo, J. L. (2005). Successful treatment of *Corynebacterium striatum* endocarditis with daptomycin plus rifampin. *Ann Pharmacother*. 39 (10): 1741-4.

Sierra, J. M., Martinez-Martinez, L., Vazquez, F., Giralt, E. & Vila, J. (2005). Relationship between mutations in the *gyr*A gene and quinolone resistance in clinical isolates of *Corynebacterium striatum* and *Corynebacterium amycolatum*, *Antimicrob Agents Chemother*. 49 (5): 1714-9.

Suzuki, E., Mochida, K. & Nakagawa, M. (1988). Naturally occurring subclinical *Corynebacterium kutscheri* infection in laboratory rats: strain and age related antibody response. *Lab Anim Sci*. 38 (1): 42-5.

Takahashi, T., Tsuji, M., Kikuchi, N., Ishihara, C., Osanai, T., Kasai, N., Yanagawa, R. & Hiramune, T. (1995). Assignment of the bacterial agent of urinary calculus in young rats by the comparative sequence analysis of the 16s rRNA genes corynebacteria. *J Vet Sci.* 57 (3): 515-7.

Tauch, A., Kassing, F., Kalinowski, J. & Pühler, A. (1995). The *Corynebacterium xerosis* composite transposon Tn*5432* consists of two identical insertion sequences, designated IS*1249*, flanking the erythromycin resistance gene ermcx. *Plasmid.* 34 (2): 119-31.

Tauch, A., Kassing, F., Kalinowski, J. & Pühler, A. (1995). The erythromycin resistance gene of the *Corynebacterium xerosis* R-plasmid pTP10 also carrying chloramphenicol, kanamycin and tetracycline resistance is capable of transposition in *Corynebacterium glutamicum.* *Plasmid.* 33 (3): 168-79.

Tauch, A., Krieft, S., Kalinowski, J. & Pühler, A. (2000). The 51,409-bp R-plasmid pTP10 from the multiresistant clinical isolate *Corynebacterium striatum* M82B is composed of DNA segments initially identified in soil bacteria and in plant, animal, and human pathogens. *Mol Gen Genet.* 263 (1): 1-11.

Tauch, A., Krieft, S., Pühler, A. & Kalinowski, J. (1999). The *tetAB* of the *Corynebacterium striatum* R-lasmid pTP10 encode an ABC transporter and confer tetracycline, oxytetracycline and oxacillin resistance in *Corynebacterium glutamicum.* *FEMS Microbiol Lett.* 173 (1): 203-9.

Tauch, A., Zheng, Z., Pühler, A. & Kalinowski, J. (1998). *Corynebacterium striatum* chloramphenicol resistance transposon Tn5564: genetic organization and transposition in *Corynebacterium glutamicum.* *Plasmid.* 40 (2): 126-39.

Troxler, R., Funke, G., von Graevenitz, A. & Stock, I. (2001). Natural antibiotic susceptibility of recently established coryneform bacteria, *Eur J Clin Microbiol Infect Dis.* 20 (5): 315-23.

Wagner, K. S, White, J. M, Neal, S., Crowcroft, N. S, Kupreviciene, N., Paberza, R., Lucenko, I., Jõks, U., Akbaş, E., Alexandrou-Athanassoulis, H., Detcheva, A., Vuopio, J., von Hunolstein, C., Murphy, P. G., Andrews, N., Members of the Diphtheria Surveillance Network & Efstratiou, A. (2011). Screening for *Corynebacterium diphtheriae* and *Corynebacterium ulcerans* in patients with upper respiratory tract infections 2007-2008: a multicentre European study. *Clin Microbiol Infect.* 17 (4): 519-25.

Weiss, K., Laverdiere, M. & Rivest, R. (1996). Comparison of antimicrobial susceptibilities of *Corynebacterium* species by broth microdilution and disc diffusion methods. *Antimicrob Agents Chemother.* 40 (4): 930-3.

Wendisch, V. F., Bott, M., Kalinowski, J., Oldiges, M. & Wiechert, W. (2006). Emerging *Corynebacterium glutamicum* systems biology, *J Biotechnol.* 124 (1): 74-92.

Williams, D. Y., Selepak, S. T., Gill, V. J. (1993). Identification of clinical isolates of nondiphterial *Corynebacterium* species and their antibiotic susceptibility patterns. *Diagn Microbiol Infect Dis.* 17 (1): 23-8.

Wilson, A. P. R. (1995). Treatment of infections caused by toxigenic and non-toxigenic strains of *Corynebacterium diphtheriae.* *J Antimicrob Chemother.* 35 (6): 717-20.

Valbuena, N., Letek, M., Ordonez, E., Atala, J., Daniel, R. A., Gil, J. A. & Mateos, L. M. (2007). Characterization of HMW-PBPs from the rod-shaped actinomecete *Corynebacterium glutamicum*: peptydoglycan synthesis in cells lacking actin-like cytoskeletal structures. *Mol Microbiol.* 66 (3): 643-57.

Vertes, A. A., Inui, M. & Yukawa, H. (2005). Manipulating Corynebacteria, from individual genes to chromosomes. *Appl Environ Microbiol.* 71 (12): 7633-42.

Von Hunolstein, C., Scopetti, F., Efstratiou, A. & Engler, K. (2002). Penicillin tolerance amongst non-toxigenic *Corynebacterium diphtheriae* isolated from cases of pharyngitis. *J. Antimicrob Chemother.* 50 (1): 125-8.

Yague Guirao, G., Mora Peris, B., Martinez-Toldos, M. C., Rodriguez Gonzalez, T., Valero Guillen, P.L. & Segovia Hernandez, M. (2005). Implication of *erm*X genes in macrolide- and telithromycin-resistance in *Corynebacterium jeikeium* and *Corynebacterium amycolatum*. *Rev Esp Quimioterap.* 18 (3): 136-242.

Yassin, A. F. and Siering, C. (2008). *Corynebacterium sputi* sp. nov., isolated from the sputum of the a patient with pneumonia. *Int J Syst Evol Microbiol.* 58 (12): 2876-9.

Yoon, S., Kim, H., Lee, Y. & Kim, S. (2011). Bacteremia caused by Corynebacterium amycolatum with a novel mutation in gyrA gene that confers high-level quinolone resistance. *Korean J Lab Med.* 31(1): 47-8.

5

Antibiotic Resistance Patterns in Faecal *E. coli*: A Longitudinal Cohort-Control Study of Hospitalized Horses

Mohamed O. Ahmed[1,3‡], Nicola J. Williams[2], Peter D. Clegg[2],
Keith E. Baptiste[4] and Malcolm Bennett[3]
*[1]Department of Microbiology and Parasitology,
Faculty of Veterinary Medicine, Tripoli university, Tripoli
[2]Department of Comparative Molecular Medicine,
[3]Department of Animal and Population Health,
[2,3]School of Veterinary Science, University of Liverpool, Leahurst,
[4]Department of Large Animal Sciences, Faculty of Life Sciences,
University of Copenhagen, Taastrup,
[1]Libya
[2,3]UK
[4]Denmark*

1. Introduction

Cross-sectional prospective surveys are a useful method for studying the effects of antimicrobials on animals (Dunowska et al., 2006; Thomson et al., 2008; Bunner et al., 2007) . However, there is a paucity of these studies in horses compared to other animals (Coe et al., 2008).

Although antibiotic consumption has been a major contributor to the antibiotic resistance phenomenon (Bunner et al., 2007) various different factors have added to the development and dissemination of antimicrobial resistance. For example, population densities among humans have been identified as risk factors for development and spread of antimicrobial resistance (Bruinsma et al., 2005; Zhang et al., 2006). Hospitalization, in humans for instance, is also associated with an increase in antibiotic resistance in pathogenic bacteria, while others have found a lack of a significant effect on the prevalence of resistance in *E. coli* (Koterba et al., 1986; Gaynes et al., 1997). A study by Dunowska and colleagues (Dunowska et al., 2006) concluded that both antimicrobial administration and hospitalization were associated with the shedding of *E. coli* resistant strains from equine faecal samples.

Certain antimicrobial administration regimes have been shown to give rise to antibiotic resistant bacteria, which then comprise a reservoir of resistant bacteria when shed into the environment (Ahmed et al., 2010; Fofana et al., 2006; Diarrassouba et al., 2007; Pallecchi et al., 2007). Linked resistance genes encoded on mobile genetic elements, can also contribute to the spread of resistance genes (Srinivasan et al., 2007), with exposure to one antimicrobial agent leading to selection for resistance against other, or multiple, antimicrobial drugs (Braoudaki et al., 2007; Schnellmann et al., 2006; Weese et al., 2006). Such genes can be maintained after antibiotic treatment, has been stopped such that removing the selective pressure does not necessarily lead to the loss of resistance (Ahmed et al., 2010; Kaszanyitzky et al., 2007; Ghidan et al.,2008). Mobile genetic elements are widely reported cause of the spread of antibiotic resistance in both *E. coli* and *Salmonella* commensals in animals bred for human consumption (Roest et al., 2007). Therefore, *E. coli* and other enteric organisms are widely used as an indicator organism (Kaneene et al., 2007; Bruinsma et al., 2003).

The purpose of this investigation was to identify changes in antibiotic resistant *E. coli* in faeces of horses entering the Philip Leverhulme Equine Hospital (PLEH), at the University of Liverpool, UK on arrival, during hospitalization, and after discharge. The dynamics affecting the prevalence of antibiotic resistant *E. coli* were used in this study in order to examine potential risk factors.

2. Materials and methods

2.1 Study design

Faecal samples were collected from horses admitted to the Philip Leverhulme Equine Hospital (PLEH) at the University of Liverpool for more than seven days at the following time points: 1st, on arrival, before treatment began; 2nd, one day; 3rd, 2-3 days after treatment had started; 4th, immediately before discharge. Further faecal samples were collected by the horse's owners, 4-8 weeks after discharge (5th), and also 6 months after discharge (6th). Horses were divided into three groups as follows: GI+, horses with gastrointestinal conditions and under antibiotic therapy; Non-GI+, horses with non-gastrointestinal conditions and under antibiotic therapy; Non-GI-, horses with non-gastrointestinal conditions and no antibiotic therapy.

2.2 Sample collection

Faecal samples were taken from stalls randomly and chosen from the firm part of the faecal balls. In total, 2-3 grams were collected and taken straight to the laboratory.

2.3 Bacterial culture

Standard microbiological methods and biochemical tests were used to isolate and confirm each *E. coli* as fully described by Ahmed et al 2010. Three single *E. coli* colonies were chosen from each sample, confirmed by biochemical testing (e.g. API system) and subjected to further susceptibility tests thereafter.

2.4 Antibiotic susceptibility tests

Antibiotic susceptibility testing was performed according to the BSAC guidelines (Andrews, 2008). Briefly, antimicrobial drugs tested for included: - ampicillin; if the isolates show resistance to ampicillin then isolates were also tested against other two cephalosporins (cefotaxime (30 µg) and ceftazidime (30µg) for extended resistance to cephalosporines and referred as potential ESBL producers (ESBLs*) for ampicillin resistant isolates), apramycin, chloramphenicol (and also against florfenicol, if chloramphenicol resistant), nalidixic acid (and also against ciprofloxacin, if nalidixic acid resistant), tetracycline and trimethoprim. Further susceptibility tests were also performed for gentamicin, spectinomycin, streptomycin and sulphamexazole for all collected resistant isolates. Isolates were considered resistant if resistance to at least one antibiotic was shown and classified as multidrug resistant isolates (MDR) if resistant to four or more classes of antibiotics (Ahmed et al., 2010). Guidelines for determining florfenicol and apramycin resistance were as followed and determined by Ahmed et al., 2010.

2.5 Identification of antibiotic resistance genes in resistant E. coli isolates

DNA was extracted by boiling: a 5μl drop of each isolate was suspended in 0.5 ml sterile water and heated for 20 minutes at 100°C. PCR assays, previously applied by Ahmed et al 2010 were also used to detect genes commonly associated with ampicillin, chloramphenicol, tetracycline and trimethoprim resistance, were carried out using modified versions of published protocols: Pitout, 1998 (Pitout et al., 1998) for ampicillin resistant genes (*tem* & *shv* genes); Vassort-Bruneau, 1996 (Vassort-Bruneau et al., 1996) and Keyes et al.,2000 (Keyes et al., 2000) for chloramphenicol resistant genes (*catI, catII catIII* & *cmlA* genes); Ng, 2001 (Ng et al., 2001) for tetracycline resistant genes (*tetA, tetB, tetC, tetD, tet E* and *tetG* genes); Gibreel & Sköld, 1998 (Gibreel et al., 1998) and Lee, 2001 (Lee et al., 2001) for trimethoprim resistant genes (*dfr1, dfr9 dfr12, dfr13, dfrA14* & *dfr17* genes).

2.6 Statistical data analysis

Data were analysed using Minitab software, in order to determine the 95% binomial confidence intervals (95%CI) and chi-square test (X^2).

2.7 Conjugation assays

Mating experiments to determine if resistance could be transferred by conjugation were carried out using a nalidixic acid resistant E. coli K12 as the recipient (as performed by Ahmed et al., 2010). The method was as following: E. coli K12 was inoculated into 20ml nutrient broths (LabM) and incubated overnight at 37°C. Resistant E. coli strains (donor strains) were inoculated into separate 3ml nutrient broths and incubated overnight; 4 ml of recipient strain was then added to the donor strain and incubated at 37°C for one hour. Broths were then streaked onto agar plates containing nalidixic acid (30μg/ml) plus ampicillin (8μg/ml). Plates were incubated for 24 hours. Successful transconjugants were subcultured onto nutrient agar for susceptibility testing by disc diffusion as previously described. The resistance profiles of the transconjugants were compared to the resistance profile of the original strains. Gene profiles of the donor isolates, characterized by PCR, were described prior to the tranconjugation experiments

3. Results

3.1 Prevalence of antibiotic resistant (AR) E. coli isolate

In total, 15 horses were used for the study: GI+ (n=6 horses), non-GI+ (n=4 horses) and non-GI- (n=5 horses). Six samples were collected from each horse (n=90 in total). The distribution of antibiotic resistance is presented in Tables 1 and 2.

Cohort group	No. of horses	No. of samples collected	No. of samples positive for AR E. coli (%)	Distribution of resistant samples(out of possible 6) for each sampling time					
				1st	2nd	3rd	4th	5th	6th
GI +	6	36	21 (58%)	2	4	5	5	3	2
NON GI +	4	24	18 (75%)	3	4	4	4	3	0
NON GI –	5	30	16 (53%)	1	3	4	4	4	0

Table 1. The number of horses, faecal samples collected and faecal samples positive for at least one antibiotic resistant (AR) E. coli isolate

Source of samples	Samples collected	Positive samples	Distributing of samples containing E. coli resistant isolates to different antibiotics									
			AMP	CEP	APR	CHL	FLO	NAL	CIP	TET	TRI	MDR
GI +	36	21	15	1	1	5	5	8	6	15	19	8
NON GI +	24	18	12	10	0	10	0	11	11	11	18	11
NON GI –	30	16	14	4	0	7	2	7	5	11	13	10

*Abbreviations: Ampicillin (AMP), Cephalosporins (CEP), Apramycin (APR), Chloramphenicol (CHL), Florfenicol (FLO), Nalidixic acid (NAL), Ciprofloxacin (CIP), Teracycline (TET), Trimethoprim (TRI), MDR (multidrug resistance i.e. resistance to four or more antimicrobials), *ESBLs* isolates show resistance to ampicillin then isolates were also tested against other two cephalosporins (cefotaxime (30 µg) and ceftazidime (30µg) for extended resistance to cephalosporines andreferred as potential ESBL producers (ESBLs*)

Table 2. Summary of horses, faecal samples, faecal samples containing resistant E. coli, and the number of faecal samples with E. coli resistant to each individual antibiotic

The proportion of samples with at least one E. coli isolate resistant to at least one antibiotic ranged from 53-75% but did not vary significantly between treatment groups (GI +, non-GI+, non GI-) (Table1). All three treatment groups also showed a similar change in prevalence of resistant isolates recovered over the duration of the study (Table1). Furthermore, there were no significant differences in the antibiotic resistance profiles of the isolates in each group (Table2). Therefore, data from the three groups were subsequently combined for the analysis of changing resistance over time. A definite pattern was observed in the prevalence of overall resistance, which increased from 40 +/-6 % at the first time point, immediately prior to admission, to 86 +/- 28 % during hospitalization (3rd time point), and decreased to 12 +/- 30 % after release (6th time point) (Figure1).

To compare the prevalence of resistant isolates before hospitalisation, immediately before discharge and 6 months after discharge (at 1st, 4th and 6th time points respectively), data was analysed by X^2 testing, analysing each individual antimicrobial as well as multidrug resistance. With the exception of ampicillin, isolates resistant to each antimicrobial drug and multidrug resistant isolates (MDR) (i.e. isolates resistant to ≥ 4 antibiotic classes), increased significantly during hospitalization and decreased after the horses had returned home (Table3). The numbers of isolates resistant to florfenicol were too low for statistical analysis.

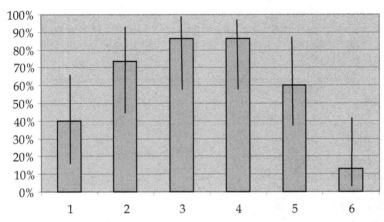

Fig. 1. Relationship between sampling time and the proportion of samples with ≥ one isolate resistant to at least one antibiotic (with 95% binomial CI); total from all three treatment groups GI+, non-GI+ and non-GI are combined (table1).

Prevalence of antibiotic resistance at sampling times	Sampling times 1 & 4		Sampling times 4 & 6	
	X^2	p	X^2	p
Resistant to at least one antibiotic	7.03	≤ 0.01	13.4	≤ 0.001
Amp	3.394	≥ 0.05	9.600	≤ 0.01
Cep	6.000	≤ 0.05	6.000	≤ 0.05
Chlo	6.136	≤ 0.05	9.130	≤ 0.01
Nal	7.500	≤ 0.01	7.500	≤ 0.01
Cip	7.500	≤ 0.01	7.500	≤ 0.01
Tet	15.000	≤ 0.001	11.627	≤ 0.001
Tri	10.995	≤ 0.001	13.393	≤ 0.001
MDR	10.909	≤ 0.001	10.109	≤ 0.001

Table 3. Two X^2 tests (2x2 analysis) to compare the effect of hospital admission and discharge on prevalence of resistance to particular antibiotic drugs.

3.2 Susceptibility testing of culture collection

In total, 138 E. coli isolates resistant to at least one antibiotic were collected. Of these, 71 (51.4%) were classified as MDR. Among these, two main distinctive MDR phenotypes (Ph_s) were found: Ph_s1;Amp,chlo,tet,tri,nal, comprising 93% of the MDR isolates, and mostly found among non-GI + samples; Ph_s2; Amp,chlo,tet,tri comprised 50% of the MDR isolates among the GI+ and the non-GI- samples. All the resistant isolates (n=138) were tested for susceptibility to further antibiotics. Overall, 38.5% were resistant to gentamicin, 71% to spectinomycin, 96% to streptomycin and 90% to sulphamexazole.

3.3 Molecular analysis of culture collection

PCRs revealed that *CatI [only](87%)*, *tem(60.8%)*, *tetA(60.8%, dfr17(50.4%)*, *dfr1(38.5%)* were identified at higher prevalence among each positive collection of resistant isolates to each antibiotic (table4). MICs were also shown at higher values of ≥256 for most isolates to the selected drugs (table4).

Antibiotic	No. of Positive Sample	No. of Positive Isolates	MICs (ug/ml)	Resistance genes
Ampicillin	41	95	128 - >256	*tem (60.8%)* *shv (2%)*
Cephalosporines	15	34		
Chloramphenicol	22	51	256 - ≥256	*catI* (only) *(87%)*
Florfenicol	7	7		*catI (71%)*
Nalidixic acid	26	65		
Ciprofloxacin	22	64	4 – 16	
Tetracycline	37	89	64 - ≥256	*tetA (60.8%)* *tetB (19%)* *tetA&tetB(11.9%)*
Trimethoprim	50	127	>256	*dfr17 (50.4%)* *dfr1 (38.5%)* *dfr12 (20%)*

Table 4. Summary of antibiotic resistance, showing levels of resistance, MIC values and resistance gene prevalence in a total of 90 faecal samples and 138 isolates.

3.4 Conjugation experiments

Mating experiments were performed on selected isolates (n=73); those exhibiting nalidixic acid resistance were excluded 16 isolates (22% of the selected isolates & 11% of the overall culture collection) were able to transfer resistance by conjugation, and these were distributed across all cohort groups. Resistance profiles of the transconjugants, determined by susceptibility testing on the transconjugant, were identical to those of the donors (Table 5).

4. Discussion

Previous studies have given rise to conflicting conclusions as to whether or not hospitalization is associated with an increase in antibiotic resistance in bacteria (Bruinsma et al., 2003; Koterba et al., 1986). Factors other than the use of antimicrobial drugs could influence the maintenance and development of antibiotic resistance of enteric bacteria in the gastrointestinal tract (Dewulf et al., 2007). The use of antibiotics in animals is of concern (Mora et al., 2005) since resistant organisms might be excreted in the faeces of animals, following administration of antimicrobials, and contribute to the reservoir of resistant bacteria in the environment (Ahmed et al., 2010). Resistant bacteria could be selected or acquired in the hospital environment and may subsequently be disseminated to the horses' home environments.

No.	Origin	Resistance phenotype	Donor genes (previously identified by PCR)
1,	NON-GI-	AMP	*Tem*
2	NON-GI-	AMP	*Tem*
3	NON-GI-	MDR	*dfr1,dfr12,tetA,tem,catI*
4	NON-GI-	MDR	*dfr1,dfr12,tetA,tem*
5	NON-GI-	MDR	*dfr1,dfr12,tetA,tem,catI*
6	NON-GI-	MDR	*tem*
7	NON-GI-	MDR	*dfr1,dfr12,tetA,tem*
8	GI+	AMP	*tem*
9	GI+	AMP,TRI	*dfr(7-17)*
10	GI+	AMP,TRI	*not identified*
11	GI+	AMP	*tem*
12	GI+	AMP	*tem*
13	GI+	AMP	*tem*
14	GI+	AMP,TRI	*dfr1*
15	GI+	AMP,TRI	*tem*
16	NON-GI +	AMP	*tem*

Table 5. Characteristics of isolates showing of transferable resistance.

This study and in contrast with others found no obvious association between antibiotic treatment, or clinical condition, and resistance profiles in faecal E. *coli*. This may be due to the relatively small sample size, or because horses entering the PLEH are largely referral cases and likely to have received antibiotic therapy prior to admission.

However, overall resistance to most individual antibiotics, and the proportion of MDR isolates increased during hospitalization and thereafter decreased during convalescence in the home environment. Recent studies by Dunowska et al, on horses, concluded that both hospitalization and antimicrobial administration were associated with the shedding of antimicrobial resistance E. *coli* strains of faecal origin (Dunowska et al., 2006). An earlier study, from a university equine hospital, found that the rate of resistance amongst E. *coli* and *Klebsiella* was higher at day seven of hospitalization compared to day one (Koterba et al., 1986). This may be due to selection during hospitalization through antibiotic therapy, and also the ready availability of resistant isolates in the hospital environment. It would be interesting to undertake PFGE analysis of the E. *coli* over time to investigate whether resistance is due to infection with resistant strains or horizontal transmission of resistance to the existing gut flora.

Antimicrobials select for resistance (Tenover et al., 2006) but the restriction of antimicrobials does not necessarily reduce antimicrobial resistance (Hoyle et al., 2006). In our study, the prevalence of resistant E. *coli* dropped markedly after discharge from the hospital, which may suggest that both the increase and decrease in resistance are due to turnover of E. *coli* between the gut and the environment.

E. *coli* with simple and multiple antimicrobial resistance (MDR) has been widely documented (Fofana et al., 2006; Ahmed et al., 2010). Bacteria can acquire or develop resistance to antimicrobials in different ways, including acquisition of resistant genes. E. *coli* has been indicated as a possible reservoir for antimicrobial resistance genes and might play a role in the spreading of such determinants to other bacteria (Ahmed et al., 2010). The flora of healthy animals has also been implicated as a reservoir of antibiotic resistance genes (De Graef et al., 2004) and resistance transfer has been shown to occur between different animal species on farm premises (Hoyle et al., 2006). *E. coli* of animal origin with resistance to antibiotics and multiple antibiotics has been widely documented (Mora et al., 2005). The importance of farm animals in the spread of resistance to human populations is increased by worldwide reports of mobile genetic elements in animals raised for human consumption (Roest et al., 2007).

Our results for MICs and the genetic determination of resistance, suggest that, resistance was due to commonly reported genes causing such resistance in *E. coli* and other bacteria. It is interesting to note, that while some MDR transferred in the conjugation studies, many transconjugants were resistant to either ampicillin alone or ampicillin and trimethoprim (table 5). This suggests that both resistance profiles are encoded on mobile genetic elements. Horses in the GI+ and non-GI+ groups were the donors for most of the Amp and Amp/Trim transconjugants, and all the horses in both groups received therapy with cephalosporin drugs. It may, therefore be that these isolates represent either an endemic strain in the hospital, or an endemic plasmid moving rapidly between horses.

Multiple drug resistance phenotypes have been shown to be related to certain antibiotic drugs such as streptomycin and tetracycline (Mora et al., 2005). Also the resistance to a single antibiotic (i.e. tetracycline), in commensal *E. coli*, is linked to other antimicrobial resistances (e.g. ampicillin, trimethoprim and sulphonamides) (Dewulf et al., 2007). The *dfrA1, dfrA12, dfrA15* and *dfrA17* genes are documented to be carried on mobile genetic elements (i.e. integron classes), harboring resistance genes to at least three antimicrobials, and thus conferring multiple resistance (Ahmed et al., 2009). Other antibiotic resistances (i.e. ampicillin resistance) although found, were not strongly related to the presence of mobile genetic elements (Hoyle et al., 2005). Our PCR results in this study revealed similar observations within our collection of *E.coli* strains to other studies, although the conjugation results show that even isolates with single resistance (to ampicillin) transferred resistance (although not MDR). Thus, mobile genetic elements could also be responsible for single resistance and antimicrobial therapy might have resulted in such selection. The type of resistance and the identified genes (i.e. ampicillin resistance) could also be related to the type of antimicrobial therapy administered (e.g. cephalosporins). Such revelations, if proven by further studies, would mean that this kind of element may acquire further resistance genes in the future and help the dissemination and development of antibiotic resistance.

The importance of mobile gene pools in the spread of antibiotic resistance has been highlighted through comprehensive genomic analysis (Fricke et al., 2008). In our survey, a high proportion of the isolates tested in conjugation experiments were able to transfer resistance. *Dfr17* was the most prevalent trimethoprim resistance gene identified among the positive PCR isolates and *dfr1* was the second most prevalent. *tetA* was the most prevalent tetracycline resistant gene. This might indicate that the *dfr17* and *tetA* resistant genes are more involved in the MDR mechanisms and most likely to be integrated within mobile genetic elements. The *tem* gene was also the most prevalent ampicillin resistant gene among the isolates and the *catI* gene was mostly found in MDR isolates. The *dfr17* is extensively reported to be involved in mobile genetic elements (Van et al., 2007). This, along with the conjugation results, suggests that these elements are present in the hospital environment or that they are already constituents of the horses' intestinal flora. The referral hospital deals with horses in the area and horses are likely to be referred more than once to this hospital, which might lead to increases in the dissemination of resistance phenotypes in horses. The similarity between MDR phenotypes among collected strains can be epidemiologically important and molecular characterization (i.e. PFGE) in future studies will enhance our understanding of the phenomena.

The florfenicol resistant isolates were positive by PCR (five out of seven were positive for *catI*) and the mechanisms of this resistance require further investigation. However florfenicol resistance has been documented in *E. coli* of animal origin (Singer et al., 2004) and it has been shown that *floR* genetic determinants and others (i.e. *cmlA, cat1, cat2*) were also largely related to florfenicol resistance (Li et al., 2007). Others have shown that *floR* mediated resistance to chloramphenicol and florfenicol is plasmid mediated and also carries resistance to other genes (Blickwede et al., 2007; Kehrenberg et al., 2008). Recent molecular analyses have suggested that florfenicol resistance is strongly due to horizontal rather than clonal dissemination (Kehrenberg et al., 2008). This correlates with our results, in that florfenicol resistance is entirely documented among MDR isolates (although not proven transconjugants by our experiments). The horses in this study had never been treated with these classes of drugs, implicating a mobile genetic system in the acquisition of resistance from other animals or the environment.

5. Conclusions

No association between therapy and resistance profile was found in this study. However, the prevalence of antimicrobial resistance, and of MDR strains, did increase during hospitalization and subsequently decreased upon release from hospital. Thus therapy and the general environment of the hospital do appear to select for resistance and resistant isolates may disseminate once horses have been discharged, leading to clinical and public health concerns.

6. Acknowledgements

Authors are grateful to all staff members at Philip Leverhulme Equine Hospital (PLEH) and the livery stables for their help and support throughout this work.

7. References

Ahmed, MO.; Clegg, P. D.; Williams, N. J.; Baptiste, K. E.; and Bennett, M.. (2010). Antimicrobial resistance in equine faecal Escherichia coli isolates from North West England. Ann.Clin.Microbiol.Antimicrob. 9:12.

Ahmed, AM.; Younis, EE.; Osman, SA.; Ishida, Y.; El-Khodery, SA.; Shimamoto, T. (2009). Genetic analysis of antimicrobial resistance in Escherichia coli isolated from diarrheic neonatal calves. *Vet Microbiol*, 136(3-4):397-402.

Andrews, JM. (2006). BSAC standardized disc susceptibility testing method (version 5). *J Antimicrob Chemother*, 58(3):511-529.

Blickwede, M.; Schwarz, S. (2004). Molecular analysis of florfenicol-resistant Escherichia coli isolates from pigs. *J Antimicrob Chemother*, 53(1):58-64.

Braoudaki, M.; Hilton, AC. (2004). Adaptive resistance to biocides in Salmonella enterica and Escherichia coli O157 and cross-resistance to antimicrobial agents. *J Clin Microbiol*, 42(1):73-78.

Bruinsma, N.; Filius, PM.; van den Bogaard, AE.; Nys, S.; Degener, J.; Endtz, HP.; Stobberingh, EE. (2003). Hospitalization, a risk factor for antibiotic-resistant Escherichia coli in the community? *J Antimicrob Chemother*, 51(4):1029-1032.

Bunner, CA.; Norby, B.; Bartlett, PC.; Erskine, RJ.; Downes, FP.; Kaneene, JB. (2007). Prevalence and pattern of antimicrobial susceptibility in Escherichia coli isolated from pigs reared under antimicrobial-free and conventional production methods. *J Am Vet Med Assoc*, 231(2):275-283.

Coe, PH.; Grooms, DL.; Metz, K.; Holland, RE. (2008). Changes in antibiotic susceptability of Escherichia coli isolated from steers exposed to antibiotics during the early feeding period. *Vet Ther*, 9(3):241-247.

De Graef, EM.; Decostere, S.; Devriese, LA.; Haesebrouck, F. (2004). Antibiotic resistance among fecal indicator bacteria from healthy individually owned and kennel dogs. *Microb Drug Resist*, 10(1):65-69.

Dewulf, J.; Catry, B.; Timmerman, T.; Opsomer, G.; de Kruif, A.; Maes, D. (2007). Tetracycline-resistance in lactose-positive enteric coliforms originating from Belgian fattening pigs: degree of resistance, multiple resistance and risk factors. *Prev Vet Med*, 78(3-4):339-351.

Diarrassouba, F.; Diarra, MS.; Bach, S.; Delaquis, P.; Pritchard, J.; Topp, E.; Skura, BJ. (2007). Antibiotic resistance and virulence genes in commensal Escherichia coli and Salmonella isolates from commercial broiler chicken farms. *J Food Prot*, 70(6):1316-1327.

Dunowska, M.; Morley, PS.; Traub-Dargatz, JL.; Hyatt, DR.; Dargatz, DA. (2006). Impact of hospitalization and antimicrobial drug administration on antimicrobial susceptibility patterns of commensal Escherichia coli isolated from the feces of horses. *J Am Vet Med Assoc*, 228(12):1909-1917.

Fofana, A.; Bada Alambedji, R.; Seydi, M.; Akakpo, AJ. (2006). Antibiotic resistance of Escherichia coli strains isolated from raw chicken meat in Senegal. *Dakar Med*, 51(3):145-150.

Fricke, WF.; Wright, MS.; Lindell, AH.; Harkins, DM.; Baker-Austin, C.; Ravel, J.; Stepanauskas, R. (2008). Insights into the environmental resistance gene pool from the genome sequence of the multidrug-resistant environmental isolate Escherichia coli SMS-3-5. *J Bacteriol*, 190(20):6779-6794.

Gaynes, R.; Monnet, D. (1997). The contribution of antibiotic use on the frequency of antibiotic resistance in hospitals. *Ciba Found Symp*, 207:47-56; discussion 56-60.

Ghidan, A.; Kaszanyitzky, EJ.; Dobay, O.; Nagy, K.; Amyes, SG.; Rozgonyi, F. (2008). Distribution and genetic relatedness of vancomycin-resistant enterococci (VRE) isolated from healthy slaughtered chickens in Hungary from 2001 to 2004. *Acta Vet Hung*, 56(1):13-25.

Gibreel, A.; Skold, O. (1998). High-level resistance to trimethoprim in clinical isolates of Campylobacter jejuni by acquisition of foreign genes (dfr1 and dfr9) expressing drug-insensitive dihydrofolate reductases. *Antimicrob Agents Chemother*, 42(12):3059-3064.

Hoyle, DV.; Davison, HC.; Knight, HI.; Yates, CM.; Dobay, O.; Gunn, GJ.; Amyes, SG.; Woolhouse, ME. (2006). Molecular characterisation of bovine faecal Escherichia coli shows persistence of defined ampicillin resistant strains and the presence of class 1 integrons on an organic beef farm. *Vet Microbiol*, 115(1-3):250-257.

Kaneene, JB.; Warnick, LD.; Bolin, CA.; Erskine, RJ.; May, K.; Miller, R. (2008). Changes in tetracycline susceptibility of enteric bacteria following switching to nonmedicated milk replacer for dairy calves. *J Clin Microbiol*, 46(6):1968-1977.

Kaszanyitzky, EJ.; Tenk, M.; Ghidan, A.; Fehervari, GY.; Papp, M. (2007). Antimicrobial susceptibility of enterococci strains isolated from slaughter animals on the data of Hungarian resistance monitoring system from 2001 to 2004. *Int J Food Microbiol*, 115(1):119-123.

Keyes, K.; Hudson, C.; Maurer, JJ.; Thayer, S.; White, DG.; Lee, MD. (2000). Detection of florfenicol resistance genes in Escherichia coli isolated from sick chickens. *Antimicrob Agents Chemother*, 44(2):421-424.

Kehrenberg, C.; Wallmann, J.; Schwarz, S. (2008) Molecular analysis of florfenicol-resistant Pasteurella multocida isolates in Germany. *J Antimicrob Chemother*, 62(5):951-955.

Koterba, A.; Torchia, J.; Silverthorne, C.; Ramphal, R.; Merritt, AM.; Manucy. (1986). Nosocomial infections and bacterial antibiotic resistance in a university equine hospital. *J Am Vet Med Assoc*, 189(2):185-191.

Lee, JC.; Oh, JY.; Cho, JW.; Park, JC.; Kim, JM.; Seol, SY.; Cho, DT. (2001) The prevalence of trimethoprim-resistance-conferring dihydrofolate reductase genes in urinary isolates of Escherichia coli in Korea. *J Antimicrob Chemother*, 47(5):599-604.

Li, XS.; Wang, GQ.; Du, XD.; Cui, BA.; Zhang, SM.; Shen, JZ. (2007). Antimicrobial susceptibility and molecular detection of chloramphenicol and florfenicol resistance among Escherichia coli isolates from diseased chickens. *J Vet Sci*, 8(3):243-247.

Mora, A.; Blanco, JE.; Blanco, M.; Alonso, MP.; Dhabi, G.; Echeita, A.; Gonzalez, EA.; Bernardez, MI.; Blanco, J. (2005). Antimicrobial resistance of Shiga toxin (verotoxin)-producing Escherichia coli O157:H7 and non-O157 strains isolated from humans, cattle, sheep and food in Spain. *Res Microbiol*, 156(7):793-806.

Ng, LK.; Martin, I.; Alfa, M.; Mulvey, M. (2001). Multiplex PCR for the detection of tetracycline resistant genes. *Mol Cell Probes*, 15(4):209-215.

Pallecchi, L.; Lucchetti, C.; Bartoloni, A.; Bartalesi, F.; Mantella, A.; Gamboa, H.; Carattoli, A.; Paradisi, F.; Rossolini, GM. (2007). Population structure and resistance genes in antibiotic-resistant bacteria from a remote community with minimal antibiotic exposure. *Antimicrob Agents Chemother*, 51(4):1179-1184.

Pitout, JD.; Thomson, KS.; Hanson, ND.; Ehrhardt, AF.; Moland, ES.; Sanders, CC. (1998). beta-Lactamases responsible for resistance to expanded-spectrum cephalosporins in Klebsiella pneumoniae, Escherichia coli, and Proteus mirabilis isolates recovered in South Africa. *Antimicrob Agents Chemother*, 42(6):1350-1354.

Roest, HI.; Liebana, E.; Wannet, W.; van Duynhoven, Y.; Veldman, KT.; Mevius, DJ. (2007). [Antibiotic resistance in Escherichia coli O157 isolated between 1998 and 2003 in The Netherlands]. *Tijdschr Diergeneeskd*, 132(24):954-958.

Singer, RS.; Patterson, SK.; Meier, AE.; Gibson, JK.; Lee, HL.; Maddox, CW. (2004). Relationship between phenotypic and genotypic florfenicol resistance in Escherichia coli. *Antimicrob Agents Chemother*, 48(10):4047-4049.

Schnellmann, C.; Gerber, V.; Rossano, A.; Jaquier, V.; Panchaud, Y.; Doherr, MG.; Thomann, A.; Straub, R.; Perreten, V. (2006). Presence of new mecA and mph(C) variants conferring antibiotic resistance in Staphylococcus spp. isolated from the skin of horses before and after clinic admission. *J Clin Microbiol*, 44(12):4444-4454.

Srinivasan, V.; Gillespie, BE.; Lewis, MJ.; Nguyen, LT.; Headrick, SI.; Schukken, YH.; Oliver, SP. (2007). Phenotypic and genotypic antimicrobial resistance patterns of Escherichia coli isolated from dairy cows with mastitis. *Vet Microbiol*, 124(3-4):319-328.

Tenover, FC. (2006). Mechanisms of antimicrobial resistance in bacteria. *Am J Med*, 119(6 Suppl 1):S3-10; discussion S62-70.

Thomson, K.; Rantala, M.; Hautala, M.; Pyorala, S.; Kaartinen, L. (2008). Cross-sectional prospective survey to study indication-based usage of antimicrobials in animals: results of use in cattle. *BMC Vet Res*, 4:15.

Van, TT.; Moutafis, G.; Tran, LT.; Coloe, PJ. (2007). Antibiotic resistance in food-borne bacterial contaminants in Vietnam. *Appl Environ Microbiol*, 73(24):7906-7911.

Vassort-Bruneau, C.; Lesage-Descauses, MC.; Martel, JL.; Lafont, JP.; Chaslus-Dancla, E. (1996). CAT III chloramphenicol resistance in Pasteurella haemolytica and Pasteurella multocida isolated from calves. *J Antimicrob Chemother*, 38(2):205-213.

Weese, JS.; Rousseau, J.; Willey, BM.; Archambault, M.; McGeer, A.; Low, DE. (2006). Methicillin-resistant Staphylococcus aureus in horses at a veterinary teaching hospital: frequency, characterization, and association with clinical disease. *J Vet Intern Med*, 20(1):182-186.

Zhang, R.; Eggleston, K.; Rotimi, V.; Zeckhauser, RJ. (2006). Antibiotic resistance as a global threat: evidence from China, Kuwait and the United States. *Global Health*, 2:6.

6

The MarR Family of Transcriptional Regulators – A Structural Perspective

Thirumananseri Kumarevel

Biometal Science Laboratory, RIKEN Spring-8 Center, Harima Institute,
Japan

1. Introduction

All living organisms have molecular systems that enable them to resist a variety of toxic substances and environmental stresses. Proteins belonging to the **M**ultiple **a**ntibiotic resistance **R**egulators (MarR) family reportedly regulate the expression of proteins conferring resistance to multiple antibiotics, organic solvents, household disinfectants, oxidative stress agents and pathogenic factors (Alekshun & Levy, 1999a; Miller & Sulavik, 1996; Aravind et al., 2005). The *marR* gene was initially identified as a component of the negative regulator encoded by the *marRAB* locus in *Escherichia coli* (George & Levy, 1983a, b). Currently, a large number of MarR-like proteins (~12,000) can be found in bacterial and archaeal domains, and the physiological role of around 100 of them have been characterized. Members of the MarR family of transcriptional regulatory proteins form a homodimer to bind to their cognate double-stranded DNA (dsDNA). The protein-DNA interactions is regulated by specific phenolic (lipophilic) compounds, such as salicylate, ethidium, carbonyl cyanide m-chlorophenylhydrazone (CCCP) and benzoate. The MarR homologues contain a winged helix-turn-helix (wHtH) motif at the DNA binding site, and this motif is well known for DNA binding in eukaryotes, prokaryotes, archaea and viruses. In this chapter, we will discuss the identification, three-dimensional structure and interactions with ligand (drug)/DNA of MarR family proteins.

2. Identification and characterization of MarR family proteins

The MarR family of transcriptional regulators was first identified in multidrug resistant strains of *E. coli* K-12 (George & Levy, 1983a, b). This MarR protein plays a key role in regulating the multiple antibiotic resistance (*marRAB*) regulon, which is responsible for the mar phenotype manifesting as resistance to a variety of structurally and medicinally important antibiotics, including sodium salicylate, tetracycline, chloramphenicol, penicillins, β-lactams, puromycin, fluoroquinolones and organic solvents (Cohen et al., 1993a). The *marA* gene encodes a transcriptional regulatory protein MarA, which is a member of the AraC protein family. As an activator of the *marRAB* operon, MarA induces the expression of over 60 genes responsible for the mar phenotype, including the AcrAB-TolC multidrug efflux system (Alekshun & Levy, 1997; Okusu et al, 1996). The *in vivo* upregulation of *marRAB* expression and the mar phenotype have been experimentally shown to be activated by a wide range of antibiotics and phenolic compounds, such as 2,4-dinitrophenol, menadione, plumbagin and salicylate (Cohen etal., 1993b; Seoane & Levy, 1995).

Similar to MarR, MexR negatively regulates an operon in *Pseudomonas aeruginosa* that, when expressed, encodes a tri-partite multidrug efflux system that results in increased resistance to multiple antibiotics, including tetracycline, β-lactams, chloramphenicol, novobiocin, sulfonamides and fluoroquinolones (Li & Poole, 1999; Srikumar et al., 2000). Analysis of the open reading frame of *mepA* reveals that the gene is part of the *mepRAB* three gene cluster, which encodes MepR, a MarR family member. MepR binds to compounds like ethidium, DAPI and rhodamine 6G. Some members of the MarR family of DNA-binding proteins, such as hypothetical uricase regulator (HucR) and organic hydroperoxide resistance regulator (OhrR), mediate a cellular response to reactive oxidative stress (ROS) (Wilkinson & Grove, 2004; 2005). The *Deinococcus radiodurans* HucR was shown to repress its own expression as well as that of a uricase. This repression is alleviated both *in vivo* and *in vitro* upon binding uric acid, the substrate for uricase. As uric acid is a potent scavenger of reactive oxygen species, and *D. radiodurans* is known for its remarkable resistance to DNA-damaging agents, these observations indicate a novel oxidative stress response mechanism (Hooper et al., 1998; Kean et al., 2000; Ames et al., 1981). Similar to HucR, the OhrR protein of *Bacillus subtilis* also mediates a response to oxidative stress; however, for OhrR, it is oxidation of a lone cysteine residue by organic hydroperoxides that abrogates DNA binding (Fuangthong et al., 2001; Fuangthong & Helmann, 2002).

2.1 Crystal structure of MarR homologues

Recently, much structural information have become available for MarR homologues. The MarR proteins exist as homodimers in solution, and as mentioned above each monomer consists of a wHtH DNA binding motif. We have recently solved one of the MarR regulators, ST1710 in the absence (apo)/presence (complex) of salicylate and in the presence of the putative DNA promoter. The overall structure of ST1710 indicates that it belongs to the α/β family of proteins and resembles those of the MarR family of proteins. It consists of six α-helices and two β-strands, arranged in the order of α1-α2-α3-α4-β1-β2-α5-α6 in the primary structure. The asymmetric subunit contains one molecule of ST1710. Two monomers of ST1710 are related by a crystallographic 2-fold symmetry to form the dimer, and this is consistent with our gel-filtration analysis (Kumarevel et al., 2008) as well as with other MarR family proteins (Alekshun et al., 2001; Lim et al., 2002; Liu et al., 2001; Wu et al., 2003; Hong et al., 2005) (Fig. 1). The N- and C-terminal residues located at the helices of each monomer are closely intertwined and form a dimerization domain, which is stabilized by hydrophobic and hydrogen bonding interactions between the residues located within these regions. Apart from the dimerization domain, as observed in many DNA binding transcriptional regulators, the residues located within the α2-α3-α4-β1-β2 structure form the wHtH DNA binding motif (Alekshun et al., 2001; Hong et al., 2005; Bordelon et al., 2006; Newberry et al., 2007; Saridakis, et al., 2008). The residues involved in dimerization play a key role in maintaining the distance between the DNA recognition helices in the wHtH loops, which can ultimately affect the fidelity and strength of the protein-DNA interactions. Mutagenesis of the residues involved in the dimeric interface has been shown to cause low DNA binding affinity (Andresen et al., 2010). Furthermore, C-terminal deletion in MarR homologs decreases the ability to form dimers, which correlates with the attenuated DNA binding affinity and increased phenotypic resistance in *E. coli* (Linde et al., 2000).

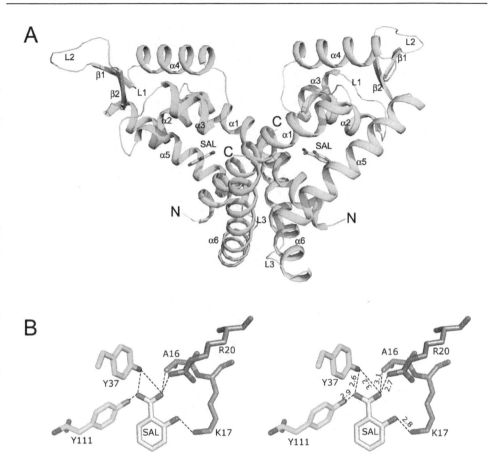

Fig. 1. Crystal structure of ST1710, a member of MarR family proteins. (A) A ribbon diagram of ST1710-salicylate complex dimer is shown. The secondary structure assignments and the N- /C-termini are labeled on the structure. (B) Close-up stereo view of salicylate binding site interactions with protein residues is shown. The hydrogen bonds are indicated by broken lines.

2.2 Structural comparison of MarR homologues

In a search for proteins with structural similarity to ST1710 protein within the known structures available in the Protein Data Bank (www.pdb.org) using the Dali program (Holm and Sander, 1996), we have identified many other protein structures within the MarR superfamily with good Z-scores. The highest ranked among those proteins is a Syla-like protein from *Enterococcus faecalis* (pdb id, 1lj9, Z-score=17.7, sequence identity=22%), which has been shown to up-regulate the expression of molecular chaperones, acid-resistance proteins and cytolysin, as well as to down-regulate several biosynthetic enzymes (Wu et al., 2003). The second highest ranked protein is a hypothetical regulator from *P. aeruginosa* (pdb ids, 2fbh, 2nnn, 2fbi), and the third one is OhrR from *B. subtilis*, an organic hydroperoxide-resistance regulator that controls the expression of the organic hydroperoxide resistance (*ohr*) gene by binding to *ohrA* promoter elements (Hong et al., 2005). Many proteins (1jgs, 1s3j, 2a61, 2nyx, 2hr3, 1xma, 3f3x, 2eth, 3nqd, 3nrv, 3bpv, 3bpx, 3s2w, 3deu, 3q5f, 3fm5, 3oop, 3cdh, 3cjn, 3e6m, 3k0l, 3bro, 3eco, 3jw4, 3bj6, 3g3z, 1lnw, 3bja, 3qww, 3kp6, 3bdd, 1z91, 2pex, 2bv6, 3hrm, 1ub9) were identified with Z-scores between 10-16. All of these proteins adopt a similar topology (rmsd between 1 to 4 Å), despite the low (~15-25%) sequence identities between them, and these sequence dissimilarities are reflected throughout the secondary structural elements (Figs. 2, 3). In addition, the high flexibility of the DNA binding domains displayed in the different crystals provides indirect evidence of the ability of this wHtH motif to adapt in order to recognize various DNA targets. In addition, a sequence homology search against ST1710 (Q96ZY1 from *Sulfolobus tokodaii*) in the non-redundant protein database using fasta revealed that many archaeal species have conserved motifs resembling MarR family regulatory sequences, including *Sulfolobus acidocaldarius*, *Sulfolobus solfataricus*,

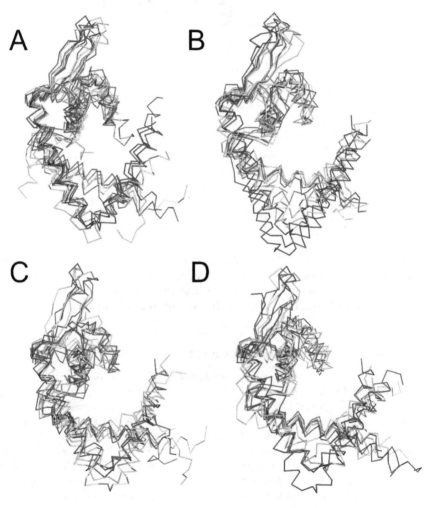

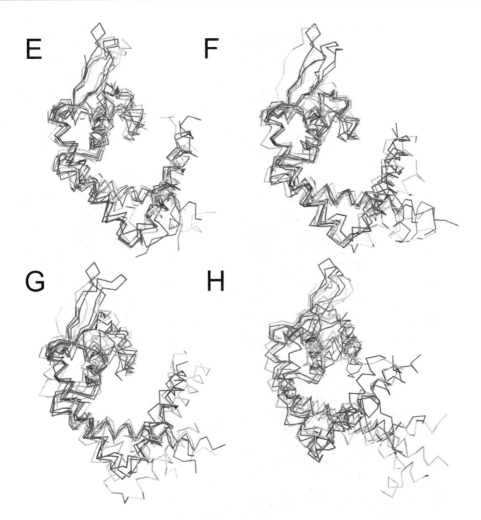

Fig. 2. Three-dimensional structural comparison of ST1710. Superposition of ST1710 with related MarR family proteins. (A) ST1710, 1JGS, 1LJ9, 1LNW, 1S3J, 1UB9 and 1XMA are colored in red, green, blue, yellow, majenta, cyan and orange, respectively. (B) ST1710, 1Z91, 2A61, 2BV6, 2ETH and 2FBH are colored in red, green blue, yellow, majenta and cyan, respectively. (C) ST1710, 2FBI, 2FNP, 2HR3, 2NNN and 2NYX are colored in red, green blue, yellow, majenta and cyan, respectively. (D) ST1710, 2PEX, 2QWW, 3BDD, 3BJ6 and 3BJA are colored in red, green blue, yellow, majenta and cyan, respectively. (E) ST1710, 3BPV, 3BPX, 3BRO, 3CDH and 3CJN are colored in red, green blue, yellow, majenta and cyan, respectively. (F) ST1710, 3DEU, 3E6M, 3ECO, 3F3X and 3FM5 are colored in red, green blue, yellow, majenta and cyan, respectively. (G) ST1710, 3G3Z, 3HRM, 3JW4, 3KOL and 3KP6 are colored in red, green blue, yellow, majenta and cyan, respectively. (H) ST1710, 3NQO, 3NRV, 3OOP, 3Q5F and 3S2W are colored in red, green blue, yellow, majenta and cyan, respectively.

A

```
             1        10        20        30        40        50        60        70        80        90       100
             |----+----+----+----+----+----+----+----+----+----+----+----+----+----+----+----+----+----+----+----|
3GF2                        MLESNENRIQIMSTIAKIYRAMSRELNRRLGEL-NLSYLDFLVLRATS---DGPKTHAYLANRYFVTQSAITASVDKLEEMGLVV
3F3X                        MQKIDEKLQLHNTIAKIYRGSIKEFNNRLGKLHNLSYLDFSILKATS---EEPRSHVYLANRYFVTQSAITAAVDKLEAKGLVR
2ETH                        HGSDKIHHHHHHHDALEIFKTLFSLVHRFSSYLPSNEEISDHKTTELYAFLYVAL--FGPKKHKEIAEFLSTTKSNVTVVDSLEKRGLVV
3NQO                        GHDYSNELKELFLMNQTYATLFILTNKIQIEGDKYFG--ILTSRQYMTILSILHLPEEETTLNNIARKHGTSKQNINRLVANLEKNGYYD
3NRV                        SNAMQKINIDRHATAQINHLANKLMLKSSTAYTGQKFGIGNTEWRIISVLS-SASDCSVQKISDILGLDKQAVSRTVKKLEEKKYIE
1LJ9                        TDILREIGHIARALDSISNIEFKELSLTRGQYLYLVRV-C-ENPGIIQEKIAELIKVDRITAARAIKRLEEQGFIY
3BPV                        IPLKGLLSIILRSHRVFIGRELGHLNLTDAQVACLLRI-H-REPGIKQDELATFFHVDKGTIARTLRRLEESGFIE
3BPX          GSHHHDR----DIPLKGLLSIILRSHRVFIGRELGHLNLTDAQVACLLRI-H-REPGIKQDELATFFHVDKGTIARTLRRLEESGFIE
3S2W   SNAHNTTEFDGISHREGLCD---KEFIGKRISYLYRYGQIYIGKKIEPYGISGQFPFLMRL-Y-REDGINQESLSDYLKIDKGTIARRIQKLVDEGYVF
2FBH          GHHAQTD--KHYFGTLLAQTSRAWRAELDRRLSHLGLSQARHLVLLHLAR-HRDSPTQRELAQSVGVEGPTLARLLDGLESQGLVR
3DEU   HGHHHHHHHHHHSSGHIEGRHHLESPLGSDLARLVRIHRALIDHRLKPLELTQTHAVTLHNIHQ-LPPDQSQIQLAKAIGIEQPSLVRTLDQLEDKGLIS
305F          SNAHESPLGSDLARLVRIHRALIDHRLKPLELTQTHAVTLHNIHQ-LPPDQSQIQLAKAIGIEQPSLVRTLDQLEDKGLIS
3FH5          GHHAESQALSDDIGFLLSRVGGHVLGAVNKALVPTGLRVRSYSYSVLVLACE-QAEGVNQRGVAATHGLDPSQIVGLVDELEERGLVV
300P          SNAHRGYYDEISFDVNTTAKKHHLFLHRSIRSYDVTPEQHSVLEGI-E-ANEPISQKEIALHTKKDTPTVNRIVDVLLRKELIV
3CDH          SNAHNDTPDDTFVSGYLLYLLARSSEERSAQFHDHIRAQGLRVPEHRVLACL-V-DNDAHNITRLAKLSLHEQSRHTRIVDQHDARGLVT
3CJN   SNAHAESTDQTEQLRELAEIG-LEGYAPYLHNRIHGRYNANLRKEHTALGLSTAKHRALAIL-S-AKDGLPIGTLGIFAYVEQSTLSRALDGLQADGLVR
3E6H   SNAHTEARKIPKPSFPYGSPGELNSFLPYLLTRITHIHSSELNQRLASEKLPTPKLRLLSSL-S-AYGELTVGQLATLGVHEQSTTSRTVDQLVDEGLAA
3KOL   SNAHLRSSSVDRKREEEPR---------LSYHIARVDRIISKYLTEHLSALEISLPQFTALSVL-A-AKPNLSNAKLAERSFIKPQSANKILQDLLANGKIE
3BRO          SNAHSRDLGRLLKIASNQHSTRFDIFAKKYDLTGTQHTIIDYLSRNKNKEVLQRDLESEFSIKSSTATVLLQRHEIKKLLY
3ECO          HEFTYSYLFRHISHEHKQKADQKLEQFDITNEQQHTLQYLDQTGQLTQNDIAKALQRTGPTVSNLLRNKEIKKLLY
3J44          SNAHKESNHLHDTPYSYLIRSIGHKLKTSADARLAELGLNSQQGRHIGYIYENQESGIIQKDLAQFFGRRGHSTSHLQGLEKKGYIE
2HR3          HPTHQDLQLAAHLRSQVTTLTRRLRREAQADPVQFSQLVVLGAIDR-LGGDVTPSELAARERHRSSNLAALLRELERGGLIV
3BJ6   SNAHTHETDQLYQRVQATRPLLRNITAAVERGTLREGVTVGQRAILEGLSL-TPGATAP-QLGAALQHKRQYISRILQEVQRAGLIE
2NNN          HSRTTPYRLDDQIGFILR-QANQRYAALFANGIGNGLTPTQHAALVRLGE-T-GPCPQNQLGRLTAHDAHTIKGYVERLQKRGLIQ
363Z          GPHHQLDQLGTRINLICNVFDKHIGQQDLNYHLFAVLYTLAT--EGSRTQKHIGEKHSLPKQTVSGYCKTLAGQGLIE
1LNW          HNYPVNPDLHIPALHAVFQHVRTRIQSELDCQ--RLDLTPPDVHVLKLIDE--QRGLNLQQLGRQHCRDKHLLTRKIRELEGRNLVR
1S3J          HKSADQLHSDIQLSLQALFQKIQPEHLESHEKQ-----GVTPAQLFVLASLKK--HGSLKVSEIAERHEVKPSAVTLHADRLEQKNLIR
2NYX   HHPTEYPATAEESVDVITDALLTASRLLVAISAHSIAQVD-E-----NITIPQFRTLVILSN--HGPINLATLATLLGVQPSATGRHVDRLVGAELID
2A61          GSHKQPFERILREICFHVKVEGRKVLRDF-----GITPAQFDILQKIYF--EGPKRPGELSLLGVAKSTVTGLVKRLEARDGYLT
3BJA          GHNNRELYGNIRDVYHLLQKNLDKAIEQY------DISYVQFGVIQVLAK--SGKVSHSKLIENHGCVPSHHTTHIQRHKRDGYVH
2FBI          GHHSTPRPSLTLTLLQAREHAHSFFRPSLNQH------GLTEQQHVRILRQ--GQGEHESYQLANQACILRPSHTGVLARLERDGLVR
2QWW          GHVGINTDTENISELLKTYHSIQRISAGYADQNARSLGLTIQQLAHINVIYS---TPGISVQDLTKRLIITGSSAAANVDQLISLGLVV
3KP6          HVRRIEDHISFLEKFINDVNTLTAKLLKDLQTEYGISAEQSHVLNHL-S--IEALTVGQITEKQGVNKAAVSRRVKKLLNAELVK
1J6S          LFNEIIPLGRLIHHVNQKKDRLLNEY-----LSPLDITRAQFKYLCSIRC--RACITPVELKKVLSVDLGALTRHLDRLVCKGHVE
3BDD          GHQEHEDLLYRLKVADETISNLF-----EKQLGISLTRYSILQTLLK--DAPLHQLALQERLQIDRHAVTRHLKLLEESGYII
1291          HENKFDHHKLENQLSFLLYASSREHTKQYKP-LLDKLNITYPQYLALLLUE--HETLTVKHGEQLYLDSGTLTRHLRHEQQGLIT
2PEX          HDTTTATTARTDTLLQLDNQLSFALYSANLAHHKLYRG-LLKALDLTYPQYLVHLVLHE--TDERSVSEIGERLYLDSATLTPLLKRLQAAGLVT
2BVG          GSHHHLKQLCFLFYVSSKEIIKKYTN-YLKEYDLTYTGYIVLHAIEN--DEKLNIKKLGERVFLDSGTLTPLLKKLEKKDYVV
3HRH          GSHHYLSKQLCFLFYVSSKEIIKKYTN-YLKEYDLTYTGYIVLHAIEN--DEKLNIKKLGERVFLDSGTLTPLLKKLEKKDYVV
2FNP          HAITKINDCFELLSHVTYADKLKSLIKKEFSISFEEFAVLTYISENKEKEYYFKDIINHLNYKQPQVVKKKILSQEDYFD
1XHA   HGSSHHHHHHSSGLVPRGSQSTSLYKKAGLHVISSDVIRGYVDTIILSLLIEGDSYGYEI---------SKNIRIKTDELYYIKETTLYSAFARLAKSYIN
1UB9          HEELKEIHKSHILGHPVRLGIHIFLLPRRKAPFSQIQKVLDLTPGHLDSHIRVLERNGLVK
Consensus                                                   q...l...........l.............*e..gl..
```

```
             101       110       120       130       140       150       160       170       180
             |----+----+----+----+----+----+----+----+----+----+----+----+----+----+----+----+|
3GF2   RVRD--REDRRKILIEITEKGLETFNKGIEIYKKLANEVTGQLSEDEVILYLDKISKILKRIEEISQ
3F3X   RIRD--SKDRRIVIVEITPKGRQVLLEAHEVLRNLVNEHLSDVENVEELL--EGLNKILSRIGSSKD
2ETH   REHD--PVDRRTYRVVLTEKGKEIFGEILSHFESLLKSVLEKFVSEGFHRHVEALSREGR
3NQO   VIPS--PHDKRAINVKVTDLGKKVHVTCSRTGINFHADVFHEFTKDELETLWSLLKKHYRFNGEEQDGFEEDAN
3NRV   VNGH--SEDKRTYRINLTEHGQELYEVASDFAIEREKQLLEEFEEREKDQLFILLKLRNKVDQH
1LJ9   RQED--ASNKKIKRIYATEKGKNVYPIIVRENQHSNQYALQGLSEVEISQLADYLVRHRKNVSEDHEFVKKG
3BPV   REQD--PEHRRRYILEVTRRGEEIIPLILKVEERHEDLLFRDFTEDIERKLFRKHCRRLAEEAVRHR
3BPX   REQD--PEHRRRYILEVTRRGEEIIPLILKVEERHEDLLFRDFTEDIERKLFRKHCRRLAEEAVRHRGEH
3S2W   REQD--EKDRRSYRVFLTEKGKKLEPDHKKIASEHGEILFSSFDDRQRREITNSLEIHFENGLKIH
2FBH   RLAV--AEDRRAKHIVLTPKADVLIADIEAIAASVRNDVLTGIDESEQALCQQVLLRILANLENR
3DEU   RQTC--ASDRRARKIKLTEKAEPLIAEHEEVIHKTRGEILAGISSEEIELLIKLIAKLEHNIHELHSHD
305F   RQTC--ASDRRARKIKLTEKAEPLIAEHEEVIHKTRGEILAGISSEEIELLIKLIAKLEHNIHELHSHD
3FH5   RTLD--PSDRRNKLIAATEEGRRLRDDAKARVDAAHGRYFEGIPDTVVNQHRDTLQSIAFPTFVEGS
300P   REIS--TEURRISLLSLTDKGRKETTELRDIVERSCEKHFAGVTRTDLEQFTAILKNISNIE
3CDH   RVAD--AKDKRRVRVRLTDDGRALAESLVASARAHETRLLSALADTDAARIKGVLRTLLDVLDRPRESR
3CJN   REVD--SDDQRSSRVYLTPAGRAVYDRLHPHHRASHDRHFQGITPQRQRFLATLNKHLANIRVHEI
3E6H   RSIS--DADQRKRTVYLTRKGKKKLAEISPLINDFHAELVGNVDPDKLQTCIEVLGEILKGKTDY
3KOL   KAPD--PTHGRRILVTVTPSGLDKLNQCNQVVQQLEAQHLQGVEIVHIALFLIRNNLELHVKNLSTFSSLDQSKE
3BRO   RKVS--GKDSRQKCLKLTKKANKLETIILSYHDSDQSQHTSGLNKEEVVFLEKILKRHIESD
3ECO   RYVD--AQDTRRKNIGLTTSGIKLVEAFTSIFDEHEQTLVSQLSEEIKRVQVLEITDYRIQSYTSKL
3J44   RRIP--ENHQRQKNIYVLPKGAALVEEFNNIFLEVEESITKGLTKDEQKQLHSIILKVNRSH
2HR3   RHAD--PQDGRRTRVSLSSEGRRNLYGNRAKREEHLVRAHHACLDESERALLAAAGPLLTRLAQFEEP
3BJ6   RRTN--PEHARSHRYHLTPRGEAIITAIRADEHAKLALFSEGFSSVELTAYHKVQLALTRFFADLAKER
2NNN   RSAD--PDDGRRLLVSLSPAGRAELEAGLAAAREINRQALAPLSLQEQETLRGLLARLI
363Z   HQEG--EQDRRKRLLIETGKAYAAPLTESAQEFSDKVFATFGDKRTTRLFADLDALAEVHEKTISENKK
1LNW   RERN--PSDDRSFQLFLTDEGLAIHQHAEAIHSRVHDELFAPLTPVEQATLVHLLDQCLAAQPLEDI
1S3J   RTHN--TKDRRVIDLSLTDGDIKFEEVLAGRKAIHARYLSFLTEEEHLQAAH--ITAKLAQAAETDEKQNHKRGNG
2NYX   RLPH--PTSRRELLAALTKRGRDVVRQVTEHRRTEIARIVEQHAPAERHGLVRALTAFTEAGGEPDARYEIERSHHHHHH
2A61   RTPD--PADRRAYFLVITRKGEVIEKVIERRENFIEKITSDLGKEKSSKILDYILKELKGVHERNFSKQ
3BJA   TEKN--PNDQRETLVYLTKKGEETKKQVDVQYSDFLKENCGCFTKEEEGILEDLLLKHKKHLN
2FBI   RWKA--PKDQRRVYYNLTEKGQQCFVSHSGDHEKNYQRIQERFGEEKLAQLLELLNELKKIKP
2QWW   KLNKTIPNDSHDLTLKLSKKGED--LSKRSTANAFHYKAHHKVFENLTENEIEELIRL-NKKVETLLKKSK
3KP6   LEKPDSNTDQRLKILSNKGKKYIKERKAIHSHIASDHTSDFDSKIEKVRQVLEIIDYRIQSYTSKL
1J6S   RLPN--PNDKRGVLVKLTTGGAAIC-----EQCHALVGQ--DLHQELTKNLTADEVATLEYLLKKVLP
3BDD   RKRN--PDHQREVLVWPTEQAREALITNPSAHHQAIKT--SHNQILTVEESEQFLATLDKLLIGLQNLPI
1291   RKRS--EEDERSVLILTEDGALLKEKRAVDIPGTILGL--SKQSGEDLKQLNELRQLNGLQPLETLHQKN
2PEX   RTRA--ASDEROVIIALIETGRALRSKAGAVPEQVFCA--SACSLDELRQLKQELEKLRSSLGAG
2BVG   RERS--EVDQREVFIHLTDKSETIRPELSNASDKVASA--SSLSQDEVKELNRLLGLVHAFDE
3HRH   RTRE--EKDERNLQISLTEQGKRAIKSPLAEISVKVFNE--FNISERASDIINNLRNFVSKNF
2FNP   KKRN--EHOERTVLILVNAQQRKKIESLLSRVNKRITEANNEIEL
1XHA   SYYGEETQGKRRTYYRITPEGIKYYKQKCEEHELTKKVINKFVKELESNGDN
1UB9   TYKV--IADRPRTVVEITDFGHEEAKRFLSSLKAVIDGLDL
Consensus   r....d.R....lt..g...................e........l..........
```

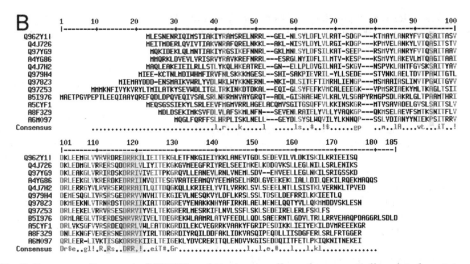

Fig. 3. Sequence alignment of ST1710 and its structurally and sequenctially related proteins from different species. (A) Structurally related proteins to ST1710, based on the Dali Zscore. (B) Sequentially related proteins from the non-redundant sequence database. The highly redundant proteins are removed. The ligand and DNA binding residues are highlighted with yellow and green shades, respectively.

Metallosphaera sedula, Thermoplasma acidophilum, Thermoplasma volcanium, Streptomyces sviceus, Pelotomaculum thermopropionicum, Thermotoga lettingae, Clostridium beijerinckii and others. Among these, the amino acid sequence of ST1710 displays about 50% identity to the *S. acidocaldarius* (Chen et al., 2005) (17) and *S. solfataricus* (She et al., 2001) sequences, 41% identity to the M. sedula sequence (Copeland et al., 2006) and approximately 30-40% identity to others (Fig. 3).

2.1.1 Interactions between MarR homologues and ligands

MarR homologues are known to bind a variety of lipophilic compounds, including salicylate, ethidium and CCCP (Table 1). These bound molecules control interaction between protein-DNA molecules. Sodium salicylate is a well-known example of a compound that can inhibit MarR activity both *in vitro* and *in vivo* at millimolar concentrations (Alekshun and Levy, 1999b). Three different MarR proteins have been solved with the salicylate ligand, including ST1710 from *S. tokodaii*, MarR from *E. coli* and MTH313 from *Methanobacterium thermoautotrophicum*. Among these, ST1710 is the only MarR homologue solved in the apo form, complexed with salicylate ligand and complexed with a putative promoter DNA (Kumarevel et al., 2009). One salicylate ligand is identified and located at the interface between the helical dimerization and wHtH DNA-binding domains in ST1710 (Fig. 1A&B), and the bound salicylate ligand shows many interactions with the surrounding protein residues. In particular, the O2′ of salicylate is bonded to the side chain oxygens of Tyr37 and Tyr111. In addition, the side chain oxygen of Tyr37 is also bonded to the O1′ of the salicylate ligand molecule. The ligand oxygen O1′ is hydrogen bonded to the amino group (NH2) of residue Arg20, while the O2 of the ligand molecule is hydrogen bonded to the side chain nitrogen of

Lys17. The latter two interactions are from the symmetrically related molecule. Notably, all of the ST1710 residues that interact with the ligand are highly conserved among closely related species (>40% identity) (Fig. 3).

In contrast to ST1710, *E. coli* MarR was solved with two salicylate molecules per dimer, and both of them are highly exposed to the solvent. These salicylate binding sites are also not comparable to that of ST1710. The bound salicylate is hydrogen bonded with some of the MarR residues (Ala70, Thr72, Arg77, Arg86); however, the physiological relevance of either salicylate binding site could not be determined (Fig. 4). It seems that salicylate may stabilize the crystal packing, since in its absence, the crystals cannot be used for structure determination in the case of *E. coli* MarR (Alekshun et al., 2001). Analyses of another MarR homolog from *M. thermoautotrophicum* MTH313, which was also solved in the free (apo) form and complexed with salicylate, revealed a large asymmetrical conformational change that is mediated by the binding of sodium salicylate to two distinct locations in the dimer (Saridakis et al., 2008) (Fig. 4). The bound salicylate has two direct and one water mediated interactions with MTH313. Although the ligand binding sites in ST1710 and MTH313 are comparable, we have not found any conformational changes in ST1710 between the apo and ligand bound complexes, as observed in MTH313.

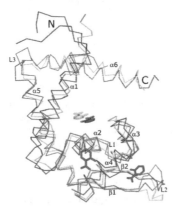

Fig. 4. Salicylate binding analysis in MarR homologues. Superposition of the ST1710-salicylate complex with other known MarR family of protein crystallized in the presence of salicylate. The ST1710, *E. coli* MarR and *M. thermoautotrophicum* MTH313 are shown in green, blue and red, respectively.

Meanwhile, eight salicylate molecules are bound to *Staphylococcus epidermidi*s of TcaR (Chang et al., 2010). Among these eight molecules, two are bound similarly to that with MTH313, while the other two were observed in the more shallow binding pocket in each monomer. The remaining ligands are highly exposed to the solvent. TcaR has also been crystallized with four different antibiotics (ampicillin, kanamycin, methicillin and penicillin), revealing their interactions with the protein (Chang et al., 2010). The available biochemical and biophysical results suggest that the MarR regulators modulate the DNA binding affinity in the presence of ligands or drug molecules. However, more ligand bound complexes are required to generalize the binding pocket properties as well as to understand how these MarR regulators allosterically change their conformation in the presence of vaious drugs/ligands to mediate the protein-DNA interactions.

Protein	Organism	Footprint (DNA)	K_d (nM)	Ligand	K_d	Reference
ST1710	*Sulfolobus tokodaii*	30	200 ~ 1500	Salicylate, Ethidium Bromide, CCCP	~2-25 µM	Kumarevel et al., 2008 & 2009 Yu et al., 2009
MepR	*Staphylococcus aureus*	27,44	6.3	Ethidium, DAPI, Rhodamine 6G	~3-63 µM	Kumaraswami et al., 2009
MarR	*Escherichia coli*	21	1	Salicylate, Plumbagin, 2,4-dinitrophenol, menadione	0.5 – 1 mM	Martin & Rosner 1995; Cohen et al., 1993b; Seoane & levy, 1995; Alekshun & Levy 1999b; Alekshun et al, 2001
EmrR	*Escherichia coli*	42	-	Salicylate, Caronyl cyanide m-chlorophenylhydrozone, 2,4,-dinitrophenol, ethidium bromide	1.3 -11.1 µM	Xiong et al. 2000; Brooun et al., 1999
MexR	*Pseudomonos aeruginosa*	28	-	β-lactamin		Evans et al., 2001.
CbaR	*Comamonas testosteroni*	22	-	3-chlorobenzoate, protocatechuate		Providenti & Wyndham, 2001
CinR	*Butyrivibro fibrisolvens*	-	-	Cinnamic acid sugar esters		Dalrymple & Swadling, 1997
HpaR	*Escherichia coli*	27	-	4-hydroxyphenyl-acetic acid, 3-hydroxyphenyl acetic acid, 3,4-hydroxyphenyl acetic acid		Galan et al., 2003
ExpG	*Sinorhizobium meliloti*	21	0.58-1.3			Bartels et al, 2003; Baumgarth et al., 2005
PecS	*Erwinia chrysanthemi*	45	4-200			Reverchon et al., 2002; Rouanet et al., 2004
SlyA	*Salmonella typhimurium*	25	-			Stapleton et al., 2002
OhrR	*Xanthomonas campestris*	44	-	Tert-butyl hydroperoxide, cumene hydroperoxide		Mongkolsuk et al., 2002
OhrR	*Bacillus subtilis*	42	5	Tert-butyl hydroperoxide, cumene hydroperoxide		Fuangthong et al., 2001; Fuangthong & Helmann, 2002; Panamanee et al., 2002
HucR	*Deinococcus radiodurans*	21	0.29	Uric acid, Salicylate	11.6 µM	Wilkinson & Grove, 2004; 2005

Table 1. DNA and ligand binding data for MarR homologues.

2.1.1 Interactions between MarR proteins and DNA

It is well-known that members of the MarR family of regulatory proteins bind to their cognate double-stranded DNA by their winged HtH motif (Alekshun et al., 2001; Hong et al., 2005; Kumarevel et al., 2009). Footprinting analyses suggested that different MarR regulators recognize promoters of different lengths with different affinities (Table 1). In an earlier study, we have used the *OhrR* promoter sequence as a search model to identify the putative promoter DNA sequence for ST1710 from the *S. tokodaii* genomic sequence (Kumarevel et al., 1998). We have also shown the binding constant for DNA to be around 15 µM using gel mobility shift assays. Yu et al. (2009) subsequently showed by fluorescence spectroscopy that the affinity of the same DNA promoter we identified is increased significantly with increasing temperature. The affinity was shown to be approximately double from 10°C (K_d = 618 ± 34 nM) to 30°C (K_d = 334 ± 15 nM) and from 30°C to 50°C (K_d = 189 ± 9 nM). We later crystallized ST1710 along with two different DNA promoters (30-mer and 26-mer) and revealed the protein-DNA interactions and mode of binding as summarized below (Kumarevel et al., 2009).

The overall structure of the ST1710-DNA complex is shown in Fig. 5A & B. The bound DNA adopts a B-form right-handed structure, passing over the protein molecule by only contacting at the winged HtH loop regions. The wHtH domains recognize the promoter DNA (TAACAAT) (15-21) region, consistent with the -10 region of the OhrR-*ohrA* operator complex. The 4 and 3 bases at the 5' and 3'-ends are highly disordered and hence not modeled. Of the bound 46 nucleotides, only 22 nucleotides were found to be involved in 36 contacts with six protein molecules. The critical protein-DNA contacts observed in this complex are as follows: Ser65 - Thy5'; Arg84 - G13' and Ade17; Arg89 - Thy14'; Arg90 - Cyt18; Asp88 – Cyt18 (two salt bridge contacts); Lys91 - Ade19; Ile91 - Ade20. The observed salt bridge may be important in fixing the conformation of residue Arg90 in order to make contact with the nucleic acid base, Cyt18. Thus, the following residues Ser65, Arg84, Asp88, Arg89, Arg90, Lys91 and Ile92 interact with the bound promoter DNA. As further clarification of these protein-DNA interactions, our analysis of three mutant proteins (Arg89Ala, Arg90Ala, Lys91Ala) at the DNA binding loop region in gel mobility shift assays clearly support that these positively charged residues are important for DNA binding (Kumarevel et al., 2009). The DNA-binding residues in ST1710 are highly conserved among the closely related proteins Fig. (3). The winged loop region connecting the strands β1 and β2 apparently plays a major role in modulating their conformation for binding to the DNA molecule, and this mode of recognition is anticipated for the proteins closely related to ST1710 as well as those in the family of MarR regulators.

In our earlier report, we noticed only a small difference at the loop region connecting strands β1 and β2 in the protein conformers crystallized in two different space groups, but the overall structures are otherwise identical (Kumarevel et al., 2008). Similarly, we have not observe any conformational changes in comparisons of the ST1710-salicylate complex and native structure crystallized under the same conditions, and the subunits in the dimer are identical. In contrast to these observations, a significant conformational change has been observed between subunits (A, B chains) in the ST1710-DNA complex, although the overall structural topology remains identical. Specifically, the C-terminal helix and the winged HtH motif region show displacement relative to the other. The DNA binding motif is elevated

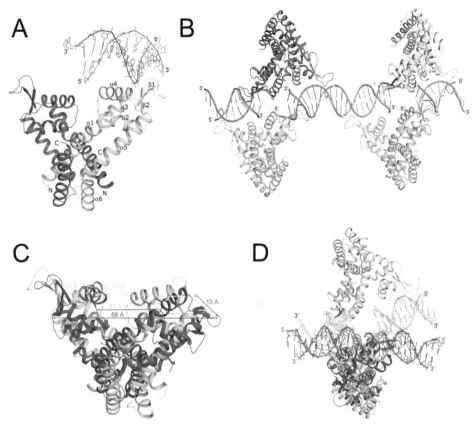

Fig. 5. Structure of ST1710-DNA complex and it's structural comparison with OhrR-*OhrA* complex. (A) ST1710-DNA complex observed in the aymmetric unit. The secondary structural assignments, N-/C- termini ends are labeled in one of the dimeric monomers. The complexed nucleic acids are shown as stick representations. (B) Part of the packing diagram. The 5'- and 3'- ends of each nucleotide chain is labeled. (C, D) Superposition of the OhrR-*OhrA* complex on the ST1710-DNA complex is shown without (A) and with nucleic acids (B). The protein and nucleic acids are shown in St1710-DNA complex are in cyan and green; while those in OhrR-*OhrA* complex are shown in blue and red, respectively.

compared to the other chain, while the C-terminal helix α6 is lower down. It is noteworthy to mention that the distances between the wHtH domains in the dimer are reduced by ~10 Å for the ST1710-DNA complex, compared to the native and salicylate complexes. These observed conformational changes are required in order to facilitate the DNA-binding and thus would explain the conformational flexibility of MarR homologues.

Another member of the MarR family of regulators that has been solved in complex with a promoter sequence is the *B. subtilis* OhrR. The OhrR was crystallized in the presence of a 29-mer duplex containing the -10 region of the cognate DNA. In the OhrR-*OhrA* complex, the wHtH motif contacts the DNA promoter sequence with substantial widening and deepening of the major groove that results from insertion of the recognition helix (α4) of the wHtH motif. The wHtH and recognition helices make many contacts with the DNA directly or mediated through water. The wHtH domain is important for the DNA interaction as evidenced by several mutagenic analyses, which show that the positively charged residues (Arg94) located at the terminals are important for the DNA contacts in *E. coli* MarR. In the OhrR-*ohrA* complex, the distance between wHtH loops is around 67 Å, and the distance between the recognition helices (α4) is about 20 Å, although the wings of the subunits are translocated about 16 Å compared to the structure of reduced OhrR (Hong et al., 2005) (Fig. 5C). In an attempt to clarify the binding mechanism of MarR regulators, a comparative analysis of our ST1710-DNA complex with the OhrR-*ohrA* complex (Fig. 5C & D) was performed, which revealed large conformational changes between these two complexes. Interestingly, we also observed unique conformational changes in the mode of DNA recognition. In contrast to the OhrR-*OhrA* complex, the bound promoter DNA passed over the wHTH motif without deepening the structure through the 2-fold axis in the ST1710-DNA complex. Despite their differences, it is interesting to note that the protein contacting residues are highly conserved between these two proteins and among the MarR family of regulators. This unexpected mode of DNA-binding in ST1710 is caused by one of the subunits translocated around 13 Å towards the 2-fold axis, reducing the distance between the recognition helix of the subunits to 13 Å. Thus, the mode of DNA binding observed in the OhrR-*ohrA* operator complex would be impossible for that of ST1710. Such unique conformational changes observed in these complexes explain how the MarR homolog regulators can modulate the DNA-binding affinity based on the cognate promoter or ligand molecules.

3. Conclusion

The MarR family of regulatory proteins in bacteria and archaea regulate a variety of biological functions, including those associated with the development of antibiotic resistance, a growing global health problem. Based on the existing crystal structures, it seems that members of the MarR family of proteins adopt similar topology, despite variations in sequence similarities among them. We have solved the crystal structure of ST1710 in three different forms (apo-form, ST1710-salicylate and ST1710-DNA complex) and demonstrated the functional importance of the ligand binding and DNA binding residues. The ligand or drug binding to the MarR regulators may regulate their promoter binding abilities as evidenced with MarR, ST1710 and MTH313. Furthermore, the promoter DNA is also recognized by the protein in a unique fashion as observed in OhrR-*OhrA* and ST1710-DNA complexes. Taken altogether, the current evidence describe the MarR regulators containing wHTH motifs as being prone to binding DNA through their positively charged residues located in their loops, and the mode of DNA binding depends on the subunit organization as observed in the MarR family of proteins (ST1710, OhrR). Through further structural and functional studies on MarR-DNA binding, we will be better poised to develop new drugs to specifically target those interactions that confer drug resistance to pathogenic organisms.

4. Acknowledgment

The author would like to thank Dr. T. Ishikawa for his moral support and encouragement.

5. References

Alekshun, M.M. & Levy, S.B. (1999a). Regulation of chromosomally mediated multiple antibiotic resistance: the mar regulon. *Antimicrob. Agents Chemother.* 41, 2067-2075.

Alekshun, M.N. & Levy, S.B. (1999b). Alteration of the repressor activity of MarR, the negative regulator of the *Escherichia coli marRAB* locus, by multiple chemicals *in vitro. J. Bacteriol.* 181, 4669-4672.

Alekshun, M.N.; Levy, S.B.; Mealy, T.R.; Seaton, B.A. & Head, J.F. (2001). The crystal structureof MarR, a regulator of multiple antibiotic resistance, at 2.3 Å resolution. *Natue Struct. Biol.* 8, 710-714.

Ames, B.N.; Cathcart, R.; Schwiers, E. & Hochstein, P. (1981). Uric acid provides an antioxidant defense in humans against oxidant- and radical-caused aging and cancer: a hypothesis. *Proc. Natl. Acad. Sci. USA* 78, 6858–6862.

Alekshun, M.N. & Levy, S.B. (1997). Regulation of chromosomally mediated multiple antibiotic resistance:the *mar* operons. *Antimicob Agents Chemother.* 41, 2067-2075.

Andresen, C.; Jalal, S.; Aili, D.; Wang, Y.; Islam, S.; Jarl, A.; Liedberg, B.; Wretlind, B.; Martensson, L.G. & Sunnerhagen, M. (2010). Critical biophyscial properties in the *Pseudomonas aeruginosa* efflux gene regulator MexR are targeted by mutations conferring multidrug resistance. *Protein Sci.* 19, 680-692.

Aravind, L.; Anantharaman, V.; Balaji, S.; Mohan Babu, M. & Iyer, L.M. (2005). The many faces of the helix-turn-helix domain: transcription regulation and beyond. *FEMS Microbiol. Rev.* 29, 231-262.

Bartels, F.W.; Baumgarth, B.; Anselmetti, D.; Ros, R. & Becker, A. (2003). Specific binding of the regulatory protein ExpG to promoter regions of the galactoglucan biosynthesis gene cluster of *Sinorhizobium meliloti* –a combined molecular biology and force spectroscopy investigation. *J. Struct. Biol.* 143, 145-152.

Baumgarth, B.; Bartels, F.W.; Anselmetti, D.; Becker, A. & Ros, R. (2005). Detailed studies of the binding mechanism of the *Sinorhizobium meliloti* transcriptional activator ExpG to DNA. *Microbiology* 151, 259-268.

Bordelon, T.; Wilkinson, S.P.; Grove, A. & Newcomer, M.E. (2006). The crystal structure of the transcriptional regulator HucR from *Deinococcus radiodurans* reveals a repressor preconfigured for DNA binding. *J. Mol. Biol.* 360, 168-177.

Brooun, A.; Tomashek, J.J. & Lewis, K. (1999). Purification and ligand binding of EmrR, a regulator of a multidrug transporter. *J. Bacteriol.* 181, 5131-5133.

Chang, Y.M.; Jeng, W.Y.; Ko, T.P.; Yeh, Y.J.; Chen, C.K. & Wang, A.H. (2010). Strutural study of TcaR and ist complexes with multiple antibiotics from *Staphylococcus epidermidis. Proc. Natl. Acad. Sci. USA.* 107, 8617-8622.

Chen, L.; Bruegger K.; Skovgaard, M.; Redder P.; She, Q.; Torarinsson, E.; Greve, B.; Awayez, M.; Zibat, A.; Klenk, H.P. & Garrett, R.A. (2005). The genome of *Sulfolobus acidocaldarius*, a model organism of the *Crenarchaeota. J. Bacteriol.* 187, 4992-4999.

Cohen, S.P.; Hachler, H. & Levy, S.B. (1993a). Genetic and functional analysis of the multiple antibiotic resistance (mar) locus in *Escherichia coli. J. Bacteriol.* 175, 1484-1492.

Cohen , S.P.; Levy, S.B.; Foulds, J. & Rosner, J.L. (1993b). Salicylate induction of antibiotic resistance in *Escherichia coli*: activation of the *mar* operon and a *mar* independent pathway. *J. Bacteriol.* 175, 7856-7862.

Copeland, A.; Lucas, S.; Lapidus, A.; Barry, K.; Glavina, del Rio, T.; Dalin, E.; Tice, H.; Bruce, D.; Pitluck, S. & Richardson, P. (2006). Sequencing of the draft genome and assembly of *Metallosphaera sedula* DSM 5348. Submitted (NOV-2006) to the EMBL/GenBank/DDBJ databases.

Dalrymple, B.P. & Swadling, Y. (1997). Expression of a *Butyrivibrio fibrisolvens* E14 gene (*cin*B) encoding an enzye with cinnamoyl ester hydrolase activity is negatively regulated by the product of an adjacent gene (*cin*R). *Microbiology* 143, 103-1210.

Evans, K.; Adewoye, L. & Poole, K. (2001). MexR repressor of the *mexAB-oprM* multidrug efflux operon of *Pseudomonas aeruginosa*: identification of MexR binding sites in the *mexA-mexR* intergenic region. *J. Bateriol.* 183, 807-812.

Fuangthong, M.; Atichartpongkul, S.; Mongkolsuk, S. & Helmann, J. D. (2001). OhrR is a repressor of *ohrA*, a key organic hydroperoxide resistance determinant in *Bacillus subtilis*. *J. Bacteriol.* 183, 4134-4141.

Fuangthong, M. & Helmann, J. D. (2002). The OhrR repressor senses organic hydroperoxide resistances by reversibile formation of a cyteine-sulfenic acid derivative. *Proc. Natl. Acad. Sci. USA* 99, 6690-6695.

Galan, B.; Kolb, A.; Sanz, J.M.; Garcia, J.L. & Prieto, M.A. (2003). Molecular determinants of the *hpa* regulatory system of *Escherichia coli*: the Hpa repressor. *Nucleic Acids Res.* 31, 6598-6609.

George, A.M. & Levy, S.B. (1983a). Amplifiable resistance to the tetracycline, chloramphenicol, and other antibiotics in *Escherichia coli*: Involvement of a nonplasmid –determined efflux of tetracycline. *J. Bacteriol.* 155, 531-540.

George, A.M. & Levy, S.B. (1983b). Gene in the major cotransduction gap of the *Escherichia coli* K-12 linkage map required for the expression of chromosomal resistance to tetracycline and other antibiotics. *J. Bacteriol.* 155, 541-548.

Holm, L. & Sander, C. (1996). A review of the use of protein structure comparison in protein classification and function identification. *Science* 273, 595-602.

Hong, M.; Fuangthong, M.; Helmann, J. D. & Brennan, R. G. (2005). Structure of an OhrR-ohrR operator complex reveals the DNA binding mechanism oft he MarR family. *Mol. Cell.* 20, 131-141.

Hooper, D.C.; Spitsin, S.; Kean, R.B.; Champion, J.M.; Dickson, G.M.; Chaudhry, I. & Koprowski, H. (1998). Uric acid, a natural scavenger of peroxynitrite, in experimental allergic encephalomyelitis and multiple sclerosis. *Proc. Natl Acad. Sci. USA* 95, 675–680.

Kean, R.B.; Spitsin, S.V.; Mikheeva, T.; Scott, G.S. & Hooper, D.C. (2000). The peroxynitrite scavenger uric acid prevents inflammatory cell invasion into the central nervous system in experimental allergic encephalomyelitis through maintenance of blood-central nervous system barrier integrity. *J. Immunol.* 165, 6511–6518.

Kumaraswami, M.; Schuman, J.T.; Seo, S. M.; Kaatz, G.W. & Brennan, R.G. (2009). Structural and biochemical characterization of MepR, a multidrug binding transcription regulator oft he *Staphylococcus aureus* multidrug efflux pump MepA. *Nucleic Acids Res.* 37, 1211-1224.

Kumarevel, T.S.; Tanaka, T.; Nishio, M.; Gopinath, S.C.B.; Takio, K.; Shinkai, A.; Kumar, P.K.R. & Yokoyama, S. (2008). Crystal structure oft he MarR family regulatory protein, ST1710, from *Sulfolobus tokodaii* strain 7. *J. Struct. Biol.* 16, 9-17.

Kumarevel, T.S.; Tanaka, T.; Umehara, T. & Yokoyama, S. (2009). ST1710-DNA complex crystal structure reveals the DNA binding mechanism oft he MarR family of regulators. Nucleic Acids Res. 37, 4723-47-35.

Li, X.Z. & Poole, K. (1999). Organic solvent tolerant mutants of *Pseudomonas aeruginosa* display multiple antibiotic resistance. *Can. J. Microbiol.* 45, 18-22.

Linde, H.J.; Notka, F.; Metz, F.; Kochanowski, B.; Heisig, P. & Lehn, N. (2000). In vivo increase in resistance to ciprofloxacin in *Escherichia coli* associated with deletion oft he C-terminal part of MarR. *Antimicrob.Agents Chemother.* 44, 1865-1868.

Yu, L.; Fang, J. & Wie, Y. (2009). Characterization oft he ligand and DNA binding properties of a putative archaeal regulators, ST1710. *Biochemistry* 48, 2099-2108.

Martin, R.G. & Rosner, J.L. (1995). Binding of purified multiple antibiotic-resistance repressor protein (MarR) to *mar* operator sequences. *Proc. Natl. Acad. Sci. USA.* 92, 5456-5460.

Miller, P.F. & Sulavik, M.C. (1996). Overlaps and parallels in the regulation of intrinsic multiple-antibiotic resistance in *Escherichia coli*. *Mol. Microbiol.* 21, 441-448.

Mongkolsuk, S.; Panmanee, W.; Atichartpongkul, S.; Vattanaviboon, P.; Whangsuk, W.; Fuangthong, M.; Eiamphungporn, W.; Sukchawalit, R. & Utamapongchai, S. (2002). The repressor for an organic peroxide-inducible operon is unlikely regulated at multiple levels. *Mol. Microbiol.* 44, 793-802.

Newberry, K.J.; Fuangthong, M.; Panmanee, W.; Mongkolsuk, S. & Brennan, R.G. (2007). Structural mechanism of organic hydroperoxide induction oft he transcription regulator OhrR. *Mol. Cell* 28, 652-664.

Okusu, H.; Ma, D. & Nikaido, H. (1996). AcrAB efflux pump plays a major role in the anibiotic resistance phenotype of *Escherichia coli* multiple antibiotic resistance(mar) mutants. *J. Bacterial.* 178, 306-308.

Panmanee, W.; Vattanaviboon, P.; Eiamphungporn, W.; Whangsuk, W.; Sallabhan, R. & Mongkolsuk, S. (2002). OhrR, a trancription repressor that senses and responds to changes in organic peroxide levels in *Xanthomonas campestris* pv. Phaseoli. *Mol. microbiol.* 45, 1647-1654.

Providenti, M.A. & Wyndham, R.C. (2001). Identification and functional chracterization of cbaR, a MarR-like modulator oft he *cbaABC*-encoded chlorobenzoate catabolism pathway. *Appl. Environ. Microbiol.* 67, 3530-3541.

Reverchon, S.; Rouanet, C.; Expert, D. & Nasser, W. (2002). Characterization of indigoidine biosynthetic genes in *Erwinia chrysanthemi* and role of this blue pigment in pathogenicity. *J. Bacteriol.* 184, 654-665.

Rouanet, C.; Reverchon, S.; Rodionov, D.A. & Nasser, W. (2004). Definition of a consensus DNA-binding site for PecS, a global regulator of virulence gene expression in *Erwinia chrysanthemi* and identification of new members oft he PecS regulon. *J. Biol. Chem.* 279, 30158-30167.

Saridakis, V.; Shahinas, D.; Xu, X. & Christendat, D. (2008). Structural insight on the mechanism of regulation oft he MarR family of proteins: high-resolution crystal structure of a transcriptional repressor from *Methanobacterium thermoautotrophicum*. *J. Mol. Biol.* 377, 655-667.

Seoane, A.S. & Levy, S.B. (1995). Characterization of MarR, the repressor oft he multiple antibiotic resistance (mar) operon in *Escherichia coli*. *J. Bacteriol.* 177, 3414-3419.

She, Q.; Singh, R.K.; Confalonieri, F.; Zivanovic, Y.; Allard, G.; Awayez, M.J.; Chan-Weiher, C. C. Y.; Clausen, I.G.; Curtis, B.A.; et al. (2001). The complete genome oft he crenarchaeon *Sulfolobus solfataricus* P2. *Proc. Natl. Acad. Sci. U.S.A.* 98, 7835-7840.

Srikumar, R.; Pau, C.J. & Poole, K. (2000). Influence of mutants in the mexR repressor gene on expression oft he MexA-MexB-oprM multidrug efflux system in *Pseudomonas aeruginosa*. *J. Bacteriol*. 182, 1410-1414.

Stapleton, M.R.; Norte, V.A.; Read, R.C. & Green, J. (2002). Interaction of the *Salmonella typhimurium* transcription and virulrnce factor SlyA with target DNA and identification of members of the SlyA regulon. *J. Biol. Chem*. 277, 17630-17637.

Wilkinson, S.P. & Grove, A. (2004). HucR, a novel uric acid responsive member of the MarR family of transcriptional regulators from *Deinococcus radiodurans*. *J. Biol. Chem*. 279, 51442-51450.

Wilkinson, S.P. & Grove, A. (2005). Negative cooperativity of uric acid Binding to the transcriptional regulator HucR from *Deinococcus radiodurans*. *J. Mol. Biol*. 350, 617-630.

Wu, R.Y.; Zhang, R.G.; Zagnitko, O.; Dementieva, I.; Maltzev, N.; Watson, J. D.; Laskowski, R.; Gornicki, P. & Joachimiak, A. (2003). Crystal structure of *Enterococcus faecalis* Syla-like transcriptional factor. *J. Bio. Chem*. 278, 20240-20244.

Xiong, A.; Gottman, A.; Park, C.; Baetens, M.; Pandza, S. & Martin, A. (2000). The EMrR protein represses the *Escherichia coli emrRAB* multidrug resistance operon by directly binding to ist promoter region. *Antimicrob. Agents Chemother*, 44, 2905-2907.

7

Clinical Impact of Extended-Spectrum β-Lactamase-Producing Bacteria

Yong Chong

Department of Blood and Marrow Transplantation, Hara-Sanshin Hospital, Fukuoka, Japan

1. Introduction

We have been forced to fight against the newly acquired antibiotic resistance of various bacteria. By the end of the 1970s, most *Escherichia coli* (*E. coli*) and *Klebsiella pneumoniae* (*K. pneumoniae*) strains contained plasmid-mediated, ampicillin-hydrolyzing β-lactamases, such as TEM-1, TEM-2, and SHV-1, and could be eliminated by the use of third-generation cephalosporins. [1] TEM-1 and TEM-2 were detected mainly in *E. coli*, and SHV-1 was mainly detected in *K. pneumoniae*. [2] The emergence of *K. pneumoniae* strains with a gene encoding β-lactamase that hydrolyzes the extended-spectrum cephalosporins was first reported by a study from Germany in 1983. [3] The gene encoding the new β-lactamase harbored a single-nucleotide mutation, as compared to the parental *bla*SHV-1 gene. In 1986, *K. pneumoniae* strains resistant to the third-generation cephalosporins were detected in France. [4] The resistance was attributed to a new β-lactamase gene, which was closely related to TEM-1 and TEM-2. These newly detected β-lactamases capable of hydrolyzing extended-spectrum β-lactam antibiotics were named extended-spectrum β-lactamases (ESBLs). [5] In 1989, the CTX-M type was reported as a new ESBL family member not belonging to either the TEM or SHV types. [6] Notably, the origin of CTX-M ESBLs is totally different from that of TEM or SHV ESBL. [7] Until the end of the 1990s, most of the ESBLs detected were either the TEM or SHV types and were usually associated with nosocomial outbreaks caused by *K. pneumoniae*. [1] In the new millennium, the worldwide spread of CTX-M-producing *E. coli* has been dramatic, and they are now considered to be the primary ESBL producers that are almost always associated with community-acquired infections. [8] ESBL-producing *E.coli* and *Klebsiella* spp. are now listed as one of the six drug-resistant pathogens for which few potentially effective drugs are available. [9] This chapter will outline the genetic aspects of TEM, SHV, and CTX-M ESBLs, including molecular epidemiology and mobile elements. In addition, we will also consider the impact of their genetic evolution on clinical aspects, including mode of infection and antibiotic resistance.

2. ESBL definition/classification

There is no exact definition of ESBLs. ESBLs are generally defined as β-lactamases that confer resistance to bacteria against the penicillins, the first-, second-, and third-generation cephalosporins, and to aztreonam by hydrolyzing these antibiotics, and are inhibited by β-lactamase inhibitors. [1] Most of ESBLs are classified as class A on the basis of the scheme devised by Ambler et al. [10] Class A ESBLs form a heterogeneous molecular group, which comprises β-lactamases sharing various identities, and consists of three major groups: the TEM, SHV, and CTX-M types. [7] TEM and SHV ESBLs genetically evolved from TEM-1, TEM-2, and SHV-1 progenitors (non-ESBLs), and CTX-M ESBLs developed independently from TEM and SHV ESBLs. Additional ESBL types, such as PER, VEB, and BES, are uncommon. [10] More than 130 TEM types and more than 50 SHV types are currently known. [10] The most common group of ESBLs not belonging to the TEM or SHV types is CTX-M, the name derives from the potent hydrolytic activity against cefotaxime. [1] More than 40 CTX-M types are now recognized and can be divided into five subgroups, CTX-M1, 2, 8, 9, and 25, according to their amino acid sequence similarities. [7]

3. Global epidemiology: dissemination of ESBLs

ESBLs were first detected in the first half of the 1980s in Europe, and they later disseminated worldwide. [1] Until the 1990s, the main producer of ESBLs was K. pneumoniae and nosocomial outbreaks caused by the organism were often reported. [1] The number of ESBL-producing E. coli isolates has been dramatically increasing during the 21st century. [11] A recent global surveillance database collected from Europe, North and South America, and Asia, showed that the detection frequencies for ESBL-producing K. pneumoniae and E. coli isolates were 7.5-44% and 2.2-13.5%, respectively. [12] The prevalence of ESBL-producing isolates increased to a greater degree, particularly in Asia than in other regions, and one study conducted in 2007 showed that the frequencies of ESBL-producing K. pneumoniae and E. coli isolates exceeded 30% in both bacterial populations. [13] A recent surveillance using samples collected from nine Asian countries showed ESBL producers accounted for 42.2% of K. pneumoniae isolates detected from patients with hospital-acquired pneumoniae. [14] Our data collected from one institution in Japan showed that the detection rate of the E. coli isolates increased first, followed by increased detection rates of the K. pneumoniae and P. mirabilis isolates. [15] (Figure1) These data suggest that K. pneumoniae, as well as E. coli, has been an important ESBL producer even in the last few years.

In the analysis of ESBL genotypes, TEM and SHV were predominantly observed until the 1990s, and it was most reported that SHV-producing K. pneumoniae strains showed clonal dissemination in hospitals. [1] Recent studies show that TEM and SHV types have been frequently detected up to the present day. Interestingly, in some cases, SHV has been found in isolates expressing other ESBL types, such as TEM and CTX-M. [16] Our study showed that multiple types of ESBLs, including TEM, SHV, and CTX-M, were most frequently detected in K. pneumoniae and E. coli. [15] (Table1) These findings suggest that the genetic mechanism underlying dissemination of ESBL genes has become more divergent and complicated. After the first half of the 2000s, it was often reported that the number of CTX-M ESBLs detected was on the rise, that the main carrier was E. coli, and that most of the CTX-M-producing E. coli strains were acquired in the community, not in hospitals. [11] The detection rate of CTX-M ESBLs has been dramatically rising, especially in the last 5 years. [17] The mechanism behind the spread of blaCTX-M genes differs from that observed in the case of blaTEM and blaSHV genes. blaTEM and blaSHV ESBL genes are associated with the dissemination of particular clones, known as an "epidemic" pattern; however, the mechanism by which blaCTX-M ESBL genes disseminate reflects the simultaneous spread of multiple specific clones, known as an "allodemic" pattern. [18] It has been indicated that various CTX-M-type ESBLs have spread

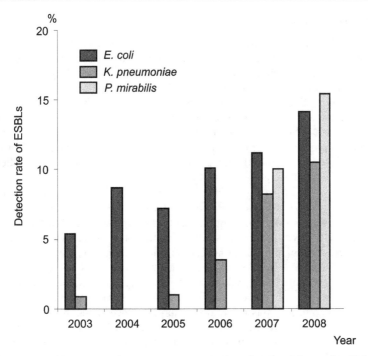

Fig. 1. Frequencies of ESBL-producing organisms at Hara-Sanshin Hospital in Fukuoka (Japan)

worldwide, and that specific CTX-M subgroups have been characterized in different geographic areas. [15,18,19] In contrast, CTX-M-15 ESBLs, which belong to the CTX-M-1 group, have been found worldwide. [18] Unlike in other countries, in the USA, ESBLs were rarely detected, until the first half of the 2000s; however, CTX-M ESBLs, specifically CTX-M-15, have frequently been encountered over the last 5 years. [20,21]

Year	Total no. of isolates	TEM/SHV	CTX-M	TEM/SHV+CTX-M
2003	11	0(0.0)	4 (36.4)	7(63.6)
2004	15	1(6.7)	5 (33.3)	9(60.0)
2005	15	0(0.0)	5(33.3)	10(66.7)
2006	20	0(0.0)	5 (25.0)	15(75.0)
2007	18	2(11.1)	7 (38.9)	9(50.0)
2008	25	5(20.0)	9(36.0)	11(44.0)
Total	104	8(7.7)	35(33.7)	61(58.6)

Table 1. Genotypes of ESBL-producing *Eschrichia coli* isolated from hospitalized patients

4. Genetic characteristics

Genes harboring ESBLs are associated with several specific genetic structures. A variety of mobile genetic elements, such as transposons, insertion sequences, and integrons, play important roles in the dissemination of ESBL genes. *bla*TEM-type ESBL genes are acquired by the mutation of plasmid-mediated, parent *bla*TEM-1 and *bla*TEM-2 genes, and the main producer of TEM-type ESBLs is *E. coli*; these genes occur within the earliest bacterial transposons identified. [2,22] *bla*SHV-type ESBL genes are the derivatives of chromosomal, parent *bla*SHV-1 genes, which occur mainly in *K. pneumoniae*,[23] and are likely acquired by the role of insertion sequences from chromosome to plasmid. [22] Notably, *bla*TEM-type and *bla*SHV-type ESBL genes located in the integron structures have never been identified. [22] The spread of *bla*CTX-M-type ESBL genes is associated with more complicated mobile elements, compared to that of *bla*TEM and *bla*SHV ESBL genes. *bla*CTX-M ESBL genes are not derivatives of *K. pneumoniae* or *E. coli* that contain original genes, as compared to *bla*TEM or *bla*SHV ESBL genes. *bla*CTX-M genes originate from the chromosomal β-lactamase genes of *Kluyvera* species, which are environmental bacteria found worldwide, and are captured mainly by insertion sequence elements translocated from chromosome to plasmid. [18] Original β-lactamase genes of *Kluyvera* species are identified in most CTX-M subgroups. [18] This differential origin might be involved in the characteristic spread of *bla*CTX-M ESBL genes, that is, an "allodemic" pattern of spread. All *bla*CTX-M genes are associated with insertion sequences. Well-studied, CTX-M-associated insertion sequence elements include IS*Ecp1* and IS*CR1*, which are involved in the mobilization of *bla*CTX-M genes by a transposition mechanism. [24,25,26] In addition, integron structures bearing insertion sequences and *bla*CTX-M genes can be linked to transposon elements, such as from the Tn*21* family, which has been intensively studied. Transposons of the Tn*21* family are disseminated worldwide in both environmental and clinical bacteria.[18,24] These highly efficient mobile genetic elements may have influenced the rapid and easy dissemination of *bla*CTX-M ESBL genes.

An antibiotic resistance plasmid itself is responsible for the efficiency of gene transfer, as well as the mobile genetic elements described above. It has been shown that ESBL gene-bearing plasmids can be transferred to different bacterial species by conjugation. [27,28] Previous studies have shown that *bla*TEM and *bla*SHV ESBL genes are associated with plasmids belonging to a few specific incompatibility (Inc) groups.[18] In contrast, *bla*CTX-M ESBL genes are carried by plasmids belonging to a variety of Inc groups including narrow- and broad-host-range types. [18,29] *bla*CTX-M-15 genes are located mainly on plasmids belonging to the IncF group. [29] Interestingly, a recent study has described the diversity of ESBL gene-bearing plasmids, including SHV types. [30] It was reported that a mosaic plasmid has been identified from a clonal CTX-M-producing *E. coli* isolate, suggesting genetic interactions among different plasmids. [31] In ESBL gene-bearing plasmids, the genetic diversity has been constantly increasing through the mechanism of gene transfer and gene shuffling.

5. Clinical impact

5.1 The mode of infection

5.1.1 Nosocomial infection

Up to the end of the 1990s, clinical infections caused by ESBL-producing bacteria were associated with nosocomial outbreaks, where the chief ESBL producer was *K. pneumoniae*, but not *E. coli*. In addition, the ESBL genotypes detected in the nosocomial setting were almost always TEM and SHV, but not CTX-M types. [1] SHV-producing *K. pneumoniae* strains were intensively examined in the analysis of clonal dissemination in hospitals. Clonally related SHV-4-producing *K. pneumoniae* isolates were shown to have spread to multiple hospitals within the specific region. [32] This phenomenon indicates that, at that time, the mode of spread for SHV-producing *K. pneumoniae* was the dissemination of particular clones, that is to say, an "epidemic" pattern. The number of nosocomial outbreaks caused by TEM- or SHV-producing *K. pneumoniae* strains have been decreased during this century; however, as observed in many studies, these organisms are frequently identified in many hospitals worldwide. Interestingly, the derivatives of TEM and SHV types have been reported to be more divergent in *K. pneumoniae* strains isolated in European hospitals. [16,33] Moreover, the new variants of *bla*SHV genes were detected from an Algerian hospital. [34]

5.1.2 Community-acquired infection

The mode of ESBL-related infection has dramatically changed since the 2000s. Community-acquired infections caused by ESBL-producing bacteria have been increasingly documented. [8] CTX-M-producing E. coli strains are chiefly responsible for community-acquired infections, which are related to an increase in the number of ESBL carriers in the general population. [11,35] One report describes a significant increase in the prevalence of ESBL carriers in a specific population from 2001 to 2006. [36] The interfamilial dissemination of ESBL-producing bacteria has also been suggested. [37] Notably, animals used as food and or pets are reported to carry CTX-M ESBLs, [38,39,40,41] and this finding may explain the dramatic spread of ESBLs in the community. The community-onset dissemination of ESBLs in both humans and animals may suggest that *bla*CTX-M ESBL genes detected in pathogenic bacteria are acquired from environmental bacteria. Branger et al showed that many CTX-M ESBLs were associated with the phylogenetic group D2 that lacked a virulence factor. [42, 43] The specific features may be related to the colonization and spread among the general population. The spread of ESBLs in the community is linked to the emergence of ESBL-related infections in outpatients, in whom urinary tract infections are most often reported along with bacteremia. [44,45, 46] One study has described the detection of CTX-M-producing *K. pneumoniae* in outpatients, [33] A nosocomial outbreak was caused by CTX-M-producing *K. pneumoniae* isolates from foods, suggesting the influx of ESBL-producing *K. pneumoniae* into a hospital. [47] These reports may account for the dissemination of CTX-M ESBL genes from *E. coli* to other bacteria in the community.

5.2 Antibiotic resistance

Antibiotic resistance is of utmost importance for the clinical impact of ESBL-producing bacteria. A meta-analysis showed increased mortality and delay in effective antibiotic use in ESBL-related bacteremia, [48] indicating the importance of constant surveillance for an antibiotic resistance pattern in organisms with ESBLs. ESBL-producing bacteria are resistant to almost all β-lactam antibiotics, except carbapenems, as indicated by their definition. In addition, most ESBL-producing bacteria, particularly those with the TEM, SHV, and CTX-M genotypes, exhibit co-resistance to aminoglycosides, tetracyclines, and sulfonamides. [18] Organisms with CTX-M genotypes, such as those with CTX-M-9, -14, and -15, are reported to be resistant to fluoroquinolones. [18] This additional resistance is induced by the main mechanism that *bla*CTX-M genes are directly linked to quinolone resistance genes, *qnr* genes. IS*CR1*, a mobile element for *bla*CTX-M genes, is associated with *qnr* genes, [26] indicating an effective transfer of quinolone resistance genes together with *bla*CTX-M genes. This genetic finding is interesting for clinical reasons. Selective pressure by the use of fluoroquinolones may induce the emergence of CTX-M ESBL-producing bacteria. As a consequence, the therapeutic options for infections caused by ESBL-producing bacteria may be more limited. Tigecycline has been shown to be microbiologically active against ESBL-producing *E. coli* and *K. pneumoniae*, [49,50] whereas, fosfomycin has been reported to be effective against urinary tract infections caused by ESBL-producing *E. coli*. [51,52]

6. Spread of CTX-M-15-producing ST131 *E. coli* clones

The dissemination of CTX-M-15 producing *E. coli* strains has become a major concern of research in antibiotic resistance. The first isolation of CTX-M-15-type ESBLs was reported in India in 2001. [53] CTX-M-15 is derived from CTX-M-3, belonging to the CTX-M-1 group, differing by one amino acid substitution. *bla*CTX-M-15 genes are transferred mainly by the IncF group plasmids, which are well adapted to *E. coli* and have acquired many antibiotic resistance genes. [54,55,56] Recently, Mnif et al reported that the IncF plasmids carrying *bla*CTX-M-15 genes contained many addiction systems, which could contribute to their maintenance in *E. coli* host strains. [57] The detection rate of the CTX-M-15 producing *E. coli* strains with multidrug resistance has been dramatically increasing worldwide since the 2000s. [56] This CTX-M-15-producing *E. coli* strain is often thought to be associated with ST131 clones. [56] Most of the CTX-M-15-producing *E. coli* strains isolated from three continents were O25:H4-ST131 clones that show highly similar PFGE profiles, suggesting a recent emergence of these clones. [58] The emergence of the CTX-M-15-producing ST131 *E. coli* clones is highly related to the recent dissemination of ESBLs in the USA. [59, 60] The worldwide spread of the multi-drug-resistant ST131 *E. coli* clones can be explained by the acquisition of IncFII plasmids harboring *bla*CTX-M-15 genes and many other antibiotic resistance genes. Interestingly, these ST131 *E. coli* clones belong to the highly virulent, phylogenetic group B2. [56] Over the past 5 years, CTX-M-15-producing ST131 *E. coli* clones have become an important causative agent for community-acquired ESBL infections, mainly urinary tract infections and bacteremia. [45]

7. Clinical impact on immunodeficient patients

The sufficient therapy for ESBL-related infections is important, especially in immunodeficient patients. One study has shown that approximately 13% of *E. coli*-related bacteremia cases detected in patients with cancer and neutropenia were caused by ESBLs, that CTX-M types were predominant among the ESBLs, and that the bacteremia induced by ESBL-producing *E. coli* strains was linked to inadequate empirical antibiotic therapy. [61] In our institution, the detection rate of ESBL-related bacteremia has been increasing in febrile neutropenic patients with hematological malignancies, and consequently, we have been forced to use carbapenems for the therapy. [62,63] In immunodeficient patients, such as those undergoing chemotherapy, serious ESBL-related infections may result in a poor prognosis owing to the failure of the initial therapy. Recently, M. D. Anderson Cancer Center has reported an interesting finding that pyomyositis was caused by ESBL-producing *E. coli* strains in neutropenic patients with hematological malignancies, and that the *E. coli* strains were ST131 clones belonging to phylogenetic group B2. [64] This notable finding implies that ESBL-producing ST131 *E. coli* clones cause fatal damage in the case of immunodeficient patients because of their high virulence.

8. Conclusions

The spread of ESBL-producing bacteria in the community has begun influencing outpatient therapy. Community-acquired bacteremia, due to ESBL-producing *E. coli* strains, is becoming a critical concern for outpatients, because inappropriate use of empirical antibiotics, such as cephalosporins and fluoroquinolones, has resulted in high mortality. [65,66] One study has shown that the resistance of CTX-M-15-producing ST131 *E. coli* strains isolated from the community to fosfomycin has increased. [67] In the near future, we may be forced to use carbapenems as the first choice for the empirical therapy of patients with community-acquired infections due to ESBL-producing bacteria. The identification of carbapenemase-producing *E coli* and *K. pneumoniae* strains has been frequently documented as evidence for additional β-lactamases-producing bacteria other than the ESBL-producing bacteria. [68] The study of NDM-1-type carbapenemase-producing *E coli* and *K. pneumoniae* is currently a topic of much interest in multidrug-resistant bacteria research. Notably, some of the NDM-1-type-producing *E coli* and *K. pneumoniae* strains express *bla*CTX-M-15 ESBL genes in a single isolate. [69,70,71] A worldwide surveillance recently showed that many NDM-1-producing bacteria detected carried additional ESBL genes. [72] The acquisition of efficient mobile elements has accelerated the transfer of various antibiotic resistance genes. Potentially, a "super bug," resistant to almost all licensed antibiotics, may emerge in the future. Constant and careful worldwide surveillance for multidrug-resistant bacteria is urgently warranted.

9. References

[1] Paterson DL, Bonomo RA. Extended-spectrum beta-lactamases: a clinical update. *Clin Microbiol Rev* 2005; 18: 657-86.

[2] Livermore DM. beta-Lactamases in laboratory and clinical resistance. *Clin Microbiol Rev* 1995; 8: 557-84.

[3] Knothe H, Shah P, Krcmery V, Antal M, Mitsuhashi S. Transferable resistance to cefotaxime, cefoxitin, cefamandole and cefuroxime in clinical isolates of Klebsiella pneumoniae and Serratia marcescens. *Infection* 1983; 11: 315-7.

[4] Brun-Buisson C, Legrand P, Philippon A, Montravers F, Ansquer M, Duval J. Transferable enzymatic resistance to third-generation cephalosporins during nosocomial outbreak of multiresistant Klebsiella pneumoniae. *Lancet* 1987; 2: 302-6.

[5] Philippon A, Labia R, Jacoby G. Extended-spectrum beta-lactamases. *Antimicrob Agents Chemother* 1989; 33: 1131-6.

[6] Bauernfeind A, Grimm H, Schweighart S. A new plasmidic cefotaximase in a clinical isolate of Escherichia coli. *Infection* 1990; 18: 294-8.

[7] Bonnet R. Growing group of extended-spectrum beta-lactamases: the CTX-M enzymes. *Antimicrob Agents Chemother* 2004; 48: 1-14.

[8] Pitout JD, Laupland KB. Extended-spectrum beta-lactamase-producing Enterobacteriaceae: an emerging public-health concern. *Lancet Infect Dis* 2008; 8: 159-66.

[9] Talbot GH, Bradley J, Edwards JE, Jr., Gilbert D, Scheld M, Bartlett JG. Bad bugs need drugs: an update on the development pipeline from the Antimicrobial Availability Task Force of the Infectious Diseases Society of America. *Clin Infect Dis* 2006; 42: 657-68.

[10] Jacoby GA, Munoz-Price LS. The new beta-lactamases. *N Engl J Med* 2005; 352: 380-91.

[11] Oteo J, Perez-Vazquez M, Campos J. Extended-spectrum [beta]-lactamase producing Escherichia coli: changing epidemiology and clinical impact. *Curr Opin Infect Dis* 2010; 23: 320-6.

[12] Reinert RR, Low DE, Rossi F, Zhang X, Wattal C, Dowzicky MJ. Antimicrobial susceptibility among organisms from the Asia/Pacific Rim, Europe and Latin and North America collected as part of TEST and the in vitro activity of tigecycline. *J Antimicrob Chemother* 2007; 60: 1018-29.

[13] Hawser SP, Bouchillon SK, Hoban DJ, Badal RE, Hsueh PR, Paterson DL. Emergence of high levels of extended-spectrum-beta-lactamase-producing gram-negative bacilli in the Asia-Pacific region: data from the Study for Monitoring Antimicrobial Resistance Trends (SMART) program, 2007. *Antimicrob Agents Chemother* 2009; 53: 3280-4.

[14] Lee MY, Ko KS, Kang CI, Chung DR, Peck KR, Song JH. High prevalence of CTX-M-15-producing Klebsiella pneumoniae isolates in Asian countries: diverse clones and clonal dissemination. *Int J Antimicrob Agents* 2011; 38: 160-3.

[15] Chong Y, Yakushiji H, Ito Y, Kamimura T. Clinical and molecular epidemiology of extended-spectrum beta-lactamase-producing Escherichia coli and Klebsiella pneumoniae in a long-term study from Japan. *Eur J Clin Microbiol Infect Dis* 2011; 30: 83-7.

[16] Canton R, Novais A, Valverde A, Machado E, Peixe L, Baquero F et al. Prevalence and spread of extended-spectrum beta-lactamase-producing Enterobacteriaceae in Europe. *Clin Microbiol Infect* 2008; 14 Suppl 1: 144-53.

[17] Rossolini GM, D'Andrea MM, Mugnaioli C. The spread of CTX-M-type extended-spectrum beta-lactamases. *Clin Microbiol Infect* 2008; 14 Suppl 1: 33-41.

[18] Canton R, Coque TM. The CTX-M beta-lactamase pandemic. *Curr Opin Microbiol* 2006; 9: 466-75.

[19] Suzuki S, Shibata N, Yamane K, Wachino J, Ito K, Arakawa Y. Change in the prevalence of extended-spectrum-beta-lactamase-producing Escherichia coli in Japan by clonal spread. *J Antimicrob Chemother* 2009; 63: 72-9.

[20] Lewis JS, 2nd, Herrera M, Wickes B, Patterson JE, Jorgensen JH. First report of the emergence of CTX-M-type extended-spectrum beta-lactamases (ESBLs) as the predominant ESBL isolated in a U.S. health care system. *Antimicrob Agents Chemother* 2007; 51: 4015-21.

[21] Sidjabat HE, Paterson DL, Adams-Haduch JM, Ewan L, Pasculle AW, Muto CA et al. Molecular epidemiology of CTX-M-producing Escherichia coli isolates at a tertiary medical center in western Pennsylvania. *Antimicrob Agents Chemother* 2009; 53: 4733-9.

[22] Poirel L, Naas T, Nordmann P. Genetic support of extended-spectrum beta-lactamases. *Clin Microbiol Infect* 2008; 14 Suppl 1: 75-81.

[23] Babini GS, Livermore DM. Are SHV beta-lactamases universal in Klebsiella pneumoniae? *Antimicrob Agents Chemother* 2000; 44: 2230.

[24] Novais A, Canton R, Valverde A, Machado E, Galan JC, Peixe L et al. Dissemination and persistence of blaCTX-M-9 are linked to class 1 integrons containing CR1 associated with defective transposon derivatives from Tn402 located in early antibiotic resistance plasmids of IncHI2, IncP1-alpha, and IncFI groups. *Antimicrob Agents Chemother* 2006; 50: 2741-50.

[25] Poirel L, Lartigue MF, Decousser JW, Nordmann P. ISEcp1B-mediated transposition of blaCTX-M in Escherichia coli. *Antimicrob Agents Chemother* 2005; 49: 447-50.

[26] Toleman MA, Bennett PM, Walsh TR. ISCR elements: novel gene-capturing systems of the 21st century? *Microbiol Mol Biol Rev* 2006; 70: 296-316.

[27] Palucha A, Mikiewicz B, Hryniewicz W, Gniadkowski M. Concurrent outbreaks of extended-spectrum beta-lactamase-producing organisms of the family Enterobacteriaceae in a Warsaw hospital. *J Antimicrob Chemother* 1999; 44: 489-99.

[28] Baraniak A, Fiett J, Sulikowska A, Hryniewicz W, Gniadkowski M. Countrywide spread of CTX-M-3 extended-spectrum beta-lactamase-producing microorganisms of the family Enterobacteriaceae in Poland. *Antimicrob Agents Chemother* 2002; 46: 151-9.

[29] Carattoli A. Resistance plasmid families in Enterobacteriaceae. *Antimicrob Agents Chemother* 2009; 53: 2227-38.

[30] Diestra K, Juan C, Curiao T, Moya B, Miro E, Oteo J et al. Characterization of plasmids encoding blaESBL and surrounding genes in Spanish clinical isolates of Escherichia coli and Klebsiella pneumoniae. *J Antimicrob Chemother* 2009; 63: 60-6.

[31] Lavollay M, Mamlouk K, Frank T, Akpabie A, Burghoffer B, Ben Redjeb S et al. Clonal dissemination of a CTX-M-15 beta-lactamase-producing Escherichia coli strain in the Paris area, Tunis, and Bangui. *Antimicrob Agents Chemother* 2006; 50: 2433-8.

[32] Yuan M, Aucken H, Hall LM, Pitt TL, Livermore DM. Epidemiological typing of klebsiellae with extended-spectrum beta-lactamases from European intensive care units. *J Antimicrob Chemother* 1998; 41: 527-39.

[33] Valverde A, Coque TM, Garcia-San Miguel L, Baquero F, Canton R. Complex molecular epidemiology of extended-spectrum beta-lactamases in Klebsiella pneumoniae: a long-term perspective from a single institution in Madrid. *J Antimicrob Chemother* 2008; 61: 64-72.

[34] Ramdani-Bouguessa N, Manageiro V, Jones-Dias D, Ferreira E, Tazir M, Canica M. Role of SHV {beta}-lactamase variants in resistance of clinical Klebsiella pneumoniae strains to {beta}-lactams in an Algerian hospital. *J Med Microbiol* 2011; 60: 983-7.

[35] Valverde A, Coque TM, Sanchez-Moreno MP, Rollan A, Baquero F, Canton R. Dramatic increase in prevalence of fecal carriage of extended-spectrum beta-lactamase-producing Enterobacteriaceae during nonoutbreak situations in Spain. *J Clin Microbiol* 2004; 42: 4769-75.

[36] Woerther PL, Angebault C, Lescat M, Ruppe E, Skurnik D, Mniai AE et al. Emergence and dissemination of extended-spectrum beta-lactamase-producing Escherichia coli in the community: lessons from the study of a remote and controlled population. *J Infect Dis* 2010; 202: 515-23.

[37] Rodriguez-Bano J, Lopez-Cerero L, Navarro MD, Diaz de Alba P, Pascual A. Faecal carriage of extended-spectrum beta-lactamase-producing Escherichia coli: prevalence, risk factors and molecular epidemiology. *J Antimicrob Chemother* 2008; 62: 1142-9.

[38] Kojima A, Ishii Y, Ishihara K, Esaki H, Asai T, Oda C et al. Extended-spectrum-beta-lactamase-producing Escherichia coli strains isolated from farm animals from 1999 to 2002: report from the Japanese Veterinary Antimicrobial Resistance Monitoring Program. *Antimicrob Agents Chemother* 2005; 49: 3533-7.

[39] Carattoli A, Lovari S, Franco A, Cordaro G, Di Matteo P, Battisti A. Extended-spectrum beta-lactamases in Escherichia coli isolated from dogs and cats in Rome, Italy, from 2001 to 2003. *Antimicrob Agents Chemother* 2005; 49: 833-5.

[40] Ho PL, Chow KH, Lai EL, Lo WU, Yeung MK, Chan J et al. Extensive dissemination of CTX-M-producing Escherichia coli with multidrug resistance to 'critically important' antibiotics among food animals in Hong Kong, 2008-10. *J Antimicrob Chemother* 2011; 66: 765-8.

[41] Leverstein-van Hall MA, Dierikx CM, Cohen Stuart J, Voets GM, van den Munckhof MP, van Essen-Zandbergen A et al. Dutch patients, retail chicken meat and poultry share the same ESBL genes, plasmids and strains. *Clin Microbiol Infect* 2011; 17: 873-80.

[42] Deschamps C, Clermont O, Hipeaux MC, Arlet G, Denamur E, Branger C. Multiple acquisitions of CTX-M plasmids in the rare D2 genotype of Escherichia coli provide evidence for convergent evolution. *Microbiology* 2009; 155: 1656-68.

[43] Branger C, Zamfir O, Geoffroy S, Laurans G, Arlet G, Thien HV et al. Genetic background of Escherichia coli and extended-spectrum beta-lactamase type. *Emerg Infect Dis* 2005; 11: 54-61.

[44] Ben-Ami R, Schwaber MJ, Navon-Venezia S, Schwartz D, Giladi M, Chmelnitsky I et al. Influx of extended-spectrum beta-lactamase-producing enterobacteriaceae into the hospital. *Clin Infect Dis* 2006; 42: 925-34.

[45] Pitout JD, Gregson DB, Campbell L, Laupland KB. Molecular characteristics of extended-spectrum-beta-lactamase-producing Escherichia coli isolates causing bacteremia in the Calgary Health Region from 2000 to 2007: emergence of clone ST131 as a cause of community-acquired infections. *Antimicrob Agents Chemother* 2009; 53: 2846-51.

[46] Meier S, Weber R, Zbinden R, Ruef C, Hasse B. Extended-spectrum beta-lactamase-producing Gram-negative pathogens in community-acquired urinary tract infections: an increasing challenge for antimicrobial therapy. *Infection* 2011.

[47] Calbo E, Freixas N, Xercavins M, Riera M, Nicolas C, Monistrol O et al. Foodborne nosocomial outbreak of SHV1 and CTX-M-15-producing Klebsiella pneumoniae: epidemiology and control. *Clin Infect Dis* 2011; 52: 743-9.

[48] Schwaber MJ, Carmeli Y. Mortality and delay in effective therapy associated with extended-spectrum beta-lactamase production in Enterobacteriaceae bacteraemia: a systematic review and meta-analysis. *J Antimicrob Chemother* 2007; 60: 913-20.

[49] Morosini MI, Garcia-Castillo M, Coque TM, Valverde A, Novais A, Loza E et al. Antibiotic coresistance in extended-spectrum-beta-lactamase-producing Enterobacteriaceae and in vitro activity of tigecycline. *Antimicrob Agents Chemother* 2006; 50: 2695-9.

[50] Kelesidis T, Karageorgopoulos DE, Kelesidis I, Falagas ME. Tigecycline for the treatment of multidrug-resistant Enterobacteriaceae: a systematic review of the evidence from microbiological and clinical studies. *J Antimicrob Chemother* 2008; 62: 895-904.

[51] Falagas ME, Kastoris AC, Kapaskelis AM, Karageorgopoulos DE. Fosfomycin for the treatment of multidrug-resistant, including extended-spectrum beta-lactamase producing, Enterobacteriaceae infections: a systematic review. *Lancet Infect Dis* 2010; 10: 43-50.

[52] Rodriguez-Bano J, Alcala JC, Cisneros JM, Grill F, Oliver A, Horcajada JP et al. Community infections caused by extended-spectrum beta-lactamase-producing Escherichia coli. *Arch Intern Med* 2008; 168: 1897-902.

[53] Karim A, Poirel L, Nagarajan S, Nordmann P. Plasmid-mediated extended-spectrum beta-lactamase (CTX-M-3 like) from India and gene association with insertion sequence ISEcp1. *FEMS Microbiol Lett* 2001; 201: 237-41.

[54] Boyd DA, Tyler S, Christianson S, McGeer A, Muller MP, Willey BM et al. Complete nucleotide sequence of a 92-kilobase plasmid harboring the CTX-M-15 extended-spectrum beta-lactamase involved in an outbreak in long-term-care facilities in Toronto, Canada. *Antimicrob Agents Chemother* 2004; 48: 3758-64.

[55] Marcade G, Deschamps C, Boyd A, Gautier V, Picard B, Branger C et al. Replicon typing of plasmids in Escherichia coli producing extended-spectrum beta-lactamases. *J Antimicrob Chemother* 2009; 63: 67-71.

[56] Peirano G, Pitout JD. Molecular epidemiology of Escherichia coli producing CTX-M beta-lactamases: the worldwide emergence of clone ST131 O25:H4. *Int J Antimicrob Agents* 2010; 35: 316-21.

[57] Mnif B, Vimont S, Boyd A, Bourit E, Picard B, Branger C et al. Molecular characterization of addiction systems of plasmids encoding extended-spectrum beta-lactamases in Escherichia coli. *J Antimicrob Chemother* 2010; 65: 1599-603.

[58] Nicolas-Chanoine MH, Blanco J, Leflon-Guibout V, Demarty R, Alonso MP, Canica MM et al. Intercontinental emergence of Escherichia coli clone O25:H4-ST131 producing CTX-M-15. *J Antimicrob Chemother* 2008; 61: 273-81.

[59] Peirano G, Costello M, Pitout JD. Molecular characteristics of extended-spectrum beta-lactamase-producing Escherichia coli from the Chicago area: high prevalence of ST131 producing CTX-M-15 in community hospitals. *Int J Antimicrob Agents* 2010; 36: 19-23.

[60] Johnson JR, Johnston B, Clabots C, Kuskowski MA, Castanheira M. Escherichia coli sequence type ST131 as the major cause of serious multidrug-resistant E. coli infections in the United States. *Clin Infect Dis* 2010; 51: 286-94.

[61] Gudiol C, Calatayud L, Garcia-Vidal C, Lora-Tamayo J, Cisnal M, Duarte R et al. Bacteraemia due to extended-spectrum beta-lactamase-producing Escherichia coli (ESBL-EC) in cancer patients: clinical features, risk factors, molecular epidemiology and outcome. *J Antimicrob Chemother* 2010; 65: 333-41.

[62] Chong Y, Yakushiji H, Ito Y, Kamimura T. Cefepime-resistant Gram-negative bacteremia in febrile neutropenic patients with hematological malignancies. *Int J Infect Dis* 2010; 14 Suppl 3: e171-5.

[63] Muratani T, Kobayashi T, Matsumoto T. Emergence and prevalence of beta-lactamase-producing Klebsiella pneumoniae resistant to cephems in Japan. *Int J Antimicrob Agents* 2006; 27: 491-9.

[64] Vigil KJ, Johnson JR, Johnston BD, Kontoyiannis DP, Mulanovich VE, Raad, II et al. Escherichia coli Pyomyositis: an emerging infectious disease among patients with hematologic malignancies. *Clin Infect Dis* 2010; 50: 374-80.

[65] Rodriguez-Bano J, Navarro MD, Romero L, Muniain MA, de Cueto M, Rios MJ et al. Bacteremia due to extended-spectrum beta -lactamase-producing Escherichia coli in the CTX-M era: a new clinical challenge. *Clin Infect Dis* 2006; 43: 1407-14.

[66] Rodriguez-Bano J, Picon E, Gijon P, Hernandez JR, Ruiz M, Pena C et al. Community-onset bacteremia due to extended-spectrum beta-lactamase-producing Escherichia coli: risk factors and prognosis. *Clin Infect Dis* 2010; 50: 40-8.

[67] Oteo J, Orden B, Bautista V, Cuevas O, Arroyo M, Martinez-Ruiz R et al. CTX-M-15-producing urinary Escherichia coli O25b-ST131-phylogroup B2 has acquired resistance to fosfomycin. *J Antimicrob Chemother* 2009; 64: 712-7.

[68] Bush K. Alarming beta-lactamase-mediated resistance in multidrug-resistant Enterobacteriaceae. *Curr Opin Microbiol* 2010; 13: 558-64.

[69] Poirel L, Al Maskari Z, Al Rashdi F, Bernabeu S, Nordmann P. NDM-1-producing Klebsiella pneumoniae isolated in the Sultanate of Oman. *J Antimicrob Chemother* 2010.

[70] Poirel L, Lagrutta E, Taylor P, Pham J, Nordmann P. Emergence of metallo-beta-lactamase NDM-1-producing multidrug-resistant Escherichia coli in Australia. *Antimicrob Agents Chemother* 2010; 54: 4914-6.

[71] Poirel L, Revathi G, Bernabeu S, Nordmann P. Detection of NDM-1-Producing Klebsiella pneumoniae in Kenya. *Antimicrob Agents Chemother* 2011; 55: 934-6.

[72] Lascols C, Hackel M, Marshall SH, Hujer AM, Bouchillon S, Badal R et al. Increasing prevalence and dissemination of NDM-1 metallo-{beta}-lactamase in India: data from the SMART study (2009). *J Antimicrob Chemother* 2011.

8

Antimicrobial Resistance of Bacteria in Food

María Consuelo Vanegas Lopez
Universidad de los Andes,
Colombia

1. Introduction

Antibiotics are a major tool utilized by the healthcare industry to fight bacterial infections; however, bacteria are highly adaptable organisms, able develop resistance to antibiotics. Consequently, decades of antibiotic use, or rather misuse, have resulted in bacterial resistance to many modern antibiotics. This resistance can cause significant danger and suffering for many people with common bacterial infections, which were once easily treatable with this type of medication [1]. Antibiotics are widely used in human and veterinary medicine as well as in agriculture for the treatment of infections, to improve growth and for animal prophylaxis, which can generate a selection of multiresistant bacteria. However, is it not fully understood how widespread antibiotic resistant bacteria are in agricultural settings. The lack of such surveillance data is especially evident in dairy farm environments.

Over the past 6 decades, the introduction of new class or modifications of antimicrobial has been marched slowly but surely by the development of new bacterial resistance mechanisms. Since the first reports different estudies have demonstrated that increases in antimicrobial resistance among both pathogenic and commensal bacteria can be observed after introduction of antimicrobial[2]. Therefore in this chapter I will discuss some of the research which in which they reported the presence of antibiotic-resistant bacteria that are of importance in foods.

2. *Campylobacter*

Campylobacter was identified as a human diarrheal pathogen in 1973. *Campylobacter* is a major cause of disease in humans and poultry around the world and *Campylobacter* was, is the most frequently diagnosed bacterial cause for human gastroenteritis in the United States and throughout the world. Most cases of *Campylobacter* infections do not require antimicrobial treatment, being clinically mild and self-limiting [4]. Macrolides are considered the first choice drug for *C. jejuni* and *C. Coli* enteritis,erythromycin and ciprofloxacin are the drugs of choice for treatment of human campylobacteriosis and fluoroquinilones are also used. Contaminated food is the usual source of human infection; therefore, the presence of antimicrobial resistant strains in the food chain has raised concerns that the treatment of human infections will be compromised. Most disease in humans is associated with the consumption of contaminated poultry or cross-contamination with other foods [4]

This section provides a review of resistance prevalence in *C.jejuni* and *C.coli* from food. In this study, was investigated the prevalence of resistance to erythromycin and ciprofloxacin in *Campylobacter* isolates recovered from turkey carcasses at two processing plants. Ciprofloxacin and erythromycin resistance in *Campylobacter* recovered from processed turkey occurred more frequently among *C. coli* than *C. jejuni*. Molecular subtyping in this study provides further information about the relationships between antimicrobial-resistant *Campylobacter* at processing level [5]

The antimicrobial resistance profiles of *Campylobacter* isolates recovered from a series of samples of retail food (n = 374) and humans (n = 314) to eight antimicrobial compounds were investigated. High levels of resistance in isolates of *C.jejuni* were observed for ceftiofur (58%), ampicillin (25%) and nalidixic acid (17%) with lowest levels observed for streptomycin (7.9%) and chloramphenicol (8.3%). A total of 80% of isolates *of C. jejuni* were resistant to human ceftiofur, while 17% were resistant to ampicillin and nalidixic acid, 8.6% to streptomycin and 4.1% to chloramphenicol. Antimicrobial resistance of clinical relevance, such as erythromycin, ciprofloxacin and tetracycline were 6.7, 12 and 15% respectively for all food isolates and was similar to the corresponding prevalence of resistance observed in human isolates, where 6 , 4%, 12 and 13, respectively, were found to be resistant. Comparisons of strains of *C. jejuni* at each site showed a high degree of similarity although some regional variations exist. Comparison of the total populations of *C. jejuni* and *C. coli* showed minor differences, with *C. jejuni* strains resistant to ampicillin and ceftiofur. Patterns of multidrug resistance showed some profiles common to the human strains and clinical [6].

Antimicrobial resistance was evaluated in *Campylobacter* spp isolated of beef cattle in four commercial feedlots in Alberta (Canada). All calves were given chlortetracycline and oxytetracycline in food, and most animals (93%) were injected with long-acting oxytetracycline. A total of 1586 *Campylobacter* strains were isolated, these consist of *Campylobacter* coli (n = 154), *Campylobacter fetus* (n = 994), *Campylobacter jejuni* (n = 431), *Campylobacter hyointestinalis* (n = 4), and *Campylobacter lanienae* (n = 3) which were recovered and characterized [4]. Increases in the prevalence of strains resistant to tetracycline and doxycycline (56 to 89%) of *C. coli*, *C. fetus* and *C. jejuni* were observed [4]. Increased resistance to erythromycin was also found in strains of *C. coli* in the three episodes of isolation. Most isolates of *C. fetus* recovered were resistant to nalidixic acid and a relatively small number of multi-drug resistant strains were recovered. Widespread use of antimicrobial agents in meat production and possible horizontal transfer of mobile genetic elements with resistance determinants among bacteria *Campylobacter* and other taxa emphasized [4].

Campylobacter has become the leading cause of zoonotic enteric infections in developed and developing countries worlwide. Epidemiological and microbial studies show that poultry is the most important source for quinolone-susceptible and quinolone-resistant campylobacter infections in humans. Trend over time for macrolide resistance show stable low rates in most countries, and macrolides should remain the drugs class of choice for *C. jejuni* and *C. coli* enteritis. However, macrolide resitance is emerging in some countries and needs to be monitored.[7].

3. *Salmonella*

Salmonella spp. is widely distribuited in nature, colonizing a range of animal hosts. *Salmonella* entérica is recognized as one of the most common bacteria causes of food borne diarrheal illness worldwide. It had been estimated that annually there are about 1.3 billion cases of acute gastroenteritis due to nontyphoidal salmonelosis, resulting in 3 million deaths. In industrialized countries food animals are the main reservoir for human infections, the majority of which originate from contaminated meat products and eggs. It is very important the issue of antibiotic resistance of *Salmonella* spp, which has been investigated as its ecology and pathogenesis

Substantial effort has been made to disclose the genetic means by which *Salmonella* spp has evolved to resist antimicrobials. Acquired resistance arises by two ways: by mutations in chromosomally encoded genetic elements and by acquisition of exogenous mobile resistance genes by plasmids, integrons and transposons. Both mechanisms can led to rapid changes of a bacterial populations, horizontal genes transfer apppers to be most important in the evolutions of salmonella resistance.[8] In this section I summarize some examples which show the presence antimicrobial resistance *Salmonella* spp in food.

Burgos et al. isolated and identified enteric bacteria in the soil of dairy farms and found that enteric bacteria from dairy farm soil are resistant to multiple drugs and carriers of antibiotic resistance plasmids. This suggests that the surface layer of farm land plays an important role, as it is an environment that can be a reservoir for the development of bacterial resistance against antibiotics [3].

In another study undertaken in Alberta during 1996 and 1999, 209 strains of *Salmonella*, obtained from food animals were isolated and 17 antimicrobial drugs were tested and , 11.8% of strains were positive for resistance. These strains were commonly resistant to tetracycline (35.4%), streptomycin(32.5%), sulfamethoxazole (28.7%), ticarcillin (27.3%) and ampicillin (26.8%)[9]. *Salmonella* enterica serovar Heidelberg frequently causes foodborne illness in humans. The authors compared the prevalence of Salmonella serotype Heidelberg in a sampling of 20,295 meats, including chicken breast ,ground turkey, ground beef and pork ribs, collected between 2002 and 2006 a total of 298 Salmonella serovar Heidelberg isolates were recovered, representing 21.6% of all Salmonella serovars from retail meats. One hundred seventy-eight (59.7%) were from ground turkey, 110 (36.9%) were from chicken breast, and 10 (3.4%) were from pork chops; none was found in ground beef. One hundred ninety-eight isolates (66.4%) were resistant to at least one compound, and 49 (16.4%) were resistant to at least five compounds. Six strains (2.0%), all ground turkey, were resistant to at least nine antimicrobial agents. The greatest resistance in isolates from poultry was to tetracycline (39.9%), followed by streptomycin (37.8%), sulfamethoxazole (27.7%), gentamicin (25.7%), kanamycin (21.5%), ampicillin (19.8%), amoxicillin-clavulanate (10.4%) and ceftiofur (9.0%). These data indicate that *Salmonella* serovar Heidelberg is a common serovar in retail poultry meat and includes widespread clones of multidrug-resistant strains [10].

Recently, *Salmonella* Enterica *subsp. enterica* serovar *Saintpaul* has been increasingly observed in several countries, including Germany. However, the pathogenic potential and epidemiology of this serotype are not very well known. Fifty-five isolates of *S. turkey saintpaul* Germany and Turkey food products isolated from 2000 to 2007 were analyzed using an antimicrobial agent, organic solvents, and disinfectant susceptibility testing, detection of determinants of resistance, plasmid profiles, pulsed-field gel electrophoresis (PFGE) and hybridization experiments[11].The pattern of resistance was observed for ampicillin, amoxicillin-clavulanate, gentamicin, kanamycin, nalidixic acid, streptomycin, spectinomycin, and several third-generation cephalosporins (including ceftiofur and cefoxitin. This study revealed that a multiresistant S. saintpaul line Saintpaul is widespread in turkeys and turkey products in Germany.[11]

In Denmark, Skov, M et al, compared 8144 Salmonella isolates collected from meat imported or produced, as well as the Danish patients. Isolates from imported meat showed a higher rate of antimicrobial resistance, including resistance to multiple drugs, which were isolated from domestic beef. Isolates from humans showed resistance rates lower than those found in imported meat. These findings suggest that programs to control resistant *Salmonella spp.* are a worldwide problem [12]

A study in Vietnam shows that enteric bacteria in samples of raw foods contain a set of mobile genetic elements and the transfer of antibiotic resistance can easily occur between similar bacteria. This study was undertaken to examine the contamination rate and molecular characteristics of enteric bacteria isolated from a selection of food sources in Vietnam [16]. One hundred and eighty raw food samples were tested; 60.8% of the samples were from meat and 18.0% of samples of shellfish contaminated with *Salmonella* spp. More than 90% of all food sources contained *Escherichia coli*. The isolates were selected for antibiotic resistance against 15 antibiotics, and 50.5% of *Salmonella* isolates and 83.8% of isolates of *E. coli* were resistant to at least one antibiotic[13]. Isolates were screened for the presence of mobile genetic elements that confer resistance to antibiotics. Fifty-seven percent of *E. coli* and 13% of *Salmonella* isolates were found to contain integrons, and some isolates contained two integrons Plasmids were also detected in the 23 *Salmonella* isolates resistant to antibiotics and 33 isolates of *E. coli*. One hundred thirty-five *Salmonella* isolates and 76% of *E. coli* isolates contained plasmids of 95 kb, and some isolates contained two large plasmids. Conjugation experiments showed the successful transfer of all or part of the phenotypes of antibiotic resistance among isolates of *Salmonella* and *E. coli* contaminated food. The results show that enteric bacteria in raw food samples from Vietnam contain a set of mobile genetic elements and the transfer of antibiotic resistance can easily occur between similar bacteria[13]

Another study in Vietnam, was undertaken to examine the levels of *Salmonella* in samples of raw foods, including chicken, beef, pork and shellfish to determine their antibiotic resistance. A total of 180 samples were collected and analyzed, we obtained 91 isolates of *Salmonella*. Sixty-one percent of meat and 18% of shellfish samples were contaminated with *Salmonella spp.* The susceptibility of all isolates to a variety of antimicrobial agents was tested, and resistance to tetracycline, ampicillin / amoxicillin, nalidixic acid and streptomycin sulfafurazole was found in 40.7%, 22.0%, 18.7%, 16.5% and 14.3% of the isolates, respectively. Resistance to enrofloxacin, trimethoprim, chloramphenicol, kanamycin, and gentamicin was also detected (8.8 to 2.2%). About half (50.5%) of the *Salmonella* isolates were resistant to at least one of the antibiotics.[14]

4. *Escherichia coli*

E. coli is a bacterium, which very easily and frequently exchanges genetic information through horizontal gene transfer (e.g. by conjugation, transformation or transduction) with other related bacteria, such as other *E. coli* strains, *Salmonella, Shigella*. Therefore, *E. coli* strains may exhibit characteristics that have been acquired from a wide variety of sources.A recent review describes the population structure of commensal E. *coli*, the factors involved in the spread of different strains, how the bacteria can adapt to different niches, and how a commensal life style can evolve into a pathogenic one (Tenaillon et al., 2010). All humans and animals carry E. *coli* in their intestines as they are part of the normal gut flora and usually harmless. However, there are several types of E. *coli* strains that may cause gastrointestinalillness in humans. These strain types can be divided into several pathogroups These strain types can be divided into several pathogroups, resistant to ampicillin, amoxicillin/clavulanic acid,piperacillin/sulbactam, piperacillin/tazobactam, cefuroxime, etc.The strain carries plasmid-borne *bla*CTX-M-15 and a *bla*TEM-1 genes.An E. *coli* O104:H4 with a MLST ST678 was previously observed about 10 years ago in Germany in a Haemolytic Uremic Syndrome (HUS) case (Mellmann et al., 2008), the STEC O104:H4 outbreak strain shows an unusual combination of virulence factors of STEC and EAEC which has only been reported sporadically in humans before (Morabito et al., 1998) [16].

Another study analyzed the prevalence of *Escherichia coli* O157 in patients with diarrhea and surface water of some selected sources in Zaria (Nigeria), was evaluated of susceptibility to antibiotics and plasmid profiles of 184 isolates of E. *coli*, obtained from water samples of 228 and 112 diarrheal stool samples (collected from children <15 years) using standard methods. The most active antibiotics were gentamicin, chloramphenicol, and fluoroquinolones. Seventy-nine (42.9%) of 184 E. *coli* isolates were resistant to four or more antibiotics. The Multidrug Resistance (MDR) was higher among water isolates than clinical isolates. Of the 35 MDR isolates (20 of which were O157 strains), 22 (62.9%) harbored plasmids, all of which not less than 2.1 kb in size. Among the 20 strains of E. *coli* O157, only seven (35.0%) contained multiple plasmids. An E. *coli* O157 isolated from the aquatic system contains two plasmids resistant to seven drugs, including ampicillin, cefuroxime, ciprofloxacin, cotrimoxazole, nalidixic acid, nitrofurantoin and tetracycline. Loss of plasmids correlated with the loss of resistance to antibiotics (mutant) strains selected on tetracycline (50 mg / mL) in nutrient agar plates [17] .

The role of animal-based foods as vehicles for antibiotic-resistant bacteria has also been studied. One study on chickens fattening evaluated the incidence and distribution of antibiotic resistance in 197 commensal *Escherichia coli* strains. The effects of supplementation with antimicrobial agents approved bambermycin, penicillin, salinomycin and bacitracin or a combination of salinomycin more bacitracin. All isolates showed some degree of resistance to multiple antibiotics and resistance to tetracycline (68.5%), amoxicillin (61.4%), ceftiofur (51.3%), spectinomycin(47.2%), and sulfonamides (42%). These data demonstrate that the multidrug resistance of E.*coli* can be found in broilers, regardless of antimicrobial growth promoters used.

Water can also be an important vehicle for transmission of bacteria durability antibiotics, so I quote a study that was performed on wastewater from a plant to produce antibiotics which characterized the population of bacteria in surface waters of production plant of oxytetracycline (OTC). Found high levels of TBT in the wastewater (WW) and the antibiotic was still detectable at 20 Km (RWD), with undetectable levels in the water upstream (RWU). A total of 341 bacterial strains, most identified as Gammaproteobacteria. The most of the isolates (94.2% and 95.4% respectively WW and RWD) had tet (A) gene and it was the most common (67.0%), followed by tet (W), tet (C), tet (J), tet (L), tet (D), tet (y) and tet (K) (in the range between 21.0% and 40.6%). The authors propose that the strong selective pressure imposed by high concentrations of TBT contributes to the widespread dissemination of resistance genes and other genes of tetracycline resistance to antibiotics, possibly through mobile genetic elements[15]

5. *Enterococcus*

Enterococci colonize the gastrointestinal tract of the oral cavity and vaginal tract of humans and most animals [18]. The emergence of antimicrobial resistance represents the greatest threat to the treatment of human enterococcal infections. Enterococci are intrinsically resistant to a number of antimicrobial agents normally used to treat infections caused by grampositive bacteria. The enterococci have a remarkable ability to acquire new mechaninms of resistance and to transfer resistance determinans by way of conjugation [19]. In this section I focus in a review of antimicrobial resistant enterococci strains isolated from somefood.

From a medical point of view, the resistance of enterococci to vancomycin, teicoplanin and streptogramins is of special interest. In the case of vancomycin, there are identical types of groups of vanA of enterococci genes from fecal samples of animals, pet food, hospital patients, people in the community and water samples, these resistance genes may contaminate humans through the food chain [20]. Also, it was found that the most frequently isolated species are *Enterococcus faecium* (32.61%), followed by *E. faecalis* (21.74%), with high levels of resistance to streptomycin and gentamicin. These results confirm the presence of enterococci whitin the community having susceptibility profiles similar to those of strains found in hospital . [21].

A study at the Faculty of Pharmaceutical Sciences, University of Sao Paulo, Brazil, reported that 52.5% of the samples of raw and pasteurized milk, meat, cheese and vegetables were positive for enterococci; the most contaminated being the meat and the cheese. *E. faecium* was the predominant species, followed by E. faecalis, E. gallinarum and E.casseliflavus. Virulence genes were found and resistance to gentamicin, tetracycline and erythromycin in *E. faecalis* and three strains of *E. faecium* were resistant to vancomycin [22]. From the strains resistant to antibiotics, 72.4% of *E. faecalis* were able to form biofilm and 13.8% to adhere to Caco-2, which shows a virulent capacity of these types of enterococci [22].

The importance of ready-to-eat food (RTEF) and the Antibiotic Resistance (AR) gene flow has been assessed. RTEF are consumed frequently and may play a role in the acquisition of the determinants of AR in the human digestive tract. The study by Macovei et al, evaluated three RTEFs (chicken salad, a chicken burger and carrot cake) which were taken as samples from five fast food restaurants five times in the summer and 5 in the and winter. The overall concentrations of enterococci during the two seasons were similar (10^3 CFU / g), the most prevalent were *Enterococcus casseliflavus* (41.5% of isolates) and *Enterococcus hirae* (41.5%) in winter and *Enterococcus faecium* (36.8%), *E. casseliflavus* (27.6%) and *Enterococcus faecalis* (22.4%) in summer. In winter isolates were resistant mainly in to tetracycline (50.8%), ciprofloxacin (13.8%) and erythromycin (4.6%). In summer isolates were resistant mainly to tetracycline (22.8%), erythromycin (22.1%), and kanamycin (13.0%). The most common gene was *tet (M)* (35.4%) Genotyping of *E. faecalis* and *E. faecium* with pulsed-field gel electrophoresis revealed that the food contamination likely originated from various sources and is not clonal [23].

Another study from the southwestern United States, which characterized the profiles of antibiotic resistance of enterococci isolated from fresh produce harvested, found that of 185 Enterococci isolates, 97 (52%) were *Enterococcus faecium*, 38 (21%) were *Enterococcus faecalis*, and 50 (27%) were other Enterococcus species. Of clinical significance in humans is the fact that strains of *E. faecium* had a much higher prevalence of resistance to ciprofloxacin, tetracycline and nitrofurantoin than *E. faecalis*. 34% of the strains had multiple patterns of drug resistance, excluding intrinsic resistance. These data may help to elucidate the role of food in the transmission of antibiotic-resistant strains in human populations [24].

Additionally, one hundred and five VanA of the Glycopeptide-resistant enterococci (GRE) isolated from, human; animal, and food , were studied for genetic variability and molecular markers. The presence of indistinguishable *vanA* elements,mostly plasmid-borne, and virulence determinants in different species and PFGE-diverse populations suggested that all GRE might be potential reservoirs of resistance determinants and virulence traits transferable to human-adapted clusters. [25].

Research undertaken in Turkey has assessed vancomycin resistance and antibiotic resistance profiles of enterococci in different types of food purchased in local markets. Of a total of 200 samples, 50% had high levels of enterococci contamination, the greater resistance being found in samples of cream cheese. Only 4 strains were identified as resistant to vancomycin and identified as *E. faecalis*, from chicken. The results of this study emphasize the urgency of preventive measures to be taken to control antibiotic use on farms [26].

In addition, a study led by Martins et. al in Portugal whereby a total of 983 strains of enterococci were isolated from sewage sludge and effluent waste. These were tested against 10 different antibiotics. Multiresistance was found in 49.4% of the strains. Only 3.3% and 0.6% were resistant to ampicillin and vancomycin, respectively. However, observed 51.5% resistance to rifampicin, tetracycline 34.6%, 24.8% and 22.5% for erythromycin, nitrofurantoin. These results indicate that the use of antibiotics has created a large pool of resistance genes and the processes of wastewater treatment do not prevent the spread of resistant enterococci in the environment [27].

Different species of enterococci can frequently be isolated from environmental samples such as soil, water, plants or animal raw products.. In a study led by M.T. Tejedor Junco in 2009, isolated 78 strains of enterococci, from alfalfa (Medicago sativa) plant samples, drip irrigated with conventional water and a secondary effluent. *E. faecalis* (10.2%), *E. faecium* (2.6%), *E. hirae* (5.1%), *E. casseliflavus* (2.6%) and *E. mundtii* (79.5%) were isolated , In They found that all strains of enterococci, were susceptible to glycopeptides, penicillin and ampicillin. They did not detect strains with high level resistance to aminoglycosides. [28].

Additionally, the products supplied for feeding animals have been widely studied because they are potential vehicles for transmission of resistant bacteria. This has been demonstrated in a study conducted in 2006 in Portugal where 1137 enterococci strains and 163 *Escherichia coli* strains were recovered from 89 poultry feed samples, where 69.1% of enterococci isolates obtained from broiler feed were resistant to tetracycline and *E. coli* were resistant to ampicillin, tetracycline and streptomycin in 22.9%, 27.6% and 19.0% respectively. These data allow us to infer that the animal feed is a significant source of antibiotic resistant bacteria , thus leading to their introduction in the farm enviroment. The Poultry feed is at the start of the food safety chain, and might serve as a source of antimicrobial resistant bacteria present in poultry meat [29].

Some antibiotics had been used as growth promoters in Europe for several years, creating strains of resistant *E. faecium* .Resistant bacteria, have been isolated from samples of sewage, animal stools, meat products, samples from community and clinical samples from different European populations. Glycopeptide-resistant *E.faecium* (GREF), can be found in hospitals and outside them, and in the food chain by contaminated meat products.This suggests that the origin of these strains are other sources outside the hospital, probably for commercial ranching. Thus, to prevent the spread of antibiotic resistant strains such as enterococci, or transferable resistance genes, prudent use of antibiotics is necessary in human medicine and veterinary and in the animal husbandry [20].

There are no available studies about strains of enterococci resistant to antibiotics, isolated from Colombian food. Its been reported to a clinical level that the rate of vancomycin resistance in isolates of Enterococcus species by 2004 was about 7% in Brazil - Pan-American Health Organization (PAHO). In Colombia the problem is raised to similar levels and is a common source of nosocomial infections [1].

6. *Staphylococcus aureus*

S. aureus is one of the most important human and veterinary pathogens, and the epidemiology,pathology and antimicrobial resistance of this bacterium has been studied intensively in innumerable studies. *S. aureus* was one of the first bacteria in which the development of antimicrobial resistance (penicillin) was observed [2]. In human medicine, methicillin resistance is not only observed among *S. aureus*, but is also prevalent among other staphylococci as, *S. intermedius, S. epidermidis, S. hominis*,etc, have been isolated from animal sources in different studies and have been demostraded that they strains have mec A gene and are Methicillin resistan bacteria. [4]

In the United States, during 1992–2003, the number of health care–associated infections due to MRSA increased from 35.9% to 64.4% and in UK, death certificates increased by 39% [30]. In Colombia, the CA-MRSA (community-acquired, or community-associated *Staphylococcus aureus*) increased from 1% in 2001 to 5.4% in 2006 [31].

While environmental MRSA transmission has been investigated, transmission through food products has not received enough attention [32, 33]. However, Normmano et al. established the presence of *S.aureus* strains that harboured the mecA gene isolated from food samples such as bovine milk, mozzarella cheese, and pecorino cheese [33]. Other than information from that report the current prevalence of resistant bacteria in food matrices and levels of MRSA consumer exposure risks remain unknown.

Nowadays the assessment of the activity of an antibiotic is crucial to the successful outcome of antimicrobial therapy; however, the development of resistance both in human and animal bacterial pathogens has been associated with the extensive therapeutic use of antimicrobials or with their administration as growth promoters in meat production [34, 35].

In order to achieve the detection of sensitivity or resistance of *Staphylococcus aureus* strains, various techniques have been described, such as the employment of a cefoxitin 30 ug disc, using semiconfluent inoculums and overnight incubation at 35°C, resulting in a sensitivity of 100% and a specificity of 99%. In this way, disc diffusion remains the method of choice for routine screening for methicillin resistance, when the technical or economic capabilities are absent in the microbiological laboratories [36]

In addition, the most widely used molecular typing method for the study of local and global epidemiologies of MRSA is pulsed field gel electrophoresis (PFGE). This method has been used to identify MRSA clones that have a particular ability to cause major outbreaks [37, 38].

An unpublished study developed by the "Laboratorio de Ecología Microbiana y de Alimentos" (LEMA at the Universidad de los Andes), in Colombia genotyped the MRSA strain detecting *mecA* gene isolated from food samples circulating in Bogotá. Positive strains were genotyped for the identification of clonal groups using pulsed field electrophoresis (PFGE). 5 of the 149 strains were confirmed to have the *mecA* gene, indicating the presence of the SCC cassette. The electrophoretic pattern obtained by PFGE for these strains has revealed that 4 (80%) of the 5 strains belong to the Chilean clone, with 100% genetic similarity; this clone has been associated with 65% of infections associated with health care. This is the first evidence of the presence of MRSA in food in Colombia; nevertheless, this study is not published yet but is in the process of submission to publication[39].

Furthermore, a review of the resistance of gram-positive cocci in Colombia shows how our neighbors, Ecuador and Venezuela have a lower rate of resistance to that identified in our country at that time (25% vs. 47%) for coagulase-negative staphylococci-hospital in 2004 to the Pan American Health Organization (PAHO), where the frequency of *S. aureus* resistant to methicillin is much higher, with maximum values for Bogotá 60% and 70% for the 2001 to 2003 period. [40]. Reyes. J. et al, investigated the resistance profiles and mechanism of macrolide resistance in isolates of *Streptococcus pneumoniae* (1679), *Staphylococcus aureus* (348), coagulase-negative staphylococci (CoNS) (175), and *Enterococcus* spp. (123) from Colombian hospitals. The prevalence of macrolide resistance is low in Colombian pneumococci and high in MRSA (cMLS$_B$-type). [41].

7. Lactic acid bacteria (LAB)

For several decades, studies on the selection and spread of antibiotic resistance have focused mainly on clinically relevant species. However, recently several researchers have suggested that commensal bacteria such as lactic acid bacteria (LAB) may act as reservoirs of genes resistance to antibiotics similar to those found in human pathogens [42]. The main threat associated with these bacteria is that these resistance genes can be transferred to pathogenic bacteria [43].

Genes that confer resistance to tetracycline, erythromycin and vancomycin have been detected and characterized in *Lactococcus lactis*, enterococci and, recently, in lactobacilli isolated from fermented meat and milk products [1]. One example of the this resistance is the presented by lactobacilli, *pediococci* and *Leuconostoc spp.* which have been reported to have a high natural resistance to vancomycin, a property that is useful to separate them from other Gram-positive bacteria [44].

Thirty-one strains of *Lactobacillus delbrueckii* subsp. *bulgaricus* as components of yoghurt cultures showed intrinsic resistance towards mycostatin, nalidixic acid, neomycin, polymyxin B, trimethoprim, colimycin, sufamethoxazol and sulphonamides. Susceptibilities to cloxacillin, dihydrostreptomycin, doxcycline, furadantin, novobiocin, oleandomycin, oxacillin and streptomycin were prominent while kanamycin and streptomycin susceptibilities varied [45]. This has raised the discussion of new issues concerning the safety of probiotics in relation to the nature of the procurement and distribution of antimicrobial resistance genes [46].

Starter cultures of *Lactobacillus, Weissella* and *Bifidobacterium* of African and European origins were studied for their susceptibility to antimicrobials. Ouoba et al, evaluated and compared on its investigation to 24 antimicrobial, variations were observed and high levels of intrinsic resistence were found among the species studied. These authors confirmed the ability of *Lb. reuteri* from Africa to transfer by conjugation the gene erm(B), (resistance to erythromycin) to enterococci in vitro experiments [47]. Finally, they also identified a higher prevalence of phenotypic resistance to aminoglycosides in isolation from Europe. This is corroborated by recent publications in which they documented the transfer of macrolide resistance in Enterococcus from *Lactobacillus* in vivo [48] .

Pan L. et al, reported the presence of higher MICs (Minimal Inhibitory Concentration) in 14 of 202 strains of LAC, isolated from Chines fermented food. 14 strains reported the presence of multi-resistance and the presence of genes tet (M) and erm (B), mefA and aphA3 located on plasmids or chromosome. They found that lactic acid bacteria resistant to antibiotics are widespread among traditional Chinese fermented food and the incidence of this resistance was dependent on raw materials and manufacturing area of food; thus, the incidence of LAC resistance isolated during fermentation of sausages is much higher than that presented in the fermentation of vegetables. The results presented in these studies indicate the posssible role of LAC as f reservoirs for dissemination of antibiotic resistance in food and environment[49].

In Colombia there are some reports about antimicrobial resistance of bacterias responsible for human diseases, but its unkwon how frequent is the presence of these bacterias in food and its importance in human illness. The following are some comments about the problem of antimicrobial resistance in Colombia. Currently in Colombia, we have data based on antibiotic resistance of nosocomial strains, usually in intensive care units (ICU). This highlights the lack of a comprehensive study of this aspect in the Industrial and Food Process. Data record of 4008 set out the isolates from ICUs in 2003, 4,004 in 2004 and 4304 in 2005, where the most frequent were, in order: *S. aureus, E. coli, P. aeruginosa K. pneumoniae, A. baumannii* and *E. cloacae*. There was a statistically significant decrease in the number of isolates of *A. baumannii*. Salient issues that expose this study is the high resistance to ciprofloxacin (CIP) from *E. coli*, which is used as a marker, because once a gram-negative bacteria is resistant to this antibiotic it must be considered resistant to other quinolones.The resistance phenotype of this organism to third generation cephalosporins suggests the production of beta-lactamases of extended spectrum (ESBL) during the three year study. [50]. Of all the bacteria studied, *A. baumannii* showed the highest rates of multidrug resistance. Therefore, although there was a significant decrease in the number of isolates of this bacterium, in ICU this is a major concern. Among all prevalent in this study enterobacteria, *E. cloacae* could have the most ability to select resistance, including the carbapenems, to produce very high amounts of AmpC and close porins [50]. However, recent studies suggest that the prevalence of vancomycin resistance by the isolation of *Enterococcus faecium* found in South America is low (only 6%) compared to that presented in the United States [51]. Finally, according to the findings of this study, it is urgent to continue working with the national surveillance network of the resistance of both the hospital and those pathogens resistant organisms from food or water, in order to assist in the control of this public health problem of great importance [51].

8. References

[1] Mathur, S. and R. Singh, *Antibiotic resistance in food lactic acid bacteria--a review.* International Journal of Food Microbiology, 2005. 105(3): p. 281-295.

[2] Frank, A., *Antimicrobial Resistance In Bacteria of Animal Origin.* 2006, PP 160

[3] Burgos, J.M., B.A. Ellington, and M.F. Varela, *Presence of Multidrug-Resistant Enteric Bacteria in Dairy Farm Topsoil.* Journal of Dairy Science, 2005. 88(4): p. 1391-1398.

[4] Frank, A., *Antimicrobial Resistance In Bacteria of Animal Origin.* 2006 PP 269.

[5] Lutgen, E., et al., *Antimicrobial resistance profiling and molecular subtyping of Campylobacter spp. from processed turkey.* BMC Microbiology, 2009. 9(1): p. 203.

[6] Inglis, G.D., et al., *Temporal Prevalence of Antimicrobial Resistance in Campylobacter spp. from Beef Cattle in Alberta Feedlots.* Appl. Environ. Microbiol., 2006. 72(6): p. 4088-4095.

[7] Frank, A., *Antimicrobial Resistance In Bacteria of Animal Origin.* 2006 PP 284.

[8] Frank, A., *Antimicrobial Resistance In Bacteria of Animal Origin.* 2006 PP 293.

[9] Johnson J, A.R., and Lynn M. McMullen, *Antimicrobial resistance of selected Salmonella isolates from food animals and food in Alberta.* Can Vet J. , 2005. 46(2): p. 141-146.

[10] Zhao, S., et al., *Antimicrobial Resistance in Salmonella enterica Serovar Heidelberg Isolates from Retail Meats, Including Poultry, from 2002 to 2006.* Appl. Environ. Microbiol., 2008. 74(21): p. 6656-6662.

[11] Beutlich, J., et al., *A predominant Multidrug resistant Salmonella Saintpaul clonal line in German turkey and related food products.* Appl. Environ. Microbiol., 2010: p. AEM.02744-09.

[12] Skov, M., Andersen, J. , Aabo, S. , Ethelberg, S. , Aarestrup, F. , Sørensen, A. , Sørensen, G. , et al, *Antimicrobial Drug Resistance of Salmonella Isolates from Meat and Humans, Denmark.* Emerging Infectious Diseases, 2007. 13(4): p. 638-641.

[13] Van, T.T.H., et al., *Antibiotic Resistance in Food-Borne Bacterial Contaminants in Vietnam.* Appl. Environ. Microbiol., 2007. 73(24): p. 7906-7911.

[14] Van, T.T.H., et al., *Detection of Salmonella spp. in Retail Raw Food Samples from Vietnam and Characterization of Their Antibiotic Resistance.* Appl. Environ. Microbiol., 2007. 73(21): p. 6885-6890.

[15] Li, D., et al., *Antibiotic Resistance Characteristics of Environmental Bacteria from an Oxytetracycline Production Wastewater Treatment Plant and the Receiving River.* Appl. Environ. Microbiol., 2010. 76(11): p. 3444-3451.

[16] EFSA, *Urgent advice on the public health risk of Shiga-toxin producing Escherichia coli in fresh vegetables.* European Food Safety Authority, 2011. 9(6):2274.

[17] Vincent N. Chigor, V.J.U., 2 Stella I. Smith,3 Etinosa O. Igbinosa,1 and Anthony I. Okoh1, *Multidrug Resistance and Plasmid Patterns of Escherichia coli O157 and Other E.*

coli Isolated from Diarrhoeal Stools and Surface Waters from Some Selected Sources in Zaria, Nigeria. Int J Environ Res Public Health, 2010. 7(10): p. 3831-3841.

[18] B.D. Jett, M.M.H., M.S. Gilmore, *Virulence of enterococci.* Clin. Microbiol., 1994.

[19] Frank, A., *Antimicrobial Resistance In Bacteria of Animal Origin.* 2006 PP 319.

[20] Klare, I., et al., *Occurrence and spread of antibiotic resistances in Enterococcus faecium.* International Journal of Food Microbiology, 2003. 88(2-3): p. 269-290.

[21] Ronconi, *Detección de Enterococcus resistentes a altos niveles de aminoglucósidos y resistentes a glucopéptidos en Lactuca sativa (lechuga).* Enferm Infecc Microbiol Clin 2002. 20(8): p. 380-383.

[22] Gomes, B.C., et al., *Prevalence and characterization of Enterococcus spp. isolated from Brazilian foods.* Food Microbiology, 2008. 25(5): p. 668-675.

[23] Macovei, L. and L. Zurek, *Influx of Enterococci and Associated Antibiotic Resistance and Virulence Genes from Ready-To-Eat Food to the Human Digestive Tract.* Appl. Environ. Microbiol., 2007. 73(21): p. 6740-6747.

[24] Johnston, L.M. and L.-A. Jaykus, *Antimicrobial Resistance of Enterococcus Species Isolated from Produce.* Appl. Environ. Microbiol., 2004. 70(5): p. 3133-3137.

[25] Biavasco, F., et al., *VANA-TYPE ENTEROCOCCI FROM HUMANS, ANIMALS AND FOOD: species distribution, population structure, Tn1546-typing and location, and virulence determinants.* Appl. Environ. Microbiol., 2007: p. AEM.02239-06.

[26] Koluman, A., L.S. Akan, and F.P. Çakiroglu, *Occurrence and antimicrobial resistance of enterococci in retail foods.* Food Control, 2009. 20(3): p. 281-283.

[27] Martins da Costa, P., P. Vaz-Pires, and F. Bernardo, *Antimicrobial resistance in Enterococcus spp. isolated in inflow, effluent and sludge from municipal sewage water treatment plants.* Water Research, 2006. 40(8): p. 1735-1740.

[28] Tejedor J, G.M., Gómez L, Mendoza V, Grimón M, Palacios P, *Aislamiento, identificación y resistencia a antibióticos en cepas de Enterococcus aisladas de plantas de Medicago sativa regadas con agua convencional y depurada* Higiene y Sanidad Ambiental, 2009. 9: p. 418-421.

[29] da Costa, P.M., et al., *Antimicrobial resistance in Enterococcus spp. and Escherichia coli isolated from poultry feed and feed ingredients.* Veterinary Microbiology, 2007. 120(1-2): p. 122-131.

[30] Jarvis, W.R., *Prevention and control of methicillin-resistant Staphylococcus aureus: dealing with reality, resistance, and resistance to reality.* Clin Infect Dis, 2010. 50(2): p. 218-20.

[31] Manuel, G.-B., et al., *Epidemiology of meticillin-resistant Staphylococcus aureus (MRSA) in Latin America.* International journal of antimicrobial agents, 2009. 34(4): p. 304-308.

[32] Normanno, G., et al., *Coagulase-positive Staphylococci and Staphylococcus aureus in food products marketed in Italy.* International Journal of Food Microbiology, 2005. 98(1): p. 73-79.

[33] Normanno, G., et al., *Methicillin-resistant Staphylococcus aureus (MRSA) in foods of animal origin product in Italy.* Int J Food Microbiol, 2007. 117(2): p. 219-22.

[34] Normanno, G., et al., *Coagulase-positive Staphylococci and Staphylococcus aureus in food products marketed in Italy.* Int J Food Microbiol, 2005. 98(1): p. 73-9.

[35] Normanno, G., et al., *Occurrence, characterization and antimicrobial resistance of enterotoxigenic Staphylococcus aureus isolated from meat and dairy products*. Int J Food Microbiol, 2007. 115(3): p. 290-6.

[36] Skov, R., et al., *Evaluation of a cefoxitin 30 µg disc on Iso-Sensitest agar for detection of methicillin-resistant Staphylococcus aureus*. Journal of Antimicrobial Chemotherapy, 2003. 52(2): p. 204-207.

[37] Enright, M.C., et al., *Multilocus Sequence Typing for Characterization of Methicillin-Resistant and Methicillin-Susceptible Clones of Staphylococcus aureus*. J. Clin. Microbiol., 2000. 38(3): p. 1008-1015.

[38] Oliveira, D.C., A. Tomasz, and H. de Lencastre, *Secrets of success of a human pathogen: molecular evolution of pandemic clones of meticillin-resistant Staphylococcus aureus*. The Lancet Infectious Diseases, 2002. 2(3): p. 180-189.

[39] Rodriguez-Noriega, E., et al., *Evolution of methicillin-resistant Staphylococcus aureus clones in Latin America*. Int J Infect Dis, 2010. 14(7): p. e560-6.

[40] Espinosa, C., Cortés, J., Castillo, J. & Leal, A *Revisión sistemática de la resistencia antimicrobiana en cocos Gram positivos intrahospitalarios en Colombia*. Biomédica, 2011. 31: p. 27-34.

[41] Reyes, J., et al., *Characterization of macrolide resistance in Gram-positive cocci from Colombian hospitals: a countrywide surveillance*. International Journal of Infectious Diseases, 2007. 11(4): p. 329-336.

[42] Levy, S.B., Salyers, A.A. *Reservoirs of antibiotic resistance (ROAR) Network*. 2002 [cited 2011; Available from:
http://www.healthsci.tufts.edu/apua/Roar/roarhome.htm.

[43] Perreten, V., et al., *Antibiotic resistance spread in food*. Nature, 1997. 389(6653): p. 801-802.

[44] Hamilton, M. and Shah, *Vancomycin susceptibility as an aid to the identification of lactobacilli*. Letters in Applied Microbiology, 1998. 26(2): p. 153-154.

[45] Sozzi, T.S., M *Antibiotic Resistances of Yogurt Starter Cultures Streptococcus thermophilus and Lactobacillus bulgaricus*. Applied and Environmental Microbiology, 1980. 40(862-865).

[46] Çataloluk, O. and B. Gogebakan, *Presence of drug resistance in intestinal lactobacilli of dairy and human origin in Turkey*. FEMS Microbiology Letters, 2004. 236(1): p. 7-12.

[47] Gevers, D., G. Huys, and J. Swings, *In vitro conjugal transfer of tetracycline resistance from Lactobacillus isolates to other Gram-positive bacteria*. FEMS Microbiology Letters, 2003. 225(1): p. 125-130.

[48] Ouoba, L.I.I., V. Lei, and L.B. Jensen, *Resistance of potential probiotic lactic acid bacteria and bifidobacteria of African and European origin to antimicrobials: Determination and transferability of the resistance genes to other bacteria*. International Journal of Food Microbiology, 2008. 121(2): p. 217-224.

[49] Pan, L., X. Hu, and X. Wang, *Assessment of antibiotic resistance of lactic acid bacteria in Chinese fermented foods*. Food Control, 2011. 22(8): p. 1316-1321.

[50] Briceño, D.F.C., Adriana; Valencia, Carlos; Torres, Julián Andrés; Pacheco, Robinson; Montealegre, María Camila; Ospina, Diego; Villegas, María Virginia, *Actualización*

de la resistencia a antimicrobianos de bacilos Gram negativos aislados en hospitales de nivel III de Colombia: años 2006, 2007 y 2008 Biomédica, 2010. 30(3): p. 371-381.

[51] Panesso, D., et al., *Molecular Epidemiology of Vancomycin-Resistant Enterococcus faecium: a Prospective, Multicenter Study in South American Hospitals.* J. Clin. Microbiol., 2010. 48(5): p. 1562-1569.

9

Antimicrobial Resistance Arising from Food-Animal Productions and Its Mitigation

Lingling Wang[1] and Zhongtang Yu[1,2,3,*]
Department of Animal Sciences[1],
Environmental Science Graduate Program[2],
Public Health Preparedness (PHP) Program[3],
The Ohio State University,
USA

1. Introduction

Antibiotics are routinely used in livestock production to treat and prevent diseases, or more often to promote growth of animals at sub-therapeutic doses. However, the huge amount of antibiotics used selects for resistant bacteria, resulting in development of antimicrobial resistance (AMR) mostly in intestinal microbiota of food animals. Therefore, animal manure constitutes the single largest reservoir of AMR. Although most of the AMR is carried by commensal bacteria, AMR genes can be transferred to pathogens of both animals and humans through horizontal gene transfer (HGT). Therefore, animal manure is a source of AMR contamination and poses a potential risk to human health. Because animal manure is the largest reservoir of AMR, management and treatment of animal manure provide an opportunity to contain and destruct AMR arising from food animal production. Several technologies are available for management and disposal of animal manure, including lagoon storage, intensive biological treatments, composting, and land application. These technologies differ in containing and reducing AMR as they create different physiochemical and biological conditions, which affect the survival of bacteria including antimicrobial-resistant bacteria. In this chapter, we discuss the development and occurrence of AMR arising from food animal production, as well as strategies and technologies to mitigate dissemination of AMR off farms to broad environment.

2. Use of antibiotics in food animal industry and development of antimicrobial resistance

In commercial food animal production, large quantities of antimicrobials are used to treat and prevent diseases and to promote animal growth (Prescott, 2008). In the latter case, antimicrobials are added to feed or drinking water at subtherapeutic levels. The Union of Concerned Scientists (UCS) reported that 11,200 metric tons of antimicrobials were used annually in the swine, poultry, and cattle industries for nontherapeutic purposes alone (Mellon *et al.*, 2001). In the United States and other countries as well, up to 50% of the

---

* Corresponding Author

antibiotics produced annually are used in food-animal production at therapeutic and subtherapeutic (for prophylaxis and growth promotion) levels (Barton, 2000; Teuber, 2001). Antimicrobials of almost all classes have been used in animal production. Some classes are primarily used for disease treatment or prevention, such as quinolones, lincosamides, and aminoglycosides, while others are used for both growth promotion and disease treatment/prevention, such as penicillins, macrolides, polypeptides, streptogramins, and tetracyclines. A survey by the American Health Institute (AHI, 2001) showed that among the antimicrobials used also in human medicine, tetracyclines leads the usage with an assumption of 3,239 tons per year followed by a combination of macrolides, lincosamides, polypeptides, streptogramins, and cephalosporins with an annual usage of 1,937 tons (Chee-Sanford et al., 2009). Such usage of antimicrobials creates selective pressure for development of AMR.

Most of the bacteria carried by individual animals are within the intestinal tract, reaching a density of 10^{11} bacteria/g fecal content. In mammalian animals, bacteria account for about 50% of the feces. Most of the intestinal bacteria are commensal bacteria belonging to several hundred species (Andremont, 2003). Because antimicrobials were fed to animals for extended periods of time (weeks or months), intestinal bacteria are under persistent selective pressure to develop resistance to the antimicrobials used. As a result, AMR develops primarily in the intestinal tract and feces becomes the single largest reservoir of AMR arising from food animal production (Chee-Sanford et al., 2009; Chen et al., 2008). It is estimated that 180 million dry tons of livestock and poultry manure is generated annually in the US (Roe & Pillai, 2003). That can be translated into 90 dry tons of bacteria, many of which can be resistant to one or more antimicrobials. Although the majority of AMR present in animal manure is carried by commensal bacteria, the resistance genes can be transferred to bacteria pathogenic to animals and/or humans (Brody et al., 2008; Witte, 2000). Figure 1 illustrates the dissemination of AMR to broad environments through vertical gene transfer (VGT) and horizontal gene transfer (HGT).

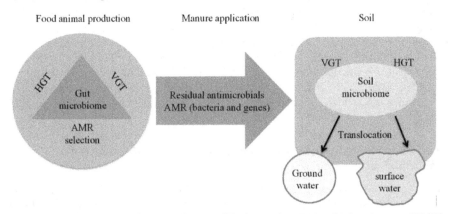

Fig. 1. Conceptualized view showing the possible fates of antimicrobial resistance (AMR) and residual antimicrobials after land application of animal manure (modified based on Chee-Sanford, et al., 2009).

It has been well documented that bacteria resistant to antimicrobials abound in the intestinal tract and manure (Chen et al., 2008). Antibiotic resistance was detected in E. coli isolated from animals soon after antibiotics were introduced to animal husbandry in the 1950s. Tetracycline-resistant *E. coli* was first found in chickens and pigs fed tetracycline in UK (Smith, 1967). With increasing use of various antimicrobials in food animals, AMR has been on the rise (Prescott, 2008). Numerous studies have been reported that examined the relationship between usage of antimicrobials and development of AMR in food animals. Although no precise quantitative relationship has been established, the accumulating body of data indicates a positive correlation between antimicrobial use and AMR development in food animals (Aarestrup *et al.*, 2008; Mathew *et al.*, 2007). As one example, in two farms where tylosin was used for growth promotion or treatment of diseases, 59% and 28%, respectively, of the *E. coli* isolates were resistant to tylosin, while only 2% of the *E. coli* isolated from an organic farm were resistant (Jackson *et al.*, 2004). In another study, as much as 71% of the *Enterococcus faecalis* isolated from swine manure was resistant to tetracycline (Haack & Andrews, 2000). These high levels of prevalence of AMR highlight the magnitude of AMR problem from animal manure.

The severity of AMR is also reflected by the wide occurrence of AMR to many drugs important to both animals and humans. Resistance has been seen to almost all kinds of veterinary antibiotics, including aminoglycoside, sulfadiazine, ampicillin, erythromycin, chloramphenicol, streptomycin, sulphonamide and tetracycline (Agustin *et al.*, 2005; Dubel *et al.*, 1982; Dunlop *et al.*, 1998; Hendriksen *et al.*, 2008; Hendriksen *et al.*, 2008; Lundin *et al.*, 2008). Additionally, AMR is distributed in many bacterial species. For example, resistance to tetracycline has been found in 26 different bacterial genera and in 60 species from swine manure (Stine *et al.*, 2007). Furthermore, with the wider use of antibiotics, multiple drug resistance often develops (Chen *et al.*, 2008; D'Lima *et al.*, 2007; Luangtongkum *et al.*, 2006). A study conducted in the 1980s on swine manure showed low levels of multiple drug resistance (Hanzawa *et al.*, 1984). However, there has been a rapid emergence of multiple drug resistance concomitant with widespread use of antimicrobials in both human medicine and animal husbandry in the past 10 to 15 years (Hawkey & Jones, 2009; Huang *et al.*, 2009).

Multiple drug resistance stems from clustering of multiple AMR genes together, primarily on mobile genetic elements. As a consequence, selection by one antibiotic drug can co-select multiple drug resistance. The selection of tetracycline resistance in beef cattle fed tylosin, a macrolide drug, (Chen *et al.*, 2008) attests this notion. Also, because multiple AMR genes are physically located on the same mobile genetic elements, multiple drug resistance can be readily transferred to other bacteria through HGT. Binh *et al* investigated the types of transferable plasmids that carry multiple AMR genes in piggery manure (Binh *et al.*, 2008) and found many of the 81 plasmids carry multiple AMR genes. Transposons and integrons were also found to carry multiple AMR genes (Barlow *et al.*, 2008; D'Lima *et al.*, 2007). This finding corroborates the potential risk posed from food animal production where antimicrobials are routinely used.

3. Impact of AMR in livestock manure on the development of AMR in environment

Animal manure from food animals is primarily applied to land either directly or after initial treatment or storage in on-farm animal facilities. Antimicrobial-resistant bacteria are, therefore, introduced to soil and disseminated to both soil and aquatic environments. Some studies have been carried out to determine the survival of manure bacteria after land application. Data from human pathogens, such as *Salmonella* and *Campylobacter*, *Yersinia enterocolitica* and *Escherichia coli* O157:H7, showed that their survival in water, soil and manure slurry varies dramatically, ranging from one day to longer than one year (Buswell *et al.*, 1998; Guo *et al.*, 2002; Santo Domingo *et al.*, 2000; Tauxe, 1997; Wang & Doyle, 1998). Although the survival of these manure bacteria remains to be determined, likely depending on the physiological and ecological features of the resistant bacteria, the resistance genes can be transferred to indigenous soil bacteria. AMR can then be further disseminated to other environments, such as groundwater and surface water through seepage and run off, respectively. Eventually, resistant bacteria can enter the food chain through crops grown on the affected land (Boehme *et al.*, 2004). There is a great interest in assessing the likelihood of AMR transfer from manure impacted soil to produce, especially ready-to-eat vegetables (Egea *et al.*, 2011; Rizek *et al.*, 2011).

The impact of AMR from animal manure to soil is also reflected at genetic level. Numerous studies have demonstrated the dissemination of AMR genes from manure to soil after land application. Although most of the manure bacteria may not survive long after manure application, the large number of manure bacteria and soil bacteria can create frequent HGT by which AMR genes are transferred to bacteria indigenous to soil (Sengeløv *et al.*, 2003). These researchers also detected increased levels of tetracycline resistance gene (*tet*) with increased application of pig manure slurry to soil. Our own data also demonstrated an increase in *tet* genes and erythromycin resistance genes (*erm*) in soil impacted by the use of antimicrobials in swine production (unpublished data).

Both surface water and groundwater can also be contaminated by AMR arising from food animal production. Groundwater downstream of a swine manure lagoon was found to contain a much higher level of *tet* genes than the groundwater upstream of the swine lagoon (Koike *et al.*, 2007). Seepage from the lagoon was responsible to the increase in *tet* genes in the groundwater. By the same token, AMR can be readily disseminated to groundwater and surface water following manure application to land and rainfall.

Significant portion (25-75%) of the antibiotic drugs consumed by food animals are excreted by the animal (Chee-Sanford *et al.*, 2009). The half-life of these excreted antimicrobials varies depending on the drugs concerned and the abiotic and biotic conditions that drugs come in contact. A few studies have found that some residual antimicrobials can persist in waste treatment systems and in the environment for long periods of time (Zilles *et al.*, 2005). It is not well understood to what extent the antimicrobials from animal manure can contribute to development of AMR in environment. However, some researchers showed that microbial populations in soil and water bodies could be affected by antimicrobial-containing manure (Campagnolo *et al.*, 2002; Kong *et al.*, 2006; Martinez, 2009).

Antimicrobial resistance is becoming an increasing health concern because antimicrobial-resistant commensal bacteria function as a huge resistance reservoir and can spread AMR to the environment and humans. Antimicrobial resistance can be transferred to human by bacteria that can survive in both animals and humans. And greater concerns come from the possibility of AMR transfer from bacteria of animal origin to those in humans. Additionally, the microbiomes present in water, soil, and crops should also be taken into consideration because the dynamics and population structure of their microbial communities can be affected by animal wastes. Although it remains to be determined if environmental AMR reservoir can serve as an intermediate between AMR genes between bacteria of animals and humans (Canton, 2009; Wright, 2010), some *in-vitro* studies did indicate possible exchange of

AMR genes between soil bacteria and bacterial of animal origin via broad host-range plasmids (Heuer & Smalla, 2007; Smalla *et al.*, 2000). Horizontal transfer of AMR genes can occur among bacteria that are not phylogenetically closely related, and such HGT aggravates the concern. In recent years, numerous studies have been reported on the emergence of multiple drug resistance and its linkage to the mobile genetic elements. Although no proof has been found of exchange of genes between environmental bacteria and human intestinal microbiota, the risk remains.

Cases of food contaminated with common pathogenic bacteria (e.g., *Campylobacter jejuni, E coli, Salmonella* and *Enterococcus faecium*) carrying resistant genes have been reported (Yan & Gilbert, 2004; Zhao *et al.*, 2003). The possible aftermath of AMR mediated via food chain could have two ramifications. First, the colonization of zoophilic resistant bacteria in human gut could compromise the therapeutic effect of treatment of human infections because most antibiotics either are used both in humans and animals or share the same resistance mechanism. Second, there is the risk of gene exchange between colonized exogenous resistant bacteria and bacteria indigenous to human intestines (Hammerum & Heuer, 2009; Luangtongkum *et al.*, 2009; Walsh & Fanning, 2008). Although it remains to be determined if colonization of pathogens of animal origin in human gut results in transfer of their resistant gene to human intestinal microbiome, the potential warrants careful examination in future studies.

Antimicrobial resistance arising from animals can also spread to humans by contact. Akwar *et al.* (Akwar *et al.*, 2007) indicated that occupational exposure of farmers to animals carrying resistant bacteria may constitute a source of AMR in humans. Ahmad *et al.* (Ahmad *et al.*, 2011) reported that insects, which can move freely over long distance, could acquire multi-drug (mainly tetracycline and erythromycin) resistant enterococci from swine manure and transfer them among animal production farms and from farms to food.

4. Mobile genetic elements and horizontal resistance gene transfer

Horizontal gene transfers (HGT), which is primarily mediated by mobile genetic elements, play an essential role in dissemination of AMR genes. Conjugative plasmids, transposons, integrons, phages, and insertion elements have all been implicated in horizontal resistance gene transfer (Barlow, 2009). Since *tet* genes were found on plasmids in the 1960s, most of the known AMR genes have been found residing on mobile genetic elements (Barlow *et al.*, 2008; Lawley *et al.*, 2000; Nandi *et al.*, 2004; Rice, 1998). By analyzing resistant strains isolated from a conventional swine farm, Stine *et al* (Stine *et al.*, 2007) found recombination of *tet* genes and multiple different *tet* genes carried in single bacterial isolates. HGT is primarily responsible for the development of multiple drug resistance (Hawkey & Jones, 2009).

It should be noted that HGT can occur between bacteria that belong to different species. As such, AMR genes can be transferred from manure bacteria to indigenous bacteria, which are adapted to the soil environment and amplify the AMR through proliferation (i.e. vertical gene transfer). Additionally, because transformation does not need a live donor, AMR released from dead bacteria can also contribute to HGT through natural transformation. Thus, AMR genes inside of dead bacteria or released from dead bacteria also constitute a portion of the AMR reservoir and should be included in risk assessment of AMR arising from animal production. Additionally, most bacteria in soil or manure are viable but not culturable. In the case of soil bacteria, as much as 99% may not be cultured (Torsvik *et al.*, 1990). Therefore, most AMR is carried by unculturable bacteria, and AMR present in both culturable and unculturable bacteria should be examined to account for the entire AMR reservoir.

5. Mitigation of AMR arising from animal production

Although antibiotics are widely thought to be the most successful drug in human medicine, risk of AMR to human health emerged from the early clinical practices (Gezon & Cryst, 1948; Rutherford *et al.*, 1946). As elaborated above, extensive use of antimicrobials in livestock production made AMR situation worse. The potential but great risk precipitated the ban, at first partially and now completely, of antimicrobials as growth promoters in Europe (Casewell *et al.*, 2003). The ban led to significant decrease in AMR though not completely eliminated AMR from animal husbandry (Dibner & Richards, 2005). Although there is much debate about the total ban of antimicrobials as growth promoters and AMR prevalence, antimicrobials are still used as growth promoters outside of Europe. Therefore, there is a need to effectively control the dissemination of AMR off animal farms, and management and disposal of animal manure provide a critical control point in containing and reducing AMR arising from animal production systems.

5.1 Lagoons

In most swine and dairy farms, animal manure is typically collected from the barn into a pit and then pumped into an on-farm lagoon. The manure is stored in the waste lagoon for extended period of time (varying from weeks to months depending on seasons) until being applied to crop land. Such lagoons are large to ensure enough capacity to store the manure from large confined animal feeding operations (CAFOs). Quite a few studies have detected high levels of AMR in animal waste lagoons (Fox, 2004; Koike *et al.*, 2007; Macauley *et al.*, 2007; Mezriouia & Baleuxb, 1994). The bottom of animal waste lagoons is rarely lined by any impermeable material, and thus lagoon water, together with some compounds, bacteria, including antimicrobial-resistant ones, can seep into the aquifer underneath and be translocated into groundwater. Thus, this type of treatment, which is thought to be improper in many aspects, can lead to serious pollutions. Several studies have examined the impact of swine lagoons on AMR in groundwater. By comparing AMR profiles of *E. coli* in groundwater underneath swine waste lagoons with those in groundwater of crop farms, Anderson *et al.* showed that swine waste lagoon dramatically increased the prevalence *E. coli* and its multiple drug resistance (Anderson & Sobsey, 2006). Using PCR assays, AMR genes arising from swine waste lagoons were also found to be disseminated to groundwater (Chee-Sanford *et al.*, 2001; Koike *et al.*, 2007). Irrigation of crop land with the lagoon water and subsequent run off can disseminate AMR further to soil and surface water.

A number of studies have examined the potential of livestock waste lagoons to reduce AMR present in the animal manure. By analyzing fecal streptococci using a cultivation-based method, several *tet* gene classes by PCR, and methylation of 23S rRNA by probe hybridization, Jindal *et al.* found that swine waste lagoons had high prevalence of AMR (Jindal *et al.*, 2006). By comparing the abundance of both *tet* and *erm* genes, between swine manure and corresponding waste lagoons, swine waste lagoons were not found to be effective in reducing AMR appreciably (Chen *et al.*, 2008; Chen *et al.*, 2007; Wang *et al.*, 2011;

Yu *et al.*, 2005). Actually, some AMR can increase during lagoon storage (Wang *et al.*, 2011). This is consistent with the previous finding that AMR can increase in lagoons that store sewage (Mezriouia & Baleuxb, 1994).

Currently, there is no regulation on animal waste lagoons, but the potential risk posed by such lagoons is of great concern. Recognizing the potential risk, several research groups have investigated reduction of manure by tertiary treatments that have been used in municipal wastewater treatments. Macauley *et al.* (Macauley *et al.*, 2006) examined the effect of chlorine, ultraviolet light and ozone on swine lagoon bacteria. They found that these treatments at enough concentration or strengths dramatically decreased total bacteria present in swine lagoons, and a combination of chlorine and tetracycline killed all bacteria. Because antimicrobial resistant bacteria have similar ecological and physiological traits than as their susceptible peers, except for their AMR ability, these treatments should equally kill antimicrobial resistant bacteria and thereby reducing AMR present in lagoons. However, additional cost associated with these tertiary treatments probably prevents them from being applied in farms. Indeed, few farms have adopted these treatments.

5.2 Aerobic and anaerobic treatments

Intensive treatments have been implemented on a few animal farms, especially swine farms. These treatments use biological and/or chemical processes to reduce organic strength of the wastewater from CAFOs. The influent and the effluent of an Ekokan upflow biofilter system implemented at a swine farm were found to contain similar levels of both *erm* and *tet* genes (Chen *et al.*, 2010; Chen *et al.*, 2007). Based on a laboratory-scale study, Chenier *et al.* also concluded that aerobic treatments were ineffective in preventing AMR from being disseminated to the environments (Chenier & Juteau, 2009; Chenier & Juteau, 2009). The survival of aerobic and facultative anaerobic resistant bacteria and HGT were suggested as possible reasons for the persistence of AMR during aerobic treatments. It should be noted, however, that aerobic treatments can alter the prevalence of individual resistant bacteria as bacterial species can differ in AMR they carry and in survival during the same aerobic treatments.

Anaerobic digestion of animal manure is increasingly being implemented. The ability of an anaerobic sequencing batch reactor (ASBR) to decrease the AMR present in swine waste was assessed by Angenent *et al.* (Angenent *et al.*, 2008). Although the anaerobic treatment was effective in reducing the tylosin present in the swine manure, both the content and the effluent of the ASBR had substantially higher levels of AMR than that the waste stream fed to this system. In a full-scale anaerobic digester, Chen *et al.* (Chen *et al.*, 2010) also found that multiple classes of *erm* genes and *tet* genes present in swine manure did not reduce substantially during anaerobic digestion even though some classes of *erm* and *tet* genes reduced to some extent. Similar results were obtained by Ma *et al.* (Ma *et al.*, 2011) who used a laboratory-scale digester to digest municipal sludge at both mesophilic and thermophilic temperatures. The similar conditions (mesophilic temperature and anaerobic environments) in anaerobic digester might explain the inability to reduce AMR. However, anaerobic digesters differ in design (complete mixed, plug-flow, etc.) and operation (organic loading rate, hydraulic retention time, temperature, etc.). More studies are warranted to examine persistence of AMR in different anaerobic digesters operated under different conditions.

5.3 Composting

Composting has been used in management and treatment of livestock manure to produce fertilizer with reduced pest and disease incidence (Deluca & Deluca, 1997; Kashmanian & Rynk, 1995; Litterick *et al.*, 2004). Compost has been shown to be effective to kill pathogens and indicator bacteria present in livestock manure (Grewal *et al.*, 2007; Grewal *et al.*, 2006; Jiang *et al.*, 2003; Lemunier *et al.*, 2005; Tiquia, 2005). In surveying abundance of a large number of *tet* genes and *erm* genes, composted manure was found to contain much less AMR genes, up to seven orders of magnitude, than fresh manure or manure treated by other technologies, including lagoon, aerobic treatment, and anaerobic treatments (Chen *et al.*, 2010; Chen *et al.*, 2007; Yu *et al.*, 2005). In a filed study using windrows of beef cattle manure, *E. coli* resistant to ampicillin and tetracycline substantially reduced in the initial two weeks (Sharma *et al.*, 2009). Multiple classes of both *tet* and *erm* genes also exhibited significant reduction in abundance, however, the magnitude of the reduction was much smaller, even after 11 weeks. Nevertheless, the *tet* and *erm* genes differed in dynamics during the 18-week composting, with *tet*(A,C) and *erm*(A) increased marginally by week 11 relative to weeks 0 and 5, while *tet*(G), RPP *tet*, *erm*(B), *erm*(C), *erm*(F), *erm*(T), and *erm*(X)) decreasing at most time points analyzed. The relatively cold ambient temperature (September to November in Alberta, Canada) prevented the temperature from reaching 55°C inside of the windrows and might have contributed to the relatively small magnitudes of decrease in the *tet* and *erm* genes.

The intensity of composting management can affect the reduction of AMR and degradation of antimicrobials during composting because composting management can dramatically affect the microbial activities within composting windrows. This was exemplified in a pilot study using horse manure (Storteboom *et al.*, 2007) where high-intensity management (including amending with alfalfa and dried leaves, and regularly watering and turning) was found to degrade antimicrobials (i.e. chlortetracycline, tylosin, and monensin) and reduce *tet*(O) gene more rapidly than low-intensity management (no amendment or watering or turning). However, *tet*(W) increased in both the composting treatments after 141 days of treatment. More classes and types of AMR genes need to be examined to determine to what extent intensities of composting management affect AMR persistence during composting treatment. By comparing the dynamics of *tet*(W) and *tet*(O) genes between beef cattle manure containing high levels of AMR and dairy manure containing low level of AMR, this pilot study also showed that manure that contains high levels of AMR requires a longer time to achieve significant reduction of AMR. Increased HGT in the presence of high levels of AMR might be one of the explanations in the observed difference in the AMR dynamics.

The temporal changes in AMR carried by both cultivated and uncultivated bacteria present in swine manure during simulated composting at 55°C (the typical temperature achieved inside of large compost windrows) were compared to a simulated lagoon treatment at room temperature in a recent study (Wang *et al.*, 2011). Over a 48-day period cultivated aerobic heterotrophic tetracycline-resistant bacteria and erythromycin-resistant bacteria decreased by more than 7 and 4 logs, respectively, in the simulated composting treatment, while only 1 to 2 logs for both resistant bacterial groups in the simulated lagoon treatment. In the above study, the dynamics of six classes each of *erm* and *tet* genes, including *erm*(A), *erm*(B), *erm*(C), *erm*(F), *erm*(T), *erm*(X), *tet*(A/C), *tet*(G), *tet*(M), *tet*(O), *tet*(T), and *tet*(W), were also monitored. Except *erm*(B) and *tet*(A/C), all the resistance gene classes analyzed declined marginally during the first 17 days of the composting treatment, but dramatically thereafter within 31 days of the composting treatment. The observed decreases in AMR were not attributed to decrease in overall bacterial population, which did not decrease in the course of the composting treatment (Wang et al., 2011). It remains to be determined why different AMR genes decreased at varying rates during composting. Two plausible explanations were offered to explain why cultured resistant bacteria decreased to a greater extent than the AMR genes analyzed: first, some resistant bacteria lost culturability or viability during composting, but their genetic materials, including the AMR genes, persisted. Second, not all the AMR genes were accounted for, as not all AMR genes could be detected by any existing real-time PCR assays. However, it is also possible that AMR might be more prevalent among culturable bacteria than among unculturable bacteria. Future studies are needed to test this hypothesis.

Different classes of *tet* or *erm* genes were found to have different persistence during composting treatment. For example, *tet*(W) was reduced slower than *tet*(O) irrespective of intensity of composting treatment of horse manure (Storteboom et al., 2007). Wang et al. also showed that *erm*(B) and *tet*(A/C) were more persistent than *erm*(A), *erm*(B), *erm*(C), *erm*(F), *erm*(T), *erm*(X), *tet*(A/C), *tet*(G), *tet*(M), *tet*(O), *tet*(T), or *tet*(W). Difference in host ranges of AMR genes and ecology and physiology of resistant bacterial hosts are major factors contributing to the variations in persistence of AMR genes. However, more detailed investigation is needed to elucidate the mechanism that affecting persistence of different AMR.

The high efficacy of composting in reducing AMR was hypothesized to be attributed to several reasons (Chen et al., 2010; Wang et al., 2011). First, livestock manure is dominated by mesophilic anaerobic bacteria, which can be killed by the thermal aerobic conditions created in compost. Second, compost has relatively low water content and thus water activity. As such, proliferation of bacteria, including antimicrobial-resistant bacteria, can be greatly reduced within compost piles or windrows. Third, horizontal transfer of resistant genes is hindered because of the phylogenetic distance between aerobic thermophiles and the anaerobic mesophiles (Chenier & Juteau, 2009; Chenier & Juteau, 2009). Indeed, Guan et al. (Guan et al., 2010; Guan et al., 2007) showed that although resistant mobile plasmids carried by E. coli could survive and be transferred during chicken manure composting, higher temperature helped prevent spread of the plasmids in the environment. The relatively low water activity and the solid state within compost matrix should also reduce HGT (Wang et al., 2011). Taken together, composting is an effective technology to reduce AMR and should help mitigate dissemination of AMR arising from animal production. .

6. Concluding remarks

Although the role(s) of AMR to bacteria is a matter of debate (Aminov, 2009; Davies, 2006; Yim et al., 2007; Yim et al., 2006), it is a fact that the widespread of AMR poses a risk to human health and livestock manure from CAFOs is a large source of AMR. Reduced use of antimicrobials in animal production is an option in decreasing development of AMR, but the perceived negative effects on productivity make it not likely, at least in the near future, to ban Antibiotic growth promoter (AGP) in many countries. Therefore, manure treatment and management should be considered as a critical control point to reduce dissemination of AMR off animal farms. Lagoon storage is probably the poorest in terms of reducing AMR present in animal manure, while compost is the most effective. Aerobic biological treatments do not effectively reduce total AMR, but shift the resistant bacterial populations. Anaerobic treatment operated at thermophilic temperature, but not at mesophilic temperature, is another option to mitigate AMR present in animal manure. However, because the current conclusions are based on studies on either a few select cultured bacteria (e.g. *E. coli*, *Enterococcus*, *Staphylococcus* and *Streptococcus*) or select AMR genes (mostly *tet* genes and *erm* genes), future studies are warranted to include more AMR so that the conclusions will be applicable to AMR in general.

Understanding the AMR genes and the corresponding resistant bacteria is essential to assess the risk posed to health of both humans and animals. DNA-based techniques (e.g. real-time PCR) enable measurement of AMR carried in both cultured and uncultured bacteria; however, these techniques typically do not allow identification of AMR-carrying bacteria. To complement this limitation cultivation-based studies are needed. Additionally, metagenomics empowered by massively parallel DNA sequencing provide an alternative in identifying the genes and bacteria in resistant populations.

No treatment technology is practical that can completely eliminate AMR present in animal manure. The surviving AMR will eventually find its way to the environments. In a recent study, we analyzed the cultured bacteria resistant to tetracyclines or erythromycin that were recovered from swine manure before and after composting treatment in a comparative manner. We observed considerable shifts in resistant bacterial populations, AMR genes (i.e. *tet* and *erm* genes), carriage of multiple AMR per isolate, and plasmids (unpublished data). This type of studies is needed to identify the surviving resistant bacteria and their ecology upon land application of composted manure.

7. References

Aarestrup, F. M., Oliver Duran, C. & Burch, D. G. (2008). Antimicrobial resistance in swine production. *Anim Health Res Rev*, 9(2), 135-148.

Agustin, A. I., Carraminana, J. J., Rota, C. & Herrera, A. (2005). Antimicrobial resistance of Salmonella spp. from pigs at slaughter in Spain in 1993 and 2001. *Letters in Applied Microbiology*, 41(1), 39-44.

Ahmad, A., Ghosh, A., Schal, C. & Zurek, L. (2011). Insects in confined swine operations carry a large antibiotic resistant and potentially virulent enterococcal community. *BMC Microbiology*, 11(1), 23.

Akwar, T. H., Poppe, C., Wilson, J., Reid-Smith, R. J., Dyck, M., Waddington, J., Shang, D., Dassie, N. & McEwen, S. A. (2007). Risk factors for antimicrobial resistance among fecal Escherichia coli from residents on forty-three swine farms. *Microb Drug Resist*, 13(1), 69-76.

Aminov, R. I. (2009). The role of antibiotics and antibiotic resistance in nature. *Environ Microbiol*, 11(12), 2970-2988.

Anderson, M. E. & Sobsey, M. D. (2006). Detection and occurrence of antimicrobially resistant E. coli in groundwater on or near swine farms in eastern North Carolina. *Water Sci Technol*, 54(3), 211-8.

Andremont, A. (2003). Commensal flora may play key role in spreading antibiotic resistance. *ASM News*, 69(12), 601-607.

Angenent, L. T., Mau, M., George, U., Zahn, J. A. & Raskin, L. (2008). Effect of the presence of the antimicrobial tylosin in swine waste on anaerobic treatment. *Water Res*, 42(10-11), 2377-84.

Barlow, M. (2009). What antimicrobial resistance has taught us about horizontal gene transfer. *Methods Mol Biol*, 532, 397-411.

Barlow, R. S., Fegan, N. & Gobius, K. S. (2008). A comparison of antibiotic resistance integrons in cattle from separate beef meat production systems at slaughter. *J Appl Microbiol*, 104(3), 651-8.

Barton, M. D. (2000). Antibiotic use in animal feed and its impact on human health. *Nutr. Res. Rev.*, 13, 279-299.

Binh, C. T., Heuer, H., Kaupenjohann, M. & Smalla, K. (2008). Piggery manure used for soil fertilization is a reservoir for transferable antibiotic resistance plasmids. *FEMS Microbiol Ecol*, 66(1), 25-37.

Boehme, S., Werner, G., Klare, I., Reissbrodt, R. & Witte, W. (2004). Occurrence of antibiotic-resistant enterobacteria in agricultural foodstuffs. *Mol Nutr Food Res*, 48(7), 522-31.

Brody, T., Yavatkar, A. S., Lin, Y., Ross, J., Kuzin, A., Kundu, M., Fann, Y. & Odenwald, W. F. (2008). Horizontal gene transfers link a human MRSA pathogen to contagious bovine mastitis bacteria. *PLoS ONE*, 3(8), e3074.

Buswell, C. M., Herlihy, Y. M., Lawrence, L. M., McGuiggan, J. T., Marsh, P. D., Keevil, C. W. & Leach, S. A. (1998). Extended survival and persistence of Campylobacter spp. in water and aquatic biofilms and their detection by immunofluorescent-antibody and -rRNA staining. *Appl Environ Microbiol*, 64(2), 733-41.

Campagnolo, E. R., Johnson, K. R., Karpati, A., Rubin, C. S., Kolpin, D. W., Meyer, M. T., Esteban, J. E., Currier, R. W., Smith, K., Thu, K. M. & McGeehin, M. (2002). Antimicrobial residues in animal waste and water resources proximal to large-scale swine and poultry feeding operations. *Sci Total Environ*, 299(1-3), 89-95.

Canton, R. (2009). Antibiotic resistance genes from the environment: a perspective through newly identified antibiotic resistance mechanisms in the clinical setting. *Clin Microbiol Infect*, 15 Suppl 1, 20-5.

Casewell, M., Friis, C., Marco, E., McMullin, P. & Phillips, I. (2003). The European ban on growth-promoting antibiotics and emerging consequences for human and animal health. *J Antimicrob Chemother*, 52(2), 159-61.

Chee-Sanford, J. C., Aminov, R. I., Krapac, I. J., Garrigues-Jeanjean, N. & Mackie, R. I. (2001). Occurrence and diversity of tetracycline resistance genes in lagoons and groundwater underlying two swine production facilities. *Appl. Environ. Microbiol.*, 67(4), 1494-1502.

Chee-Sanford, J. C., Mackie, R. I., Koike, S., Krapac, I. G., Lin, Y. F., Yannarell, A. C., Maxwell, S. & Aminov, R. I. (2009). Fate and transport of antibiotic residues and antibiotic resistance genes following land application of manure waste. *J Environ Qual*, 38(3), 1086-108.

Chen, J., Fluharty, F. L., St-Pierre, N., Morrison, M. & Yu, Z. (2008). Technical note: Occurrence in fecal microbiota of genes conferring resistance to both macrolide-lincosamide-streptogramin B and tetracyclines concomitant with feeding of beef cattle with tylosin. *J Anim Sci*, 86(9), 2385-2391.

Chen, J., Michel Jr., F. C., Sreevatsan, S., Morrison, M. & Yu, Z. (2010). Occurrence and persistence of erythromycin resistance genes (*erm*) and tetracycline resistance genes (*tet*) in waste treatment systems on swine farms. *Microbial Ecology*, 60, 479-486.

Chen, J., Yu, Z., Michel Jr., F. C., Wittum, T. & Morrison, M. (2007). Development and application of real-time PCR assays for quantification of *erm* genes conferring resistance to macrolides-lincosamides-streptogramin B in livestock manure and manure management systems. *Appl. Environ. Microbiol.*, 73(14), 4407-4416.

Chenier, M. R. & Juteau, P. (2009). Fate of chlortetracycline- and tylosin-resistant bacteria in an aerobic thermophilic sequencing batch reactor treating swine waste. *Microb Ecol*, 58(1), 86-97.

Chenier, M. R. & Juteau, P. (2009). Impact of an aerobic thermophilic sequencing batch reactor on antibiotic-resistant anaerobic bacteria in swine waste. *Microb Ecol*, 58(4), 773-85.

D'Lima, C. B., Miller, W. G., Mandrell, R. E., Wright, S. L., Siletzky, R. M., Carver, D. K. & Kathariou, S. (2007). Clonal Population Structure and Specific Genotypes of Multidrug-Resistant Campylobacter coli from Turkeys. *Appl. Environ. Microbiol.*, 73(7), 2156-2164.

Davies, J. (2006). Are antibiotics naturally antibiotics? *J Ind Microbiol Biotechnol*, 33(7), 496-9.

Deluca, T. H. & Deluca, D. K. (1997). Composting for feedlot manure management and soil quality. *Journal of Production Agriculture*, 10(2), 235-241.

Dibner, J. J. & Richards, J. D. (2005). Antibiotic growth promoters in agriculture: history and mode of action. *Poult Sci*, 84(4), 634-43.

Dubel, J. R., Zink, D. L., Kelley, L. M., Naqi, S. A. & Renshaw, H. W. (1982). Bacterial antibiotic resistance frequency of gentamicin resistant strains of *Escherichia coli* in the fecal microflora of commercial turkeys. *American Journal of Veterinary Research*, 43(10), 1786-1789.

Dunlop, R. H., McEwen, S. A., Meek, A. H., Black, W. D., Friendship, R. M. & Clarke, R. C. (1998). Prevalences of resistance to seven antimicrobials among fecal Escherichia coli of swine on thirty-four farrow-to-finish farms in Ontario, Canada. *Prev Vet Med*, 34(4), 265-82.

Egea, P., Lopez-Cerero, L., Navarro, M. D., Rodriguez-Bano, J. & Pascual, A. (2011). Assessment of the presence of extended-spectrum beta-lactamase-producing Escherichia coli in eggshells and ready-to-eat products. *Eur J Clin Microbiol Infect Dis*, 30(9), 1045-7.

Fox, J. (2004). Drug resistance at the community level and in swine lagoons, ground water. *ASM News*, 70(9), 392-393.

Gezon, H. M. & Cryst, E. E. (1948). Antibiotic studies on beta hemolytic streptococci; streptomycin resistance acquired by group A, B, and C organisms. *Proc Soc Exp Biol Med*, 68(3), 653-7.

Grewal, S., Sreevatsan, S. & Michel Jr., F. C. (2007). Persistence of *Listeria monocytogenes* and *Salmonella enterica* serovar typhimurium during simulated composting, pack storage, and aerated and unaerated liquid storage of swine manure. *Compost Sci. Util.*, 15(1), 53-62.

Grewal, S. K., Rajeev, S., Sreevatsan, S. & Michel, F. C., Jr. (2006). Persistence of Mycobacterium avium subsp. paratuberculosis and other zoonotic pathogens during simulated composting, manure packing, and liquid storage of dairy manure. *Appl Environ Microbiol*, 72(1), 565-74.

Guan, J., Chan, M. & Spencer, J. L. (2010). The fate of recombinant plasmids during composting of organic wastes. *J Environ Sci Health B*, 45(4), 279-84.

Guan, J., Wasty, A., Grenier, C. & Chan, M. (2007). Influence of temperature on survival and conjugative transfer of multiple antibiotic-resistant plasmids in chicken manure and compost microcosms. *Poult Sci*, 86(4), 610-3.

Guo, X., Chen, J., Brackett, R. E. & Beuchat, L. R. (2002). Survival of Salmonella on tomatoes stored at high relative humidity, in soil, and on tomatoes in contact with soil. *J Food Prot*, 65(2), 274-9.

Haack, B. J. & Andrews, R. E. J. (2000). Isolation of Tn916-like conjugal elements from swine lot effluent. *Canadian Journal of Microbiology*, 46(6), 542-549.

Hammerum, A. M. & Heuer, O. E. (2009). Human health hazards from antimicrobial-resistant *Escherichia coli* of animal origin. *Clin Infect Dis*, 48(7), 916-21.

Hanzawa, Y., Oka, C., Ishiguro, N. & Sato, G. (1984). Antibiotic-resistant coliforms in the waste of piggeries and dairy farms. *Japanese Journal of Veterinary Science*, 46, 363-372.

Hawkey, P. M. & Jones, A. M. (2009). The changing epidemiology of resistance. *J Antimicrob Chemother*, 64 Suppl 1, i3-10.

Hendriksen, R. S., Mevius, D. J., Schroeter, A., Teale, C., Jouy, E., Butaye, P., Franco, A., Utinane, A., Amado, A., Moreno, M., Greko, C., Stark, K. D., Berghold, C., Myllyniemi, A. L., Hoszowski, A., Sunde, M. & Aarestrup, F. M. (2008). Occurrence of antimicrobial resistance among bacterial pathogens and indicator bacteria in pigs in different European countries from year 2002 - 2004: the ARBAO-II study. *Acta Vet Scand*, 50, 19.

Hendriksen, R. S., Mevius, D. J., Schroeter, A., Teale, C., Meunier, D., Butaye, P., Franco, A., Utinane, A., Amado, A., Moreno, M., Greko, C., Stark, K., Berghold, C., Myllyniemi, A. L., Wasyl, D., Sunde, M. & Aarestrup, F. M. (2008). Prevalence of antimicrobial resistance among bacterial pathogens isolated from cattle in different European countries: 2002-2004. *Acta Vet Scand*, 50, 28.

Heuer, H. & Smalla, K. (2007). Manure and sulfadiazine synergistically increased bacterial antibiotic resistance in soil over at least two months. *Environmental Microbiology*, 9(3), 657-666.

Huang, T. M., Lin, T. L. & Wu, C. C. (2009). Antimicrobial susceptibility and resistance of chicken Escherichia coli, Salmonella spp., and Pasteurella multocida isolates. *Avian Dis*, 53(1), 89-93.

Jackson, C. R., Fedorka-Cray, P. J., Barrett, J. B. & Ladely, S. R. (2004). Effects of tylosin use on erythromycin resistance in enterococci isolated from swine. *Appl. Environ. Microbiol.*, 70(7), 4205-4210.

Jiang, X., Morgan, J. & Doyle, M. P. (2003). Fate of *Escherichia coli* O157:H7 during composting of bovine manure in a laboratory-scale bioreactor. *J. of Food Protection*, 66(1), 25-30.

Jindal, A., Kocherginskaya, S., Mehboob, A., Robert, M., Mackie, R. I., Raskin, L. & Zilles, J. L. (2006). Antimicrobial use and resistance in swine waste treatment systems. *Appl. Environ. Microbiol.*, 72(12), 7813-7820.

Kashmanian, R. M. & Rynk, R. F. (1995). Agricultural composting in the United States. *Compost Sci. & Utiliz.*, 3(3), 84-88.

Koike, S., Krapac, I. G., Oliver, H. D., Yannarell, A. C., Chee-Sanford, J. C., Aminov, R. I. & Mackie, R. I. (2007). Monitoring and source tracking of tetracycline resistance genes in lagoons and groundwater adjacent to swine production facilities over a 3-year period. *Appl. Environ. Microbiol.*, 73(15), 4813-4823.

Kong, W. D., Zhu, Y. G., Fu, B. J., Marschner, P. & He, J. Z. (2006). The veterinary antibiotic oxytetracycline and Cu influence functional diversity of the soil microbial community. *Environ Pollut*, 143(1), 129-137.

Lawley, T. D., Burland, V. & Taylor, D. E. (2000). Analysis of the complete nucleotide sequence of the tetracycline-resistance transposon Tn10. *Plasmid*, 43(3), 235-239.

Lemunier, M., Francou, C., Rousseaux, S., Houot, S., Dantigny, P., Piveteau, P. & Guzzo, J. (2005). Long-Term Survival of Pathogenic and Sanitation Indicator Bacteria in Experimental Biowaste Composts. *Appl. Environ. Microbiol.*, 71(10), 5779-5786.

Litterick, A. M., Harrier, L., Wallace, P., Watson, C. A. & Wood, M. (2004). The role of uncomposted materials, composts, manures, and compost extracts in reducing pest and disease incidence and severity in sustainable temperate agricultural and horticultural crop production - A review. *Critical Reviews in Plant Sciences*, 23(6), 453-479.

Luangtongkum, T., Jeon, B., Han, J., Plummer, P., Logue, C. M. & Zhang, Q. (2009). Antibiotic resistance in Campylobacter: emergence, transmission and persistence. *Future Microbiol*, 4(2), 189-200.

Luangtongkum, T., Morishita, T. Y., Ison, A. J., Huang, S., McDermott, P. F. & Zhang, Q. (2006). Effect of conventional and organic production practices on the prevalence and antimicrobial resistance of *Campylobacter* spp. in poultry. *Appl. Environ. Microbiol.*, 72(5), 3600-3607.

Lundin, J. I., Dargatz, D. A., Wagner, B. A., Lombard, J. E., Hill, A. E., Ladely, S. R. & Fedorka-Cray, P. J. (2008). Antimicrobial drug resistance of fecal Escherichia coli and Salmonella spp. isolates from United States dairy cows. *Foodborne Pathog Dis*, 5(1), 7-19.

Ma, Y., Wilson, C. A., Novak, J. T., Riffat, R., Aynur, S., Murthy, S. & Pruden, A. (2011). Effect of Various Sludge Digestion Conditions on Sulfonamide, Macrolide, and Tetracycline Resistance Genes and Class I Integrons. *Environ Sci Technol*.

Macauley, J. J., Adams, C. D. & Mormile, M. R. (2007). Diversity of tet resistance genes in tetracycline-resistant bacteria isolated from a swine lagoon with low antibiotic impact. *Can J Microbiol*, 53(12), 1307-15.

Macauley, J. J., Qiang, Z., Adams, C. D., Surampalli, R. & Mormile, M. R. (2006). Disinfection of swine wastewater using chlorine, ultraviolet light and ozone. *Water Res*, 40(10), 2017-26.

Martinez, J. L. (2009). Environmental pollution by antibiotics and by antibiotic resistance determinants. *Environ Pollut*, 157(11), 2893-2902.

Mathew, A. G., Cissell, R. & Liamthong, S. (2007). Antibiotic resistance in bacteria associated with food animals: a United States perspective of livestock production. *Foodborne Pathog Dis*, 4(2), 115-33.

Mellon, M., Benbrook, C. M. & Benbrook, K. L. (2001). *Hogging it: estimates of antimicrobial abuse in livestock*. UCS Publications., Cambridge, MA.

Mezriouia, N. & Baleuxb, B. (1994). Resistance patterns of *E. coli* strains isolated from domestic sewage before and after treatment in both aerobic lagoon and activated sludge. *Water Res.,* 28(11), 2399-2406.

Nandi, S., Maurer, J. J., Hofacre, C. & Summers, A. O. (2004). Gram-positive bacteria are a major reservoir of Class 1 antibiotic resistance integrons in poultry litter. *PNAS,* 101(18), 7118-7122.

Prescott, J. F. (2008). Antimicrobial use in food and companion animals. *Anim Health Res Rev,* 9(2), 127-33.

Rice, L. B. (1998). Tn916 family conjugative transposons and dissemination of antimicrobial resistance determinants. *Antimicrob Agents Chemother,* 42(8), 1871-7.

Rizek, C. F., Matte, M. H., Dropa, M., Mamizuka, E. M., de Almeida, L. M., Lincopan, N., Matte, G. R. & Germano, P. M. (2011). Identification of Staphylococcus aureus carrying the mecA gene in ready-to-eat food products sold in Brazil. *Foodborne Pathog Dis,* 8(4), 561-3.

Roe, M. T. & Pillai, S. D. (2003). Monitoring and identifying antibiotic resistance mechanisms in bacteria. *Poultry Science,* 82(4), 622-626.

Rutherford, R. H., Marquardt, G. H. & Van Ravenswaay, A. C. (1946). Resistance to antibiotic agents. *Mo Med,* 43(8), 535-8.

Santo Domingo, J. W., Harmon, S. & Bennett, J. (2000). Survival of Salmonella species in river water. *Curr Microbiol,* 40(6), 409-17.

Sengeløv, G., Agersø, Y., Halling-Sørensen, B., Baloda, S. B., Andersen, J. S. & Jensen, L. B. (2003). Bacterial antibiotic resistance levels in Danish farmland as a result of treatment with pig manure slurry. *Environment International,* 28(7), 587-595.

Sharma, R., Larney, F. J., Chen, J., Yanke, L. J., Morrison, M., Topp, E., McAllister, T. A. & Yu, Z. (2009). Selected antimicrobial resistance during composting of manure from cattle administered sub-therapeutic antimicrobials. *J Environ Qual,* 38(2), 567-75.

Smalla, K., Heuer, H., Gotz, A., Niemeyer, D., Krogerrecklenfort, E. & Tietze, E. (2000). Exogenous isolation of antibiotic resistance plasmids from piggery manure slurries reveals a high prevalence and diversity of IncQ-like plasmids. *Appl Environ Microbiol,* 66(11), 4854-62.

Smith, H. W. (1967). The effect of the use of antibacterial drugs, particularly as food additives, on the emergence of drug-resistant strains of bacteria in animals. *New Zealand Veterinary Journal,* 15(9), 153-166.

Stine, O. C., Johnson, J. A., Keefer-Norris, A., Perry, K. L., Tigno, J., Qaiyumi, S., Stine, M. S. & Morris, J. G., Jr. (2007). Widespread distribution of tetracycline resistance genes in a confined animal feeding facility. *Int J Antimicrob Agents,* 29(3), 348-52.

Storteboom, H. N., Kim, S. C., Doesken, K. C., Carlson, K. H., Davis, J. G. & Pruden, A. (2007). Response of antibiotics and resistance genes to high-intensity and low-intensity manure management. *J Environ Qual,* 36(6), 1695-703.

Tauxe, R. V. (1997). Emerging foodborne diseases: an evolving public health challenge. *Emerg Infect Dis,* 3(4), 425-34.

Teuber, M. (2001). Veterinary use and antibiotic resistance. *Curr. Opin. Microbiol.,* 4(5), 493-499.

Tiquia, S. M. (2005). Microbiological parameters as indicators of compost maturity. *Journal of Applied Microbiology,* 99(4), 816-828.

Torsvik, V., Goksoyr, J. & Daae, F. L. (1990). High diversity in DNA of soil bacteria. *Appl. Environ. Microbiol.*, 56(3), 782-787.

Walsh, C. & Fanning, S. (2008). Antimicrobial resistance in foodborne pathogens--a cause for concern? *Curr Drug Targets*, 9(9), 808-15.

Wang, G. & Doyle, M. P. (1998). Survival of enterohemorrhagic Escherichia coli O157:H7 in water. *J Food Prot*, 61(6), 662-7.

Wang, L., Oda, Y., Grewal, S., Morrison, M., F.C., M. J. & Yu, Z. (2011). Persistance of resistance to erythromycin and in swine manure during simulated composting and treatments. *Microbial Ecology*, online First.

Witte, W. (2000). Selective pressure by antibiotic use in livestock. *Int. J. Antimicrob. Agents*, 16(Sup 1), S19-S24.

Wright, G. D. (2010). Antibiotic resistance in the environment: a link to the clinic? *Curr Opin Microbiol*, 13(5), 589-94.

Yan, S. S. & Gilbert, J. M. (2004). Antimicrobial drug delivery in food animals and microbial food safety concerns: an overview of in vitro and in vivo factors potentially affecting the animal gut microflora. *Adv Drug Deliv Rev*, 56(10), 1497-521.

Yim, G., Wang, H. H. & Davies, J. (2007). Antibiotics as signalling molecules. *Philos Trans R Soc Lond B Biol Sci*, 362(1483), 1195-200.

Yim, G., Wang, H. H. & Davies, J. (2006). The truth about antibiotics. *Int J Med Microbiol*, 296(2-3), 163-70.

Yu, Z., Michel Jr., F. C., Hansen, G., Wittum, T. & Morrison, M. (2005). Development and application of real-time PCR assays for quantification of genes encoding tetracycline resistance. *Appl. Environ. Microbiol.*, 71(11), 6926-6933.

Zhao, S., Qaiyumi, S., Friedman, S., Singh, R., Foley, S. L., White, D. G., McDermott, P. F., Donkar, T., Bolin, C., Munro, S., Baron, E. J. & Walker, R. D. (2003). Characterization of *Salmonella enterica* serotype Newport isolated from humans and food animals. *J Clin Microbiol*, 41(12), 5366-71.

Zilles, J., Shimada, T., Jindal, A., Robert, M. & Raskin, L. (2005). Presence of macrolide-lincosamide-streptogramin B and tetracycline antimicrobials in swine waste treatment processes and amended soil. *Water Environ Res*, 77(1), 57-62.

10

Occurrence, Antibiotic Resistance and Pathogenicity of Non-O1 *Vibrio cholerae* in Moroccan Aquatic Ecosystems: A Review

Khalid Oufdou and Nour-Eddine Mezrioui
Laboratory of Biology and Biotechnology of Microorganisms,
Faculty of Sciences, Semlalia, Cadi Ayyad University,
Morocco

1. Introduction

The problem of water scarcity is becoming more pronounced especially in countries with arid and semi-arid climates such as Morocco. Wastewaters discharge into different aquatic ecosystems (groundwater, sea water, river, lake water...), are draining different types of microorganisms and hazardous chemicals. The microbiological risk is not negligible, especially in areas where wastewater or other contaminated water, are reused for irrigation without preliminary treatment or for direct consumption by human and animals.

The emergence of bacteria resistant to antibiotics is common in areas where antibiotics are widely used, but the occurrence of antibiotic-resistant bacteria is also increasing in aquatic environments. Some pathogenic bacteria may occur naturally with the spread of resistance genes.

Vibrio cholerae is a natural inhabitant of the aquatic environment where water plays an important role in its transmission and epidemiology (WHO 1993; Chakraborty et al. 1997). This bacterium plays a role in ecological ecosystems and it is widely distributed in bays, estuaries, coastal water, reservoirs, rivers and possible water supplies for human consumption (Pathak et al., 1992; Caldini et al., 1997; Isaac-Marquez et al., 1998; Dumont et al., 2000).

The interest in examining the non-O1 serogroup of *V. cholerae* has been accentuated at an international level, given that some recent epidemic outbreaks in India and Bangladesh have been caused by non-O1 *V. cholerae* isolated in aquatic environment (Ramamurthy et al., 1993). Currently, it is recognized that non-O1 *V. cholerae* plays an important role as the causative agent of sporadic cases of cholera-like disease and isolated outbreaks linked to the consumption of contaminated water (Yamamoto et al., 1983; Chakraborty et al., 1997; Bag et al., 2008). Non-O1 *V. cholerae* has also been implicated in extra intestinal infections, including wounds, ear, sputum, urine and cerebrospinal fluid (WHO, 1993).

Resistance of *V. cholerae* to commonly used antimicrobials is increasing both in the farm animal and public health sectors and has emerged as a global problem.

This review present a synthesis of our research works on non-O1 *V. cholerae* since 1992, in comparison to faecal indicator bacteria, in some Moroccan aquatic ecosystems especially in wastewaters and groundwaters. We will discuss and compare our works with some other studies over the world.

2. Occurrence, pathogenicity of non-O1 *V. cholerae* in some Moroccan aquatic ecosystems

2.1 Occurrence and ecology of non-O1 *V. cholerae*

The use of untreated wastewater for agriculture irrigation poses serious health problems over the world. Several treatment systems of wastewater were developed to reduce the load of pollution. The stabilization pond system was tested in Marrakech region (Mezrioui et al., 1995; Mezrioui & Oufdou, 1996; Oufdou et al. 2004). It is composed of two oval ponds linked in series, each is of 2500 m^2 in area. The first pond is anaerobic (depth of water 2.3 m) and the second pond is facultative aerobic (depth : 1.5 m). The raw sewage flow to the system is maintained at 5.4 L/sec. The total hydraulic retention time was set at about 18 days with 10.5 days in the first pond and 7.5 days in the second pond.

Non-O1 *V. cholerae* was quantified using the most probale number (MPN) method using three tubes or flasks per inoculated volume and a series of 100, 10, 1 mL, and dilutions of water. They were inoculated into the three tubes with 3 stages: (i) enrichment by culture of 100, 10 or 1 mL of the sample from the series of three tubes of alkaline peptone water (1% peptone, 1% NaCl, pH 8.6) incubated at 37 °C for 18 h. (ii) Isolation was performed by culture of 0.1 mL taken from the surface in each enrichment tube or from one of its dilutions on thiosulfate-citrate-bile-sucrose agar (TCBS), incubated at 37 °C for 24 h. (iii) Identification of the colonies assumed to be those of non-O1 *V. cholerae* was carried out according to the methodology described by Lesne *et al.* (1991), Mezrioui and Oufdou (1996), Lamrani Alaoui et al. (2008) and Lamrani et al. (2010).

The seasonal abundance of non-O1 *V. cholerae* in wastewaters before and after treatment in stabilization ponds in an arid Mediterranean climate has been undertaken. A series of stations along the two stabilization ponds were sampled during two periods. The cold (or hot) period corresponds to months when the water temperature is below (or above) 22°C. This temperature was the average water temperature for the whole period of study (16 months).

Results showed that high abundances of non-O1 *V. cholerae* were noted during the hot months and low abundances during the cold months. In treated wastewaters, high abundances of non-O1 *V. cholerae* were recorded during hot period with an average abundance of 1.7x10^3 MPN/mL. During cold periods, these densities were calculated to be 2.5x10^1 MPN mL^{-1}. These seasonal dynamics were confirmed by the autocorrelation coefficient showing the cyclic nature of non-O1 *V. cholerae* abundances (Mezrioui et al., 1995).

In contrast, the spatial-temporal dynamics of faecal coliforms (FC) were the inverse of those of non-O1 *V. cholerae* abundances. Average FC abundances at the system's inflow point were 1.7x10^5 cfu/mL, while at the seconf pond's outflow, they were 8.3x10^3 cfu/mL.

The average seasonal variation of FC abundances at the second pond's outflow point was evaluated to 8.3×10^3 cfu/mL at the cold period and 1.8×10^3 cfu/mL at the hot period (Mezrioui & Oufdou, 1996). The inverse relationship between non-O1 *V. cholerae* and FC was more pronounced at the outflow point of the second pond ($R^2 = 0.68$) than that of the first pond ($R^2 = 0.51$).

As for removal efficiency, stabilization pond system of Marrakech led to 97.97% average overall reduction in FCs, whereas this system treatment is not efficient in removing non-O1 *V. cholerae* abundances (Mezrioui et al., 1995; Mezrioui & Oufdou, 1996).

We have also followed the dynamics of non-O1 *V. cholerae* in Marrakech groundwater (in supplying well waters) in comparison with other bacteria of sanitary interest. Sixteen wells covering two regions (Tensift and Jbilet) were studied. They are situated at the North of Marrakesh city (31°36' N, 08°02' W, Morocco) (Lamrani et al., 2010).

Detectable non-O1 *V. cholerae* was present in 81% of samples and the average abundances ranged from 0 to 11100 MPN/100 mL. Detectable *P. aeruginosa* was present in 88% of samples and its abundances ranged from 0 to 1670 cfu/100 mL. The total occurrence of FC and Faecal Streptococci (FS) during the period of study was 94% and their densities varied respectively from a minimum of 0 cfu/100 mL to a maximum of 10200 cfu/100 mL for FC and 6700 cfu/100 mL for FS. The annual average densities of non-O1 *V. cholerae* were 4903 MPN/100 mL in all samples. Whereas, the annual average densities of *P. aeruginosa*, FC and FS were respectively 206 cfu/100 mL, 1891 cfu/100 mL and 1246 cfu/100 mL (Lamrani et al., 2010).

Our results demonstrated that non-O1 *V. cholerae* and the other studied bacteria, occurred in the majority of the studied wells water. These wells serve as an important natural resource for drinking water, domestic water supply and recreation for rural and suburban populations. This fact could be responsible for potential health effects on populations using this groundwater. According to WHO standards, the studied wells are completely unsuitable for drinking water and other domestic uses.

The highest abundances of studied bacteria were detected at the wells located near malfunctioning septic systems or beside a high number of pollution sources such as infiltration of wastewater, septic tanks seepage, discharge leachates or human and animal faecal materials nearby the studied wells. Moreover, the majority of the studied wells are situated at 0 m to 400 m from pollution sources. These factors led to the contamination of the groundwater.

Based on the results of the present study, it is possible to conclude that groundwater can play an important role as a transmission vehicle of non-O1 *V. cholerae* and the other studied bacteria. Isaac-Marquez et al. (1998) considered that the presence of non-O1 *V. cholerae* in water supplies might be responsible for a proportion of diarrheic diseases among population of the city of Campeche and the rural locality of Becal (Mexico). Several reports have demonstrated that gastrointestinal and extra-intestinal infections caused by non-O1 *V. cholerae* are linked with contaminated water and other activities in aquatic environments, and this bacterium could therefore pose a problem for public health (WHO, 1993; Chakraborty et al., 1997).

Our findings (Lamrani et al. 2010) are in agreement with those reported by Nogueira *et al.* (2003) and Isaac-Marquez *et al.* (1998). These authors investigated water quality at sources and points of consumption of urban and rural communities. According to these authors, water distribution system, spring water and private wells samples had high coliforms positive and high percentages of non-O1 *V. cholerae*.

The comparison of non-O1 *V. cholerae* and FC abundances, using the Spearman correlation test, has showed that there is generally a positive relationship between these bacteria in the studied wells. FC can be used to detect the presence of non-O1 *V. cholerae* in Marrakesh groundwater. However, no significant relationship was observed between the presence of non-O1 *V. cholerae* and *P. aeruginosa* (Lamrani et al., 2010).

The ecological role of *V. cholerae* in environment implies a direct influence of environmental conditions and climate on the presence, persistence and abundance of bacteria in the aquatic ecosystem. To explain this difference of behavior of these bacteria, we have established the correlation of some of these factors with non-O1 *V. cholerae* abundances. We also tested some experimental studies on the effects of some environmental factors (temperature, pH, sunlight and algae) on survival of non-O1 *V. cholerae* compared to faecal indicator bacteria (Oufdou et al., 1998; Oufdou et al., 1999; Lamrani et al., 2009; Oufdou & Oudra, 2009).

The correlation of non-01 *V. cholerae* abundances in Marrakech stabilization ponds (Spearman correlation) was carried out. A positive and very significant correlation ($p<0.01$) between water temperature and pH was observed at the system's outflow point. At this point, Spearman coefficients values were respectively 0.91 and 0.76. In the system's inflow, an extremely significant correlation was observed only with temperature (Mezrioui et al., 1995).

The experimental effects of pH, temperature and sunlight were carried out. The strains of non-O1 *V. cholerae* and *E. coli* tested were isolated from the first pond of Marrakech stabilization pond. The survival of these bacteria was studied in experimental microcosms of 500mL flasks, each contained 200mL of filtered outflow water. Each microcosm was seeded separately with a standard inoculums (approximately 10^5 cfu/mL) prepared from a bacterial suspension (non-O1 *V. cholerae* or *E. coli*) in physiological water (0.9% NaCl).

The pH values tested (6.6, 7.3, 8 and 8.8) and the temperature values tested (8, 15, 23 and 30°C) corresponded to those measured at the stabilization ponds over the year.

The effect on bacterial survival was evaluated after calculation of the die-off coefficient k which is determined in accordance with the formula:

$$N_t = N_0 \, e^{-kt}$$

Where N_0 and N_t are respectively the initial bacterial number and the number of bacteria at time t. k is the die-off coefficients expressed in hourly terms (/h) (Crane and Moore, 1986).

The effect of pH on the behaviour of non-O1 *V. choleare* differed from the effect on *E. coli*. The greatest survival of non-O1 *V. cholerae* was at pH 8 ($k = 0.0164$/h) followed by the pH 8.8 ($k= 0.0170$/h). Whereas at the pH values of 6.6 and 7.3, the die-off coefficient were respectively 0.0197/h and 0.0195/h. The alkaline pH of 8.8 promoted survival of non-O1 *V. cholerae* ($k=0.0170$/h) and reduced that of *E. coli* ($k=0.0232$/h). At neutral pH (7.3), non-O1 *V. cholerae* did not survive as well ($k= 0.0195$/h) as *E. coli* ($k=0.0124$/h).

The minor variations in pH occurring in natural environments, making pH a relatively unimportant variable compared with other environmental factors, such as sunlight, temperature... However, in aquatic ecosystems such as stabilization ponds, phytoplanktonic blooms appears systematically and increase pH values (Oufdou et al., 2004; Oufdou & Oudra, 2008). The pH is a parameter that was used to improve the isolation of *V. cholerae* environmental samples by enrichment (using alkaline peptone water at pH 8.6) (Lipp et al., 2002).

Non-O1 *V. cholerae* and *E. coli* survived longer at low temperatures. The survival of both bacteria was noticeably reduced at 23 and 30°C. This low survival rate of non-O1 *V. cholerae* did not explain the high positive correlation between the non-O1 *V. cholerae* abundances and temperature. Indeed, it would appear that the effect of temperature is a function of other factors such as nutrients. In microcosms such as flasks, where there is considerable confinement, nutrients are heavily depleted at 23 or 30°C, with a resultant decrease in bacterial survival. In the environments like wastewater, where there is no lack of nutrients, high temperatures lead to a multiplication of bacteria.

Solar radiation had a much greater effect on *E. coli* than it did on non-O1 *V. cholerae* (Mezrioui et al. 1995). This difference in bacterial survival as a result of sunlight factor could be explained by a difference in the bacterial's reaction to sunlight. Indeed, sunlight is absorber by a sensitizer that reacts with oxygen to form peroxides or hydroxyl radicals (Curtis et al., 1992). These authors indicated that damage to the membrane of an organism is ecologically important, since it makes the organism more sensitive to the effects of other factors such as the high pH values encountered in stabilization ponds. The obtained results by Mezrioui et al. (1995) showed that alkaline pH values inhibit the survival of *E. coli*, and its survival is thus less after exposure to sunlight. Non-O1 *V. cholerae*, on other hand, which survived better at pH 8 than at pH 7.3, is less sensitive to sunlight.

The effect of the cyanobacterium *Synechocystis* sp. on the survival of non-O1 *V. cholerae* was carried out (Oufdou et al., 1998 ; Oufdou et al., 2000). Blooms of this cyanobacterium occur during hot periods in wastewater stabilization ponds of Marrakech. Oufdou et al. (1998) have studied the effect of the picocyanobacterium Chroococcale: *Synechocystis* sp. on the behaviour of non-O1 *V. cholerae* in comparison to those of *E. coli* and *Salmonella* sp.. *Synechocystis* sp. was isolated from this ecosystem and cultivated in laboratory at controlled conditions of light and temperature.

Extracellular and intracellular products released by this microalga were tested on studied bacteria. Extracellular products obtained at the supernatant of algal culture in stationary phase, reduced *E. coli* and *Salmonella* sp. growth and stimulated non-O1 *V. cholerae* growth. Intracellular products obtained after lysing algal cells by ether, reduced *E. coli* and *Salmonella* sp. growth. The effect of products released by *Synechocystis* sp. was compared for axenic and non axenic strain alga. Obtained results showed that the presence of heterotrophic bacteria increased the reduction of *E. coli* and *Salmonella* sp. growth by extracellular and intracellular products of *Synechocystis* sp..

Blooms of this picocyanobacterium in Marrakech waste stabilization ponds, is among the important factors that affect the dynamics and survival of studied bacteria in this aquatic ecosystems which functions under a Mediterranean arid climate.

2.2 Pathogenicity of non-O1 *V. cholerae*

Several virulence factors such heat stable toxin (ST) (Arita et al., 1986), hemolysin (Yoh et al., 1986; Bag et al., 2008) and other cell-associated hemagglutinins (Banerjee et al., 1990) have been identified in non-O1 *V. cholerae*. Production of hemolysin and surface hemagglutinins of pathogenic bacteria, are important virulence determinants as they may serve as recognition and invasion molecules in cell-cell interaction affecting the host-pathogen relationship (Guhathakurta et al., 1999; Singh et al., 2001; Chatterjee et al., 2009). It has been demonstrated that non-O1 *V. cholerae* adheres and invades the epithelial cells of gut mucosa and starts its multiplication (Nishibuchi et al., 1983). This situation occurs only with expression of certain virulence factors as previously cited (Nishibuchi et al., 1983; O'Brien et al., 1984; Ichinose et al., 1987).

To characterize the virulence factors of the bacterial isolates in our study, hemolysis and hemagglutination with human erythrocytes were realized.

The hemagglutination and hemolytic activities of non-O1 *V. cholerae* strains isolated from wastewater and suburban and rural groundwater supplies of Marrakech region were carried out. Non-O1 *V. cholerae* strains isolated from Marrakech wastewater showed a hemagglutination rate of 55%. The distinction between the degrees of hemagglutination showed that 42.5% of non-O1 *V. cholerae* strains are able to agglutinate with a high level, red cells of human blood O group, while the percentage of strains showing hemagglutination reaction with low level is only 12.5%. As for the production of hemolysins, non-O1 *V. cholerae* strains showed 37.5% of β-hemolytic activity whereas no hemolytic activity α was noted.

In the groundwater, bacterial strains were found to be adhesive (hemagglutination), with percentages of 63.09%, 65.09%, 84.06% and 87.98% respectively for non-O1 *V. cholerae*, FS, FC and *P. aeruginosa*. Non-O1 *V. cholerae* strains had the highest percentage of hemolytic activities (production of hemolysin: α+β) (71.29%), in comparison to FS (20.71%), to FC (16.88%) and to *P. aeruginosa* strains (9.13%).

Analysis of a total of 1183 strains isolated from the studied wells, revealed that non-O1 *V. cholerae* had the highest β hemolytic activity (33.12%), while only 3.44% of FC and 4.44% of FS strains have this type of hemolysis. As for *P. aeruginosa*, β hemolytic activity was very low (1.44%). FC, FS and *P. aeruginosa* strains isolated from Marrakech groundwater expressed significantly lower hemolytic activity compared to non-O1 *V. cholerae* ($P < 0.05$, test of two proportions). Hemolysin of *V. cholerae* is suggested to be a virulence factor contributing towards pathogenesis (Nagamune et al., 1995). Guhathakurta et al. (1999) purified a bifunctional hemolysin-phospholipase C molecule from non-O1 *V. cholerae* (O139) showing enterotoxic activity, as shown by fluid accumulation in the ligated rabbit ileal loop and in the intestine of suckling mice (Pal et al., 1998).

The percentages of hemolytic isolates observed in this study are comparable to those reported by Begum et al. (2006). These authors found that 80% of the total non-O1 and non-O139 *V. cholerae* isolates were hemolysin positive. However, our results were lower than those obtained by Amaro et al. (1990). These authors showed that 97% of environmental non-O1 *V. cholerae* strains displayed hemolytic activity for human blood.

Adhesion to the intestinal mucosa represents the first step in the infectivity of bacterial pathogens such as *V. cholerae* (Booth and Finkelstein, 1986). This process is mediated by non-specific (mainly hydrophobic) and specific (binding of the bacterial adhesin with its receptor on the epithelial cell) interactions (Kabir and Ali, 1983). Agglutination of erythrocytes is among the most useful assays to test the attachment ability of potential pathogens.

Bacterial strains isolated from Marrakesh groundwater were found to be adhesive, with a range of hemagglutination activities varying from 63.09% for non-O1 *V. cholerae* to 65.09% for FS, 84.06% for FC and 87.98% for *P. aeruginosa*.

Among 317 strains of non-O1 *V. cholerae*, 60 strains (18.93%) were strongly adhesive (+2) and 140 (44.16%) were partially agglutinated (+1) to erythrocytes. On the other hand, 69.06% of FC strains and 62.02% of *P. aeruginosa* expressed complete agglutination (+2) capacity, and respectively 15% and 25.96% of them agglutinated partially (+1) to erythrocytes.

Our findings are in agreement with previous studies on hemagglutination distribution in *V. cholerae* (Amaro et al., 1990). These authors showed that 109 (78%) of the environmental non-O1 *V. cholerae* strains assayed, possessed agglutinating capacity.

Determination of several potential virulence factors in *Vibrio* spp. by Baffone et al. (2001) demonstrated that species were adhesive, with percentages ranging from 40% for *V. fluvialis* to 55-80% for *V. alginolyticus*, non-O1 *V. cholerae* and *V. parahaemolyticus*.

2.3 Antibiotic resistance of non-O1 *V. cholerae*

Among the 240 non-O1 *V. cholerae* strains isolated from Marrakech stabilization ponds, 89 (37.1%) isolates were resistant to at least one of 14 tested antibiotics (Mezrioui et al., 1995; Mezrioui & Oufdou, 1996). The levels of antibiotic resistance at the inflow and outflow points of the system were respectively 40 and 34% and were not significantly different. This antibiotic resistance level was lower than that obtained by Amaro et al. (1988). These authors showed that among 146 non-O1 *V. cholerae* strains isolated from the environment and tested for antibiotic resistance, 93% were resistant to at least one antibiotic.

It appears that in wastewater treated by Marrakech stabilization ponds treatment, non-O1 *V. cholerae* antibiotic resistance was not significantly modified. However, in the same treatment system, Hassani et al. (1992) have showed that the antibiotic resistance increased in 693 *E. coli* strains as they passed through the ponds. Levels of *E. coli* antibiotic resistance on the inflow and the outflow were 21% and 34% respectively.

Mezrioui & Oufdou (1996) have noted that non-O1 *V. cholerae* showed high resistance to ampicillin, amoxicillin and mezlocillin at all sampling points of Marrakech stabilisation pond system, followed by resistance to cefalexin, cefoperazone and amikacin.

Combined resistance to ampicillin and amoxicillin or to ampicillin and mezlocillin were the most frequently observed resistance pattern. Few isolates were resistant to cefalexin, cefoperazone or amikacin (less than 9%).

More importantly, some strains of non-O1 *V. cholerae* were found to be capable of receiving and stably maintaining plasmids conjugally transferred from *E. coli*. Antibiotic resistance can be transferred from non-O1 *V. cholerae* to other members of the *Enterobacteriaceae* family such as *E. coli* K12. Transfer frequencies in nutrient broth and filtered wastewater were respectively 3×10^{-5} and 2×10^{-8} (Mezrioui & Oufdou, 1996).

As for antibiotic resistance in groundwater of Marrakech-Tensift-Al Haouz region, antibiotic susceptibility testing revealed that the overall resistance (resistance to at least one antibiotic) of non-O1 *V. cholerae* strains was 79%, while it was 100% for *P. aeruginosa*, faecal coliforms (FC) and Faecal streptococci (FS) strains (Lamrani et al. 2010). 317, 208, 320 and 338 strains were respectively tested. The multiresistance level of non-O1 *V. cholerae* strains (69%) was significantly lower than that of FC and FS strains (95%), whereas 100% of *P. aeruginosa* strains were multiresistant. The monoresistance (resistance to one antibiotic) of non-O1 *V. cholerae* was 10% while it was 5% for FC and FS strains. Sixty six strains (21%) of non-O1 *V. cholerae* were susceptible to all antibiotics tested, while none of the isolates *P. aeruginosa*, FC and FS was susceptible to all antibiotics tested. Our results showed that among non-O1 *V. cholerae* strains resistance was most commonly observed towards sulfamethoxazole (75%), followed by streptomycin (62%) and cephalothin (60%) and trimethoprim (49%). A smaller proportion of these isolates were resistant to erythromycin (18%), kanamycin and polymyxin B (12%), cephotaxim (8%), gentamycin (7%) and tetracycline (2%). All the 317 non-O1 *V. cholerae* isolates were susceptible to chloramphenicol, nalidixic acid and novobiocin.

The obtained results showed correlation between bacteriological pollution and their antibiotic resistance and virulence.

The dominant multiresistant profiles noted for non-O1 *V. cholerae* were to seven antibiotics; of 220 strains resistant to at least two antibiotics, 53 strains (24.09%) were resistant to seven antibiotics. The maximal multiresistance was to ten antibiotics with two profiles: "Gm, Str, Km, Tpm, Smx, Amp, Amx, Cfl, Cfm, Ery" and "Gm, Str, Km, Tpm, Smx, Tc, Amp, Amx, Cfl, Cfm".

Of the antimicrobial resistant FC strains isolated, 80% were resistant to five or more antibiotics. The dominant multiresistant profile noted for FC was to eight antibiotics (11.6%). The maximal multiresistance was to fourteen antibiotics with two profiles: "Amp, Amx, Amx-clav, Cfl, Cfm, Cft, Chl, Gm, Na, PB, Smx, Str, Tc, Tpm" and "Amp, Amx, Amx-clav, Cfl, Cfm, Cft, Gm, Km, Na, PB, Smx, Str, Tc, Tpm".

3. Conclusion

Although the stabilization ponds showed considerable effectiveness in eliminating faecal coliforms, the system's final effluent contained not inconsiderable non-O1 *V. cholerae* concentrations. Their presence in treated wastewater limits their re-use in agriculture. The risks associated with the presence of non-O1 *V. cholerae* in effluent will be greater if these bacteria are multi-antibiotic resistant. The addition of a third maturation pond to Marrakech stabilization ponds may help in the reduction of bacteria.

The experimental studies on the effects of some environmental factors (temperature, pH, sunlight and the cyanobacterium; *Synechocystis*) on survival of both bacteria, showed that the alkaline pH (>8) seems to present a more bactericidal effect on FC than on non-O1 *V. cholerae*. Thus, the Cyanobacteria blooms, occurring periodically during summer in sewage stabilization ponds of Marrakech, will be considered as one of the major factors leading to high levels of non-O1 *V. cholerae* and low abundances of FC bacteria during the hot period.

Conjugative transfer of resistance genes occurred between non-01 *V. cholerae* strains and other bacteria such as *E. coli*. The high dissemination capacity for these R-factors plasmids can occur even when intergeneric transfer frequencies are relatively low.

Effluent discharged from stabilization ponds into receptor environment or re-used for irrigation purposes should be purified by more advanced methods prior to discharge in areas of greatest human impact and where antibiotic resistance could well prove to be a serious human problem in the future.

The bacteriological quality of groundwater in Marrakech region suggested that the studied wells water were heavily contaminated with FC, FS, *P. aeruginosa* and non-O1 *V. cholerae*. Their presence could have significant health risks for local population when it is used as a drinking water. According to WHO standards for drinking water, the studied well waters were unsuitable for the consumers. The characteristics of the environment of the prospected wells and their proximity from many sources of pollution as well as the lack of rigorous protection contributed to their contamination. In these wells water, the result of the interaction network underwent a high variability. This may be at the origin of a high ecological instability of the studied bacteria and physicochemical parameters. The need for guidelines to protect groundwater quality in Morocco is imperative.

Non-O1 *V. cholerae* and the other studied bacteria isolated from Marrakesh groundwater are virulent since most of them are producers of hemolysins, hemagglutinins and are multiresistant to antibiotics. These bacteria may have important public health implications. Their role in several cases of gastro-enteric and systemic pathologies noted at the local population of Marrakech area (Jbilet and Tensift region) deserve greater interest and attention.

Urgent reactions are required to apply adequate solutions such as disinfection of groundwater, protection of the wells, public awareness. This study may be considered a typical example of what is happening in other cities in the developing world and it is estimated to assist local authorities in developing plans and actions to improve groundwater quality.

4. Acknowledgment

This work is partly financed by the ifs projects n°F/2826-2 and F/2826-3F.

5. References

Amaro, C., Aznar, R., Garay, E. & Alcaid, E. (1988). R plasmids in environmental *Vibrio cholerae* non-O1 strains. *Applied and Environmental Microbiology*, 54: 277 1-2776.

Amaro, C., Toranzo, A.E., Gonzalez, E.A., Blanco, J., Pujalte, M. J., Aznar, R. & Garay, E. (1990). Surface and Virulence Properties of Environmental *Vibrio cholerae* Non-O1 from Albufera Lake (Valencia, Spain). *Applied and Environmental Microbiology*, 56: 1140-1147.

Arita, M., Takeda, T., Honda, T. & Miwatani, T. (1986). Purification and characterization of *Vibrio cholerae* non-O1 heat-stable enterotoxin. *Infection and Immunity*, 52: 45-49.

Baffone, W., Citterio, B., Vittoria, E., Casaroli, A., Pianetti, A., Campana, R. & Bruscolini, F. (2001). Determination of several potential virulence factors in *Vibrio* spp. isolated from seawater. *Food Microbiology*, 18: 479-488.

Bag, P.K., Bhowmik, P., Hajra, T.K., Ramamurthy, T., Sarkar, P., Majumder, M., Chowdhury, G. & Das, S.C. (2008). Putative Virulence Traits and Pathogenicity of

Vibrio cholerae Non-O1, Non-O139 Isolates from Surface Waters in Kolkata, India. *Applied and Environmental Microbiology*, 74 (18): 5635-5644

Banerjee, K.K., Ghosh, A.N., Dutta-Roy, K., Pal, S.C. & Ghose, A.C. (1990). Purification and characterization of a novel hemagglutinin from *Vibrio cholerae*. *Infection and Immunity*, 58: 3698-3705.

Begum, K., Ahsan, C.R., Ansaruzzaman, M., Dutta, D.K., Ahmad, Q.S. & Talukder, K.A. (2006). Toxin(s), other than cholera toxin, produced by environmental non-O1 non-O139 *Vibrio cholerae*. *Cellular and Molecular Immunology*, 3: 115-121.

Booth, B.A. & Finkelstein, R.A. (1986). Presence of hemagglutinin/protease and other potential virulence factors in O1 and non-O1 *Vibrio cholerae*. *Journal of Infectious Diseases*, 154: 183-186.

Caldini, G., Neri, A., Cresti, S., Boddi, V., Rossolini, G.M. & Lanciotti, E. (1997). High Prevalence of *Vibrio cholerae* Non-O1 Carrying Heat-Stable-Enterotoxin-Encoding Genes among *Vibrio* Isolates from a Temperate-Climate River Basin of Central Italy. *Applied and Environmental Microbiology*, 63 (7): 2934-2939.

Chakraborty, S., Nair, G.B. & Shinoda, S. (1997). Pathogenic *Vibrios* in the natural aquatic environment. *Review of Environmental Health*, 12: 63-80.

Chatterjee, S., Ghosh, K., Raychoudhuri A., Basu, A., Rajendran K., et al. (2009). Incidence, virulence factors, and clonality among clinical strains of non-O1, non-O139 *Vibrio cholerae* isolates from hospitalized diarrheal patients in Kolkata, India. *Journal of Clinical Microbiology*, 47: 1087–1095.

Crane, S. R., Moore, J. A. (1986). Modeling enteric bacteria die off: a review. *Water, Air and Soil Pollution*, 27: 411-439.

Curtis T., Mara D., Silva S. (1992). The effect of sunlight on fecal coliforms in ponds: implications for research and design. *Water Science Technology*, 26: 1729-1738.

Dumont, S., Krovacek, K., Svenson, S.B., Pasquale, V., Baloda, S.B. & Figliuolod G. (2000). Prevalence and diversity of *Aeromonas* and *Vibrio* spp. in coastal waters of Southern Italy. *Comparative Immunology Microbiology and Infectious Diseases*, 23: 53-72.

Guhathakurta, B., Sasmal, D., Pal, S., Chakraborty, S., Nair, G.B. & Datta, A. (1999). Comparative analysis of cytotoxin, hemolysin, hemagglutinin and exocellular enzymes among clinical and environmental isolates of *Vibrio cholerae* O139 and non-O1, non-O139. *FEMS Microbiology Letters*, 179: 401-407.

Hassani, L., Imziln, B., Boussaid, A. & Gauthier, M.J. (1992). Seasonal incidences of and antibiotic resistance among *Aeromonas* species isolated from domestic wastewater before and after treatment in stabilization ponds. *Microbial Ecology*, 23: 227-237.

Ichinose, Y., Yamamoto, K. & Nakasone, N. (1987). Enterotoxicity of El Tor-like hemolysin of non-O1 *Vibrio cholerae*. *Infection and Immunity*, 55: 1090-1093.

Isaac-Marquez, A.P., Lezama-Davila, C.M., Eslava-Campos, C., Navarro-Ocana, A. & Cravioto-quintana, A. (1998). Serotype of *Vibrio cholerae* non-O1 isolated from water supplies for human consumption in Campeche, Mexico and their antibiotic resistance susceptibility pattern. *Memorias do Instituto Oswaldo Cruz, Rio de Janeiro*, 93: 17-21.

Kabir, S. & Ali, S. (1983). Characterization of surface properties of *Vibrio cholerae*. *Infection and Immunity*, 39: 1048-1058.

Lamrani Alaoui, H., Oufdou, K. & Mezrioui, N. (2008). Environmental pollutions impacts on the bacteriological and physicochemical quality of suburban and rural groundwater supplies in Marrakesh area (Morocco). *Journal of Environmental Monitoring and Assessment*. 145: 195-207.

Lamrani Alaoui, H., Oufdou, K. & Mezrioui, N. (2009). Rôle de la désinfection par rayonnement solaire ou par chloration dans l'amélioration de la qualité bactériologique des eaux de puits de la région de Marrakech. *Revue Electronique de Microbiologie Industrielle Sanitaire et Environnementale*. 03 (1) : 96-124.

Lamrani Alaoui, H., Oufdou, K. & Mezrioui, N. (2010). Determination of several potential virulence factors in non-O1 *Vibrio cholerae, Pseudomonas aeruginosa*, fecal coliforms and streptococci isolated from Marrakesh groundwater. *Water Science and Technology*. 61 (7) : 1895-1905.

Lesne, J., Baleux, B., Bousaid, A. & Hassani, L. (1991). Dynamics of non-O1 *Vibrio cholerae* in experimental sewage stabilization ponds under arid Mediterranean climate. *Water Science and Technology*, 22: 387-390.

Lipp, E.K., Huq, A. & Colwell, R.R. (2002). Effects of global climate on infectious disease: the cholera model. *Clinical Microbiology Reviews*, 15: 757–770.

Mezrioui, N., Oufdou, K. & Baleux, B. (1995). Dynamics of non-O1 *Vibrio cholerae* and fecal coliforms in experimental stabilization ponds in the arid region of Marrakesh, Morocco, and the effect of pH, temperature and sunlight on their experimental survival. *Canadian Journal of Microbiology*, 41: 489-498.

Mezrioui, N. & Oufdou, K. (1996). Abundance and antibiotic resistance of non-O1 *Vibrio cholerae* strains in domestic wastewater before and after treatment in stabilization ponds in an arid region (Marrakesh, Morocco). *FEMS Microbiology Ecology*, 21: 277-284.

Nagamune, K., Yamamoto, K. & Honda, T. (1995). Cloning and sequencing of a novel hemolysin gene of *Vibrio cholerae*. *FEMS Microbiology Letters*, 128: 265-269.

Nishibuchi, M., Seidler, R.J., Rollins, D.M. & Joseph, S.W. (1983). *Vibrio* factors cause rapid fluid accumulation in suckling mice. *Infection and Immunity*, 40: 1083-1091.

Nogueira G., Celso V.N., Maria C.B.T., Benécio A.A.F., Benedito P.D.F. (2003). Microbiological quality of drinking water of urban and rural communities. *Review Saùde Pùblica*, 37: 232-236

O'Brien, A.D., Chen, M.E., Holmes, R.K., Kaper, J. & Levine, M.M. (1984). Environmental and human isolates of *Vibrio cholerae* and *Vibrio parahaemolyticus* produce a *Shigella dysenteriae* 1 (Shiga)-like cytotoxin. *Lancet*, i: 77–78.

Oufdou, K. & Oudra, B. (2009). Substances bioactives élaborées par des cyanobactéries isolées de certains écosystèmes aquatiques marocains. *Afrique Science*. 05 (2): 260-279.

Oufdou, K. & Oudra, B. (2008). Impact des blooms à cyanobactéries sur certaines bactéries d'intérêt sanitaire dans le lac-réservoir Lalla Takerkoust (Marrakech, Maroc). *Bulletin de la Société d'Histoires Naturelles de Toulouse*. 144: 35-41.

Oufdou, K., Oudra, B. & Mezrioui, N. (2004). Interactions between bacteria and cyanobacteria in the stabilisation ponds of Marrakech (Morocco): Their role in purification of wastewater. *Proceeding of 3ʳᵈ International training program TCTP' 2004 "Technologies on Waste Treatment and Environmental Pollution Control"*. INRST-LEE / JICA : 67-74.

Oufdou, K., Mezrioui, N., Ait Melloul, A., Barakate, M. & Ait Alla, A. (1999). Effects of sunlight and *Synechocystis* sp. (picocyanobacterium) on the incidence of antibiotic resistance in wastewater enteric bacteria. *World Journal of Microbiology and Biotechnology*, 15 : 553-559.

Oufdou, K., Mezrioui, N., Oudra, B., Barakate, M., Loudiki, M. & Ait Alla, A. (2000). Relationships between bacteria and cyanobacteria in the Marrakech waste stabilisation ponds. *Water Science and Technology*, 42, N° 10-11 : 553-559.

Oufdou, K., Mezrioui, N., Oudra, B. & Ouhdouch, Y. (1998). Etude expérimentale de l'effet de *Synechocystis* sp. (picocyanobactérie) sur le comportement de certaines bactéries d'intérêt sanitaire. *International Journal of Limnology*, 34, (3): 259-268.

Pal, S., Datta, A., Nair, G.B. & Guhathakurta, B. (1998). Use of monoclonal antibodies to identify phospholipase C as the enterotoxic factor of the bifunctional hemolysin phospholipase C molecule of *Vibrio cholerae* O139. *Infection and Immunity*, 66: 3974-3977.

Pathak, S.P., Gautam, A.R., Garg, N. & Bhattacharjee, J.W. (1992). Ecology and toxigenicity of *Vibrio cholerae* non-O1 isolated from tropical river water. *Journal of General Applied Microbiology*, 38: 253-262.

Ramamurthy, T., Garg, S., Sharma, R., Bhattacharya, S.K., Nair, G.B., Shimada, T., Takeda, T., Karasawa, T., Kurazano, H., Pal, A. & Takeda, Y. (1993). Emergence of novel strain of *Vibrio cholerae* with epidemic potential in southern and eastern India. *Lancet*, 341: 703–704.

Singh, D.V., Matte, M.H., Matte, G.R., Jiang, S., Sabeena, F., Shukla, B.N., Sanyal, S.C., Huq A. & Colwell, R.R. (2001). Molecular analysis of *Vibrio cholerae* O1, O139, non-O1, and non-O139 strains: clonal relationships between clinical and environmental isolates. *Applied and Environmental Microbiology*, 67 (2): 910 - 921.

WHO (1993). Epidemic diarrhea due to *Vibrio cholerae* non-O1. *Weekly Epidemiological Report*, 68: 141-142.

Yamamoto, K., Takeda, Y., Miwatani, T. & Craig, J.P. (1983). Purification and some properties of a non-O1 *Vibrio cholerae* enterotoxin that is identical to cholera enterotoxin. *Infection and Immunity*, 39: 1128-1135.

Yoh, M., Honda, T. & Miwatani, T. (1986). Purification and partial characterization of a *Vibrio hollisae* hemolysin that relates to the thermostable direct hemolysin of *Vibrio parahaemolyticus*. *Canadian Journal of Microbiology*, 32: 632-636.

11

Assessment of Antibiotic Resistance in Probiotic Lactobacilli

Masanori Fukao and Nobuhiro Yajima
Research Institute, KAGOME Co., Ltd.
Japan

1. Introduction

Probiotics are live microorganisms that confer a health benefit on the host when administered in adequate amounts (Food and Agriculture Organization of the United Nations-World Health Organization Working Group, 2002). Many microbial species have probiotic properties, but those most commonly used are lactobacilli (Salminen et al, 1998; Caplice & Fitzgerald, 1999; Leroy & De Vuyst, 2004). Lactobacilli have a long history of safe use in the production and consumption of fermented foods and beverages. Over recent decades, as awareness of the beneficial effects of probiotic strains in promoting gut and general health has grown, the development and consumption of probiotic foods has increased worldwide (Saarela et al, 2002). Thus, it is essential to thoroughly investigate the safety of lactobacilli used in probiotic products (Salminen et al, 1998; Borriello et al, 2003).

The human gut is the natural habitat for a large and dynamic bacterial community that has a great relevance for health (Spor et al, 2011). The human gut microbiota is a complex ecosystem colonized by approximately 10^{14} bacterial cells with *Bacteroides, Eubacterium, Bifidobacterium, Ruminococcus,* and *Clostridium* as the pre-dominant genera (Kurokawa et al, 2007). The huge diversity of antibiotic resistance genes detected in the human gut microbiome suggests that antibiotic resistant bacteria in the gastrointestinal tract (GIT) function as reservoir of antibiotic resistance genes (Salyers et al, 2007; Sommer et al, 2009). When probiotic strains enter the gut, they interact with the native microbiota and gene transfer can occur (Teuber et al, 1999; Mathur & Singh, 2005; Salim Ammor et al, 2007). The dissemination of antibiotic resistance genes can reduce the therapeutic possibilities in infectious diseases. It is therefore relevant to look for the presence of transferable antibiotic resistance genes in lactobacilli that are or shall be used as probiotic strains for human consumption or as starter cultures of fermented food or feed products.

This article reviews the experiments to be performed and the criteria for assessment of antibiotic resistance in probiotic lactobacilli. Due to the growing availability of whole bacterial genome sequences, sequence-based identification approaches for antibiotic resistance are also discussed.

2. Antibiotic resistance of probiotic lactobacilli

Many food production is estimated to involve microbial fermentation processes by using lactic acid bacterial (LAB) strains (Food and Agriculture Organization of the United

Nations-World Health Organization Working Group, 2002), for example, sausage, ham, cheese, and dairy products. In addition, probiotics have become available on the market, containing a single strain or a combination of strains. The proposed problem is that probiotic strains might contain acquired resistance genes. From a point of safety, it is necessary to distinguish between intrinsic and acquired resistance genes.

Antibiotic resistance profiles have recently been reported for several lactobailli. These have been found susceptible to penicillins and ampicillin (cell wall synthesis inhibitor) (Danielsen & Wind, 2003; Coppola et al, 2005) in contrast to vancomycin. Most lactobacilli have been found to be resistant to glycopeptides types of antibiotics. However, the resistance towards vancomycin has been demonstrated being as intrinsic (Tynkkynen et al, 1998). Lactobacilli are usually susceptible to chloramphenicol, erythromycin and clindamycin (protein synthesis inhibitors) (Coppola et al, 2005; Klare et al, 2007). In addition, resistance against trimethoprim (nucleic acid synthesis inhibitor), seems to be intrinsic (Ammor et al, 2007). Resistance to tetracycline has been observed more often among lactobacilli (Roberts, 2005; Korhonen et al, 2008). Resistance against neomycin, kanamycin, streptomycin and gentamicin (aminoglycosides) has been observed more frequently among lactobacilli (Coppola et al, 2005; Danielsen, 2002; Zhou et al, 2005).

Acquired resistance genes which are potentially transferable have been detected in lactobailli. These have been described in multiple studies and have been reviewed (Ammor et al, 2007). Two of the most commonly observed resistance genes in lactobacilli found so far are *tet*(M) for tetracycline resistance and *erm*(B) for erythromycin resistance, followed with *cat* genes coding for chloramphenicol resistance (Danielsen, 2002; Lin et al, 1996; Gevers et al, 2003a; Cataloluk & Gogebakan, 2004).

Acquired resistance genes of probiotic lactobacilli have been reported previously (Table 1). In the PROSAFE project, probiotic lactobacilli possessed *erm*(B) and/or *tet*(W), *tet*(M) or unidentified members of the *tet*(M) group (Klare et al, 2007). In probiotic commercial *L. reuteri* ATCC 55730, *tet*(W) and the lincosamide resistance gene *lnu*(A) were detected (Kastner et al, 2006). Hummel et al determined antibiotic resistances of probiotic lactobacilli and to verify these at the genetic level. *L. salivarius* BFE 7441 possessed an *erm*(B) gene, which was encoded on the chromosome (Hummel et al, 2007). Probiotic lactobacilli of African and European origins were studied and compared for their susceptibility to antibiotics. Acquired resistance genes encoding aminoglycoside (*aph*(3')-III, *aadA*, *aadE*) and *tet*(S) and *erm*(B) were detected (Ouoba et al, 2008). The potentially probiotic strain *L. plantarum* CCUG 43738, which displayed atypical phenotypic resistance to tetracycline and minocycline, was found to contain a *tet*(S) gene located on a plasmid of approximately 14 kb (Huys et al, 2006).

3. Evidence of potential horizontal gene transfer of probiotic lactobacilli

When probiotic strains enter the gut, they interact with the native microbiota and gene transfer can occur. Probiotics might contribute to the transfer of antibiotic resistance genes to other commensal bacteria or pathogens present in the GIT. The occurrence of large numbers of transferable resistance genes within the intestinal microbiota is undesirable due to the potential risk of acquisition by pathogens present in the GIT and subsequent antibiotic treatment failure (Licht & Wilcks, 2005).

Probiotic strains	Antibiotic phenotype	Antibiotic genotype (gene location)	Transferability	Reference
L. rhamnosus GG (ATCC 53103)	Vm^r	Not detacted	No transconjugants in mating experiment	Tynkkynen et al, 1998
L. brevis KB290	Vm^r, Tc^r, Ci^r	Not detected	No transconjugants in mating experiment	Fukao et al, 2009
L. reuteri ATCC 55730	Tc^r, Lm^r	tet(W), lnu(A) (pLR581, pLR585)	Potentially transferable	Rosander et al, 2008
L. crispatus L-295	$Em^r, Cm^{r,} Tc^r$	erm(B), tet(W)	No transconjugants in mating experiment	Klare et al, 2007
L. crispatus L-296	Em^r, Cm^r, Tc^r	erm(B), tet(W)	No transconjugants in mating experiment	Klare et al, 2007
L. plantarum L-437	Tc^r	tet(M) group	No transconjugants in mating experiment	Klare et al, 2007
L. reuteri L-285	Tc^r	tet(W)	No transconjugants in mating experiment	Klare et al, 2007
L. reuteri L-285-2	Tc^r	tet(M) group	No transconjugants in mating experiment	Klare et al, 2007
L. salivarius BFE 7441	Em^r, Ci^r, Gm^r, Sm^r	erm(B) (chromosome)	No transconjugants in mating experiment	Hummel et al, 2007
L. reuteri L4: 12002	$Ci^r, Em^r, Gm^r, Sm^r, Km^r, Nm^r, Tc^r, Vm^r$	erm(B) (plasmid)	Transferable	Ouoba et al, 2008
L. paracasei L5	$Am^r, Ci^r, Gm^r, Km^r, Sm^r, Vm^r$	aph(3')-III, aadA	No transconjugants in mating experiment	Ouoba et al, 2008
L. plantarum L7	$Am^r, Ci^r, Gm^r, Tc^r, Km^r, Sm^r, Vm^r$	aadE	No transconjugants in mating experiment	Ouoba et al, 2008
L. casei L9	$Am^r, Ci^r, Gm^r, Km^r, Sm^r, Vm^r$	aph(3')-III, aadA, aadE	No transconjugants in mating experiment	Ouoba et al, 2008
L. paraplantarm L10	Am^r, Ci^r, Tc^r, Vm^r	tet(S)	No transconjugants in mating experiment	Ouoba et al, 2008

Vancomycin (Vm), ampicillin (Am), tetracycline (Tc), erythromycin (Em), clindamycin (Cm), gentamicin (Gm), ciprofloxacin (Ci), lincosamide (Lm), Kanamycin (Km), streptomycin (Sm) and chloramphenicol (Cl)

Table 1. Systematic assessment of antibiotic resistance in probiotic lactobacilli have been reported previously

Several of these genetic determinants in lactobacilli are harboured by extrachromosomal elements which are conjugative plasmids and transposons (Mathur & Singh, 2005; Danielsen, 2002; Gevers et al, 2003a; Axelsson et al, 1988; Gfeller et al, 2003). Transfer from lactobacilli to other commensal bacteria has been documented in vitro (Feld et al, 2008;

Gevers et al, 2003b; Jacobsen et al, 2007; Sasaki et al, 1988; Schlundt et al, 1994). Studying the board-host-range conjugative plasmid pAMβ1, transfer was observed in vitro from lactobacilli (*L. plantarum*, *L. reuteri*, *L. fermentum*, and *L. murinus*) to other commensal bacteria (Ouoba et al, 2008; Tannock, 1987; Gasson & Davies, 1980; Shrago et al, 1986; West & Warner, 1985). In the diassociated model pAMβ1 has been transferred from *L. reuteri* to *Enterococcus faecalis* (Morelli et al, 1988). Interspecies conjugative transfer of tetracycline and erythromycin resistance plasmids from lactobacilli has been demonstrated previously in vitro (Gevers et al, 2003a; Ouoba et al, 2008; Feld et al, 2008). Recently, tetracycline-resistant *L. paracasei* strains were identified in samples of milk and natural whey starter cultures. A transposon *Tn916* including *tet*(M) was transferred to *E. faecalis* in vitro (Devirgiliis et al, 2009).

Transfer has been demonstrated in the GIT of rodents, both gnotobiotic (Feld et al, 2008; Jacobsen et al, 2007; Morelli et al, 1988) and those having an indigenous gut microbiota (Feld et al, 2008; Jacobsen et al, 2007; Schlundt et al, 1994; McConnell et al, 1991; Gruzza et al, 1994; Igimi et al, 1996). In addition, the in vivo transfer of vancomycin resistance has recently been shown between enterococci and probiotic lactobacilli in gnotobiotic mice (Mater et al, 2008). Recent experiments of antibiotic resistance transferability in vivo were also conducted from *L. plantarum* to *E. faecalis* (Jacobsen et al, 2007). However, the potential contribution of lactobacilli to the acquisition and dissemination of antibiotic resistance genes in the human GIT is poorly addressed for both conjugative and non-conjugative resistance plasmids. Nevertheless, conclusive documentation of transfer in the GI from probiotic lactobacilli is lacking and therefore more studies need to be carried out.

4. Systematic assessment of antibiotic resistance in probiotic lactobacilli

Antibiotic-resistance screening for lactobacilli intended for use in dairy products such as probiotics or as starters is now tending to become systematic. The European Food Safety Authority (EFSA) has taken responsibility to launch the European initiative toward a "qualified presumption of safety" (QPS) concept which, similar to the GRAS system in the United States, is aimed to allow strains with an established history and safety status to enter the market without extensive testing requirements (European Commission, 2003). The QPS approach together with the recommendations of the FEEDAP panel of EFSA will give a framework for better decision making in safety assessments of antibiotic resistance (Figure 1) (European Commission, 2005; European Food Safety Authority, 2008).

In phenotypic methods, FEEDAP requires the determination of the MICs of the most relevant antibiotics for each bacterial strain that is used as a feed additive in order to eliminate the possibility of acquired resistances. Those microbiological breakpoints define a MICs which, if exceeded, triggers the need for a more extensive investigation to define the genetic basis of the observed resistance and to assess the risk for transfer of this resistance to other bacteria. In genotypic methods, the latest literature indicates that the search for acquired resistance genes using PCR-based techniques (Klare et al, 2007; Hummel et al, 2007; Ouoba et al, 2008; Ammor et al, 2008; Devirgiliis et al, 2008; Fukao et al, 2009; Rizzotti et al, 2009; Comunian et al, 2010) or micro-arrays (Ammor et al, 2008) is a powerful tool to identify resistant LAB strains.

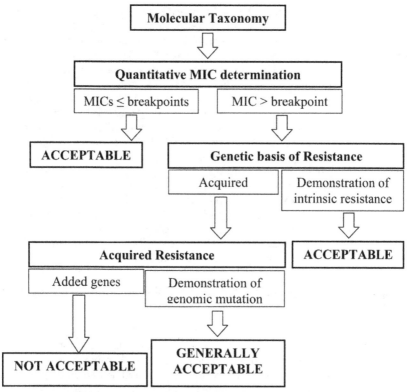

Fig. 1. Proposed scheme for the antibiotic resistance assessment of a bacterial strain (European Commission, 2005; European Food Safety Authority, 2008)

In case of suspected acquired resistance or intrinsic resistance, transferability tests are optional. Conjugation can be detected with bacterial mating experiments. The suspected donor with an antibiotic resistant phenotype is mixed with a recipient strain sensitive to the respective antibiotic, and the transfer of the resistance is subsequently checked. Frequencies of 10^{-6} to 10^{-5} of transconjugant cells are usually the highest experimentally obtainable. If transferability of the resistance is proven, then the strain will not be considered for use in microbial products and further tests are superfluous.

Systematic assessment of antibiotic resistance in some commercial probiotic lactobacilli have been reported previously (Table 1). *L. rhamnosus* GG (ATCC 53103) is a probiotic strain used in fermented dairy products in many countries. Studies have shown that the genes needed for vancomycin resistance in *L. rhamnosus* GG are not related to transferable enterococcal *van* genes and have not revealed any potential risks caused by the vancomycin resistance in this strain (Tynkkynen et al, 1998). The QPS approach was applied to determine the resistance of the probiotic strain *Lactobacillus brevis* KB290 that is used as a probiotic strain in fermented food products in Japan. The authors concluded from their investigation that the antibiotic resistance observed in *L. brevis* KB290 was due not to a potentially acquired mechanisms but to intrinsic resistance. It was concluded that according to the QPS criteria, these results provided safety assurance for the ongoing use of *L. brevis* KB290 as a probiotic (Fukao et al,

2009). In the PROSAFE project, probiotic lactobacilli displayed phenotypic resistance to tetracycline and/or erythromycin possessed *erm*(B) and/or *tet*(W), *tet*(M) or unidentified members of the *tet*(M) group. In vitro intra- and interspecies filter-mating experiments failed to show transfer of resistance determinants. *L. reuteri* ATCC 55730, a commercially available, well-documented a probiotic bacterium, has been shown to carry unusual resistances to tetracycline and lincosamides (Kastner et al, 2006). Deletion of the two plasmids was achieved by use of a protoplast-formation technique. BioGaia concluded that *L. reuteri* strain DSM 17938, except for the deletion of plasmids pLR581 and pLR585, was substantially equivalent to its parent strain *L. reuteri* ATCC 55730. Additionally, BioGaia concluded that the evidence demonstrating the safety of strain ATCC 55730 is equally applicable to strain DSM 17938 (Rosander et al, 2008). Hummel et al determined antibiotic resistances and to verify these at the genetic level according to the QPS system. *L. salivarius* BFE 7441 possessed an *erm*(B) gene, which was encoded on the chromosome and which could not be transferred in filter-mating experiments (Hummel et al, 2007). Probiotic lactobacilli of African and European origins were studied and compared for their susceptibility to antibiotics. Acquired antibiotic resistance genes encoding aminoglycoside (*aph*(3')-III, *aadA*, *aadE*) and *tet*(S) and *erm*(B) were detected. Only the *erm*(B) gene found in *L. reuteri* 12002 could be transferred in vitro to enterococci (Ouoba et al, 2008).

5. Whole genome based assessment of antibiotic resistance in probiotic lactobacilli

Due to the growing availability of whole bacterial genome sequences, sequence-based identification approaches have in recent years been intensively explored for safety evaluation such as antibiotic resistance in probiotic lactobacilli. Commercial probiotic *L. acidophilus* NCFM and *L. reuteri* DSM 17938 were assessed with whole genome and no known acquired resistance genes were detected (Agency Response Letter GRAS Notice No. GRN 000357; (Heimbach, 2008). Whole genome sequences were used to screen for acquired antibiotic resistance genes in lactobacilli strains which could be used in human nutrition (Bennedsen et al, 2011).

Moreover the overall NCBI clusters of orthologous groups (COGs) analysis is recommended (Heimbach, 2008). The COG category V (termed defense mechanisms) consists of many COGs that may have a potential safety interest, such as antibiotic resistance (Heimbach, 2008). Although it doesn't imply that these genes in COG category V are involved in antibiotic resistance, it is recommended to be assessed that there is nothing unusual about the number of COGs belonging to category V and none of the each gene was a part of a detectable mobile element such as predicted transposase genes (Heimbach, 2008). The overall COG analysis of *L. reuteri* DSM 17938 with complete genomes revealed that several COGs belonging to category V were found (Heimbach, 2008). The data indicated that there was nothing unusual about the number of COGs belonging to category V among these strains. Further analysis of each of the genes revealed that no gene was clustered with complete transposons or ISs. Thus none of the genes was a part of a detectable mobile element (Heimbach, 2008).

6. Conclusions

In this context, probiotic lactobacilli are considered to pool the resistant genes and might transfer these to pathogenic bacteria. In order to eliminate this possibility, resistance to the most relevant antibiotics for each strain used as probiotic lactobacilli, food or feed additives could be determined using the systematic QPS protocols. Moreover, due to the growing availability of whole bacterial genome sequences, sequence-based identification approaches have been enployed. These can be used to screen strains for unwanted genetic content such as antibiotic resistance. This screening supports normal safety assessment of probiotic lactobacilli.

7. References

Ammor MS, Florez AB, van Hoek AH, de Los Reyes-Gavilan CG, Aarts HJ, Margolles A, *et al.* (2008). Molecular characterization of intrinsic and acquired antibiotic resistance in lactic acid bacteria and bifidobacteria. J Mol Microbiol Biotechnol 14:6-15.

Ammor MS, Florez AB, Mayo B (2007). Antibiotic resistance in non-enterococcal lactic acid bacteria and bifidobacteria. Food Microbiol 24:559-570.

Axelsson LT, Ahrne SE, Andersson MC, Stahl SR (1988). Identification and cloning of a plasmid-encoded erythromycin resistance determinant from *Lactobacillus reuteri*. Plasmid 20:171-174.

Bennedsen M, Stuer-Lauridsen B, Danielsen M, Johansen E (2011). Screening for antimicrobial resistance genes and virulence factors via genome sequencing. Appl Environ Microbiol 77:2785-2787.

Borriello SP, Hammes WP, Holzapfel W, Marteau P, Schrezenmeir J, Vaara M, *et al.* (2003). Safety of probiotics that contain lactobacilli or bifidobacteria. Clin Infect Dis 36:775-780.

Caplice E, Fitzgerald GF (1999). Food fermentations: role of microorganisms in food production and preservation. Int J Food Microbiol 50:131-149.

Cataloluk O, Gogebakan B (2004). Presence of drug resistance in intestinal lactobacilli of dairy and human origin in Turkey. FEMS Microbiol Lett 236:7-12.

Comunian R, Daga E, Dupre I, Paba A, Devirgiliis C, Piccioni V, *et al.* (2010). Susceptibility to tetracycline and erythromycin of *Lactobacillus paracasei* strains isolated from traditional Italian fermented foods. Int J Food Microbiol 138:151-156.

Coppola R, Succi M, Tremonte P, Reale A, Salzano G, Sorrentino E (2005). Antibiotic susceptibility of *Lactobacillus rhamnosus* strains isolated from Parmigiano Reggiano cheese. Lait 85:193-204.

Danielsen M, Wind A (2003). Susceptibility of *Lactobacillus* spp. to antimicrobial agents. Int J Food Microbiol 82:1-11.

Danielsen M (2002). Characterization of the tetracycline resistance plasmid pMD5057 from *Lactobacillus plantarum* 5057 reveals a composite structure. Plasmid 48:98-103.

Devirgiliis C, Coppola D, Barile S, Colonna B, Perozzi G (2009). Characterization of the Tn*916* conjugative transposon in a food-borne strain of *Lactobacillus paracasei*. Appl Environ Microbiol 75:3866-3871.

Devirgiliis C, Caravelli A, Coppola D, Barile S, Perozzi G (2008). Antibiotic resistance and microbial composition along the manufacturing process of Mozzarella di Bufala Campana. Int J Food Microbiol 128:378-384.

European Commission (2005). Opinion of the Scientific Committee on Animal Nutrition on the criteria for assessing the safety of micro-organisms resistant to antibiotics of human clinical and veterinary importance. European Commission .

European Commission (2003). On a generic approach to the safety assessment of micro-organisms used in feed/food and feed/food production. European Commission .

European Food Safety Authority (2008). Update of the criteria used in the assessment of bacterial resistance to antibiotics of human or veterinary importance. EFSA J 732:1-15.

Feld L, Schjorring S, Hammer K, Licht TR, Danielsen M, Krogfelt K, et al. (2008). Selective pressure affects transfer and establishment of a Lactobacillus plantarum resistance plasmid in the gastrointestinal environment. J Antimicrob Chemother 61:845-852.

Food and Agriculture Organization of the United Nations-World Health Organization Working Group (2002). Guidelines for the evaluation of probiotics in foods, Report of a joint FAO/WHO working group on drafting guidelines for the evaluation of probiotics in food.

Fukao M, Tomita H, Yakabe T, Nomura T, Ike Y, Yajima N (2009). Assessment of antibiotic resistance in probiotic strain Lactobacillus brevis KB290. J Food Prot 72:1923-1929.

Gasson MJ, Davies FL (1980). Cnjugal transfer of the drug resistance plasmid pAMβ1 in the lactic streptococci. FEMS Microbiol Lett 7:51-53.

Gevers D, Danielsen M, Huys G, Swings J (2003a). Molecular characterization of tet(M) genes in Lactobacillus isolates from different types of fermented dry sausage. Appl Environ Microbiol 69:1270-1275.

Gevers D, Huys G, Swings J (2003b). In vitro conjugal transfer of tetracycline resistance from Lactobacillus isolates to other Gram-positive bacteria. FEMS Microbiol Lett 225:125-130.

Gfeller KY, Roth M, Meile L, Teuber M (2003). Sequence and genetic organization of the 19.3-kb erythromycin- and dalfopristin-resistance plasmid pLME300 from Lactobacillus fermentum ROT1. Plasmid 50:190-201.

Gruzza M, Fons M, Ouriet MF, Duval-Iflah Y, Ducluzeau R (1994). Study of gene transfer in vitro and in the digestive tract of gnotobiotic mice from Lactococcus lactis strains to various strains belonging to human intestinal flora. Microb Releases 2:183-189.

Heimbach J (2008). Generally Recognized as Safe (GRAS) determination of Lactobacillus reuteri strain DSM 17938. GRAS Notice (disclosable information) .

Hummel AS, Hertel C, Holzapfel WH, Franz CM (2007). Antibiotic resistances of starter and probiotic strains of lactic acid bacteria. Appl Environ Microbiol 73:730-739.

Huys G, D'Haene K, Swings J (2006). Genetic basis of tetracycline and minocycline resistance in potentially probiotic Lactobacillus plantarum strain CCUG 43738. Antimicrob Agents Chemother 50:1550-1551.

Igimi S, Ryu CH, Park SH, Sasaki Y, Sasaki T, Kumagai S (1996). Transfer of conjugative plasmid pAM beta 1 from Lactococcus lactis to mouse intestinal bacteria. Lett Appl Microbiol 23:31-35.

Jacobsen L, Wilcks A, Hammer K, Huys G, Gevers D, Andersen SR (2007). Horizontal transfer of tet(M) and erm(B) resistance plasmids from food strains of Lactobacillus *plantarum* to *Enterococcus faecalis* JH2-2 in the gastrointestinal tract of gnotobiotic rats. FEMS Microbiol Ecol 59:158-166.

Kastner S, Perreten V, Bleuler H, Hugenschmidt G, Lacroix C, Meile L (2006). Antibiotic susceptibility patterns and resistance genes of starter cultures and probiotic bacteria used in food. Syst Appl Microbiol 29:145-155.

Klare I, Konstabel C, Werner G, Huys G, Vankerckhoven V, Kahlmeter G, *et al.* (2007). Antimicrobial susceptibilities of *Lactobacillus*, *Pediococcus* and *Lactococcus* human isolates and cultures intended for probiotic or nutritional use. J Antimicrob Chemother 59:900-912.

Korhonen JM, Danielsen M, Mayo B, Egervärn M, Axelsson L, H uys G, *et al.* (2008). Antimicrobial susceptibility and proposed microbiological cut-off values of lactobacilli by phenotypic determination. Int J Prob Preb 3:257-268.

Kurokawa K, Itoh T, Kuwahara T, Oshima K, Toh H, Toyoda A, *et al.* (2007). Comparative metagenomics revealed commonly enriched gene sets in human gut microbiomes. DNA Res 14:169-181.

Leroy F, De Vuyst L (2004). Lactic acid bacteria as functional starter cultures for the food fermentation industry. Trends Food Sci Technol 15:67-78.

Licht TR, Wilcks A (2005). Conjugative Gene Transfer in the Gastrointestinal Environment. Adv Appl Microbiol 58C:77-95.

Lin CF, Fung ZF, Wu CL, Chung TC (1996). Molecular characterization of a plasmid-borne (pTC82) chloramphenicol resistance determinant (*cat*-TC) from *Lactobacillus reuteri* G4. Plasmid 36:116-124.

Mater DD, Langella P, Corthier G, Flores MJ (2008). A probiotic *Lactobacillus* strain can acquire vancomycin resistance during digestive transit in mice. J Mol Microbiol Biotechnol 14:123-127.

Mathur S, Singh R (2005). Antibiotic resistance in food lactic acid bacteria--a review. Int J Food Microbiol 105:281-295.

McConnell M, Mercer A, Tannock G (1991). Transfer of Plasmid pAMβ1 Between Members of the Normal Microflora Inhabiting the Murine Digestive Tract and Modification of the Plasmid in a *Lactobacillus reuteri* Host. Microbial Ecology in Health and Disease 4:343-355.

Morelli L, Sarra PG, Bottazzi V (1988). *In vivo* transfer of pAM beta 1 from *Lactobacillus reuteri* to *Enterococcus faecalis*. J Appl Bacteriol 65:371-375.

Ouoba LI, Lei V, Jensen LB (2008). Resistance of potential probiotic lactic acid bacteria and bifidobacteria of African and European origin to antimicrobials: determination and transferability of the resistance genes to other bacteria. Int J Food Microbiol 121:217-224.

Rizzotti L, La Gioia F, Dellaglio F, Torriani S (2009). Characterization of tetracycline-resistant *Streptococcus thermophilus* isolates from Italian soft cheeses. Appl Environ Microbiol 75:4224-4229.

Roberts MC (2005). Update on acquired tetracycline resistance genes. FEMS Microbiol Lett 245:195-203.

Rosander A, Connolly E, Roos S (2008). Removal of antibiotic resistance gene-carrying plasmids from *Lactobacillus reuteri* ATCC 55730 and characterization of the resulting daughter strain, *L. reuteri* DSM 17938. Appl Environ Microbiol 74:6032-6040.

Saarela M, Lahteenmaki L, Crittenden R, Salminen S, Mattila-Sandholm T (2002). Gut bacteria and health foods--the European perspective. Int J Food Microbiol 78:99-117.

Salim Ammor M, Belen Florez A, Mayo B (2007). Antibiotic resistance in non-enterococcal lactic acid bacteria and bifidobacteria. Food Microbiol 24:559-570.

Salminen S, von Wright A, Morelli L, Marteau P, Brassart D, de Vos WM, *et al.* (1998). Demonstration of safety of probiotics -- a review. Int J Food Microbiol 44:93-106.

Salyers A, Moon K, Schlesinger D (2007). The human intestinal tract - a hotbed of resistance gene transfer? Part I CM Newsletter 29:17-21.

Sasaki Y, Taketomo N, Sasaki T (1988). Factors affecting transfer frequency of pAM beta 1 from *Streptococcus faecalis* to *Lactobacillus plantarum*. J Bacteriol 170:5939-5942.

Schlundt J, Saadbye P, Lohmann B, Jacobsen BL, Nielsen EM (1994). Conjugal Transfer of Plasmid Dna between *Lactococcus-lactis* Strains and Distribution of Transconjugants in the Digestive-Tract of Gnotobiotic-Rats. Microb Ecol Health Dis 7:59-69.

Shrago AW, Chassy BM, Dobrogosz WJ (1986). Conjugal plasmid transfer (pAM beta 1) in *Lactobacillus plantarum*. Appl Environ Microbiol 52:574-576.

Sommer MO, Dantas G, Church GM (2009). Functional characterization of the antibiotic resistance reservoir in the human microflora. Science 325:1128-1131.

Spor A, Koren O, Ley R (2011). Unravelling the effects of the environment and host genotype on the gut microbiome. Nat Rev Microbiol 9:279-290.

Tannock GW (1987). Conjugal transfer of plasmid pAM beta 1 in *Lactobacillus reuteri* and between lactobacilli and *Enterococcus faecalis*. Appl Environ Microbiol 53:2693-2695.

Teuber M, Meile L, Schwarz F (1999). Acquired antibiotic resistance in lactic acid bacteria from food. Antonie Van Leeuwenhoek 76:115-137.

Tynkkynen S, Singh KV, Varmanen P (1998). Vancomycin resistance factor of *Lactobacillus rhamnosus* GG in relation to enterococcal vancomycin resistance (*van*) genes. Int J Food Microbiol 41:195-204.

West CA, Warner PJ (1985). Plasmid profiles and transfer of plasmid-encoded antibiotic resistance in *Lactobacillus plantarum*. Appl Environ Microbiol 50:1319-1321.

Zhou JS, Pillidge CJ, Gopal PK, Gill HS (2005). Antibiotic susceptibility profiles of new probiotic *Lactobacillus* and *Bifidobacterium* strains. Int J Food Microbiol 98:211-217.

12

Design, Development and Synthesis of Novel Cephalosporin Group of Antibiotics

Kumar Gaurav, Sourish Karmakar, Kanika Kundu and Subir Kundu*

*Institute of Technology & MMV, Banaras Hindu University, Varanasi,
India*

1. Introduction

Cephalosporins are β- lactam antibiotics. In cephalosporin C, four membered β- lactam ring (which is mainly responsible for the activity) is fused with six membered dihydrothiazine ring to form the basic nucleus, 7-aminocephalosporanic acid (7-ACA) and to which α-aminoadipic acid side chain is attached through an amide bond (Fig 1). (Mandell and Sande,1991)Although cephalosporin was found to be active against large number of pathogenic bacteria (Medeiros, 1997) but the main hindrance in its application is its low stability. Also, occurrence of bacterial strains that are resistant to already existing antibiotics such as methicillin resistant *Staphylococcus aureus* (MRSA) and vancomycin resistant *E. faecalis* (VRE) has led to the search of new semisynthetic cephalosporins with better solubility and new mechanism of action. Only cephalosporin C is found naturally, so it's chemical modification allowed production of a whole series of semisynthetic cephalosporins which can be used as therapeutics to fight organisms that have become penicillin resistant. Chemical modifications of cephalosporin C resulted in new cephalosporin derivatives. These semisynthetic cephalosporins are classified based on their activity profile, the antibacterial spectrum. Each newer generation of cephalosporin has significantly greater Gram –ve antimicrobial properties than the preceding generations, (Stan,2004; Jones,1994; Jacoby,2000; Babini and Livermore, 2000) in most cases with decreased activity against Gram +ve organism. Fourth generation cephalosporins are known to have true broad spectrum activity. (Wilson,1998; Tzouvelekis et al., 1998) In the past decade, even though the cephalosporin antibiotics have made remarkable progress and contribution in the treatment of acute diseases originated from pathogenic infection in clinics, many efforts still exist to achieve the well balanced broad spectrum and to improve beta-lactamase stability. 7α-formamido cephalosporins were isolated as fermentation product of various gram negative bacteria. The development of a new antibiotic focuses mainly with the study and characterization of its mechanism of its activity (Table 1). The β-lactam antibiotics like penicillin, cephalosporins, vancomycin, etc. are specific inhibitor working against bacterial cell wall (peptidoglycan) synthesis but newer strains have β-lactamase activity which destroys most of the β-lactam antibiotics and thus make them resistant to it. However, cephalosporins proved to be more stable to β-lactamase. Cephalosporin-C (CPC) shows similarity to in structure with the penicillin in having an acyl side chain attached to an

---

* Corresponding Author

amino group of a double ring nucleus (Figure 1). The side chain was identical to that of penicillin N, *i.e.* D-α-aminoadipic acid. Although both the types have the four membered β-lactam group, cephalosporin-C have a six membered dihydrothiazine ring in place of the five membered thiazolidine ring system which is a characteristic of penicillins. But these antibiotics are not that effective to be used for clinical purposes. The cephalosporin nucleus, 7-aminocephalosporanic acid (7-ACA) is derived from cephalosporin-C, prove to be more effective. Modification of 7-ACA side chains resulted in the development of newer generations of useful antibiotic agents, which leaded to various generations of cephalosporins.

Antibiotics	Source	Mode of action
Antibacterial antibiotics		
Bacitracin	*Bacillus subtilis*	Cell-wall synthesis
Cephalosporin	*Cephalosporium sp.*	Cell-wall synthesis
Chloramphenicol	*Streptomyces venezuelae*	Protein synthesis
Cycloserin	*Streptomyces leavendulae*	Cell-wall synthesis
Erythromycin	*Streptomyces erythraeus*	Protein synthesis
Kanamycin	*Streptomyces kanomycetoius*	Protein synthesis
Neomycin	*Streptomyces fradiae*	Protein synthesis
Novobiocin	*Streptomyces sp.*	DNA synthesis
Penicillin	*Penicillium sp.*	Cell-wall synthesis
Polymixin	*Bacillus polymyxa*	Cell membrane
Streptomycin	*Streptomyces griseus*	Protein synthesis
Tetracycline	*Streptomyces aureofaciens*	Protein synthesis
Vancomycin	*Streptomyces orientalis*	Cell-wall synthesis
Antiprotozoan antibiotics		
Fumagilin	*Aspergillus fumigatus*	Protein synthesis
Antifungal antibiotics		
Amphotericin B	*Streptomyces nodosus*	Membrane function
Cycloheximide	*Streptomyces griseus*	Protein synthesis
Griseofulvin	*Penicillium griseofulvum*	Cell-wall, microtubules
Nystatin	*Streptomyces noursei*	Damages cell-membrane

Table 1. Different mode of activity/ action of major antibiotics. (Gaurav *et al.*, 2011)

The β-lactam antibiotics like penicillin, cephalosporins, vancomycin, etc. are specific inhibitor working against bacterial cell wall (peptidoglycan) synthesis but newer strains have β-lactamase activity which destroys most of the β-lactam antibiotics and thus make them resistant to it. However, cephalosporins proved to be more stable to β-lactamase. Cephalosporin-C (CPC) shows similarity to in structure with the penicillins in having an acyl side chain attached to an amino group of a double ring nucleus (Figure 1). The side chain was identical to that of penicillin N, *i.e.* D-α-aminoadipic acid. Although both the types have the four membered β-lactam group, cephalosporin-C have a six membered dihydrothiazine ring in place of the five membered thiazolidine ring system which is a characteristic of penicillins. But these antibiotics are not that effective to be used for clinical purposes. The cephalosporin nucleus, 7- aminocephalosporanic acid (7-ACA) is derived from cephalosporin-C, prove to be more effective. Modification of 7-ACA side chains resulted in the development of newer generations of useful antibiotic agents, which leaded to various generations of cephalosporins.

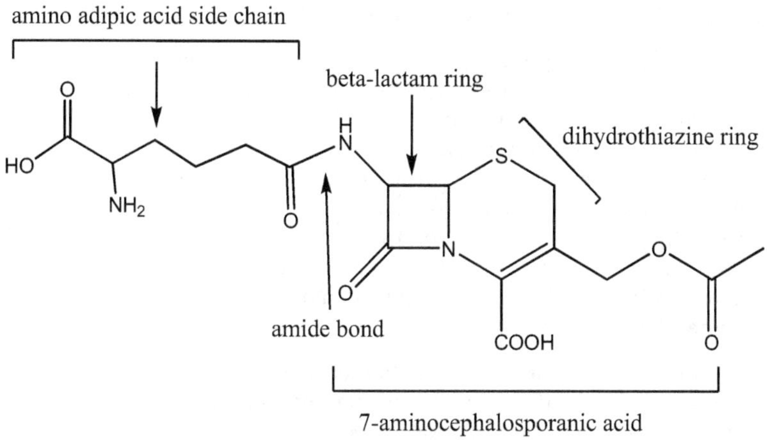

Cephalosporin C

Fig. 1. The structure of Cephalosporin

Cephalosporins are nowadays more suggested for the prophylaxis and treatment of bacterial infections caused by susceptible microorganisms. First generation cephalosporins are predominantly effective against gram positive bacteria and successive generations (Table 2) have further enhanced the activity against the gram negative bacteria too (Essack, 2001) However, the synthesis of different generations of cephalosporins are only possible either by microbial routes or by enzymatically converting cephalosporin-C. Hence, a brief discussion on microbial synthesis of cephalosporin-C is quite needed.

Various Generation	Example
First generation Cephalosporins	Cephalothin
	Cephaloridine
	Cephazolin
	Cephradine
	Cefroxadine
Second generation Cephalosporins	Cephamandole
	Cefuroime
	Ceforanide
	Cefotiam
Third generation Cephalosporins	Cefotaxime
	Ceftazidime
	Ceftizoxime
	Ceftriaxone
	Cefixime
	Ceftibuten
Fourth generation Cephalosporins	Cefipime
	Cefpirome

Table 2. Various Generations of Cephalosporin group of antibiotics

2. Microbial synthesis of cephalosporin-C

The biosynthesis of cephalosporin-C is carried only by few microorganisms, viz. fungi, *Streptomyces* sp. and bacteria. It can produced by free and immobilized microbial cells (Kundu et al., 2000) using various cultivation modes of batch and continuous strategy (Mahapatra et al., 2002). In batch mode of fermentation, Cephalosporin-C is produced in stirred tank bioreactors (Srivastava et.al, 1996) as well as in air lift bioreactor (Srivastava et al., 1995; 1999).In continuous mode of fermentation, it can be produced both by packed bed bioreactor using different types of immobilization processes and in continuous stirred tank bioreactor. As it's a highly aerobic process in nature, cephalosporin-C is also produced by immobilized microbial cells utilizing symbiotic mode (*in-situ* oxygen production) in a packed bed bioreactor. (Kundu et al., 1993)

In order to fulfill the need of large quantity of semi-synthetic cephalosporin, the key intermediates should be produced in large quantity through very efficient and cheap production routes. But the chemical production of the intermediates generates large quantities of wastes and requires expensive and hazardous chemicals and reaction conditions. In order to overcome these problems, enzymes are used to perform the required reactions. Cephalosporin C is converted to 7-ACA in a two step enzymatic process. First the side chain is deaminated by a D-amino oxidase, resulting in an α-keto acid that spontaneously loses carbon dioxide in the presence of hydrogen peroxide to form glutaryl-7-ACA. Subsequent enzymztic deacylation of the glutaryl side chain yields 7-ACA. The enzyme used, cephalosporin acylase, removes a charged aliphatic side chain without damaging the β- lactam nucleus. These enzymatic processes have the advantage of generating less waste and requiring less expensive chemicals. Thus, cephalosporin-C is directly converted to 7-ACA by cephalosporin-C acylase enzyme. (Zhang and Xu, 1993)

2.1 Production strategy of cephalosporin C (primary precursor)

Microbial production of Cephalosporin C, a secondary metabolite, occurs in late stationary phase (Idio-phase) of growth. So the main strategy of the production is to grow the culture to saturation level and then control the flow of nutrient to maintain the stationary phase. (Srivastava et al., 2006) Cephalosporin C fermentation always requires highly aerobic condition to maintain uniform yield. Hence, maximum focus is given on oxygenation of the media. There are different processes involved using various modes of bioreactors, *viz.* conventional and non conventional Bioreactors. The conventional mode of bioreactors involves in batch or continuous stirred tank bioreactors whereas non conventional mode involves in packed bed bioreactors, airlift bioreactors and the like. (Srivastava et al., 1996)

2.1.1 Cephalosporin C production by conventional mode of bioreactors

Conventional mode involves production by batch bioreactor or continuous stirred tank reactor (Kundu et al., 1993). Surface liquid culture and solid state fermentation are not very much favorable as there is high probability of oxygen limitation. There are some research occurring in the field but the stable process involved is the stirred tank batch bioreactors. They have special attachment for oxygen sparging and agitation for making the oxygen more available to microorganisms (Srivastava et al., 1996).The morphological characteristics of the mold change under high agitation which in turn affects the yield of the Cephalosporin C. (Kundu et al., 1993)

Continuous mode involves various continuous stirred tank bioreactors. The first type is where the oxygen is being sparged in the reactor fitted with an agitator (Figure 2 A). The second process involves addition of highly oxygenated media in the bioreactor (Figure 2 B). The continuous processes have advantages but there are several parameters which are to be maintained. Due to the microorganism, being filamentous and taking long time to reach stationary phase microorganism are first allowed to grow under batch condition and then continuous mode of operation is started. (Srivastava *et al.*, 2006)

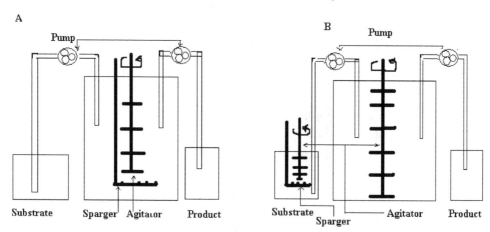

Fig. 2. A) Continuous Bioreactor with oxygen Sparger B) Continuous Bioreactor with oxygen enriched fresh substrate

2.1.2 Cephalosporin C production by Non conventional mode of bioreactors

The non conventional mode involves in either Packed bed bioreactor or Airlift bioreactor. Various modes of immobilized microorganisms are used in packed bed reactors. The main advantage of packed bed reactor is that it can be operated in batch or continuous mode. The residence time and microorganism reusability is high in case of packed bed reactors. There are reported studies involving silk sachets for holding the immobilized beads with significant increase in production. (Kundu et al., 2000)

Cephalosporin C fermentation is a highly aerobic process. The major problem which arises with aerobic fermentation are the mass transfer limitation of oxygen to immobilized cell. (Mishra *et al.*, 2005) Even with addition of highly oxygenated media, the beads packed in depth doesn't have enough oxygen to carry out cephalosporin C production, instead they produce Penicillin N, which is not desirable. There is a reported study where mixed culture technique for improving the oxygen supply to the immobilized cells. In such system, the products of metabolism of one microorganism are utilized by the second microorganism. Photoautotrophic algae (*Chlorella* sp.) which produce oxygen *in situ* are coupled with fungi (*Cephalosporium acremonium*) which in turn produce the Cephalosporin C. (Figure 3) (Kundu and Mahapatra, 1993; Kundu *et al.*, 2003) The algae absorb CO_2 from air and media producing free oxygen which not only removes the anaerobic condition prevailing in packed bed reactor but also adds up oxygen to the media. Co-immobilization of whole cells were reported to be carried out by using various immobilizing agents, *viz.* Bagasse, Silk sachets, calcium/Barium/strontium alginate and the same coated with poly-acrylamide resin.

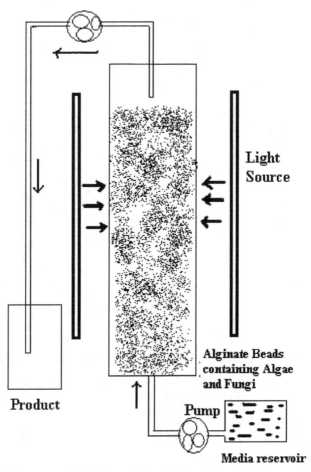

Fig. 3. Packed Bed Reactor with Co-immobilized microbial cells (Algae and Fungi) for enhanced oxygenation

Airlift Bioreactors are the most favorable reactors for production as it completely solve the oxygenation issue. There are two types of Airlift bioreactors. Internal air loop reactors have inner draft tube (Figure 4) while the external bioreactors have external tube as downcomer. They both have significant production values. (Srivastava and Kundu, 1999; Srivastava *et al.*, 1995)The air lift reactor ensures proper oxygenation and agitation. They are also gentle on filamentous fungi imparting low shear than any other conventional process agitator, improving production. Though, the process is costlier and tough but it ensures high cephalosporin C production. Figure 4 shows the airlift bioreactors involved in cephalosporin C production. The internal loop airlift reactors have better oxygenation and are preferred above external loop bioreactor.

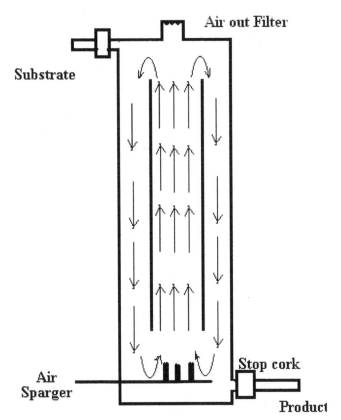

Fig. 4. Internal air-loop reactor for Cephalosporin C production

2.2 Production strategy of 7- amino cephalosporanic acid (secondary precursor)

Biosynthesis of 7- Amino cephalosporanic acid (7-ACA) is an important process which involves the use of free and immobilized microbial cells. This can be single step or multi-step microbial enzymatic process (Gaurav *et al.*, 2007). There are lots of advantages of single step over the multi-step process (Nigam *et al.*, 2005). Cephalosporin C acylase enzyme is involved in the conversion of Cephalosporin C to 7- ACA in single step mode of conversion. The microorganisms used for the synthesis of this enzyme are *Pseudomonas diminuta, Bacillus megaterium* and *E. coli* (Nigam and Kundu, 1999). There is also study on continuous production of 7-ACA by loading immobilized microbial cell in a packed bed bioreactor at optimum cells to carrier ratio and at an optimum flow rate (Nigam *et al.*, 2005).

3. Different generations Cephalosporins

Cephalosporins can usually be classified into four different generations though newer generations are in active research, developed in response to a specific clinical need for a drug with different characteristics than the previous generation. Table 2 narrates the examples of various generation of Cephalosporins group of antibiotics.

3.1 First generation cephalosporins

The first generation cephalosporins were first introduced in the mid-1960s and were stable to the β-lactamases known at that time. They permeated the outer membrane of gram-negative bacilli quicker than the penicillins. The first generation drugs include Cephalothin, Cephaloridine and Cefazolin (Figure 5). Cephalothin was synthesized by biochemically using different processing strategies [Gaurav et.al., 2007]. Cephalexin and Cefeclor are both used as oral treatment drugs, and have broad activity against both gram-positive and gram-negative microorganisms. However, they are inactive against *Enterococci* as they don't bind well to PBPs of the *Enterococci* having slight difference.

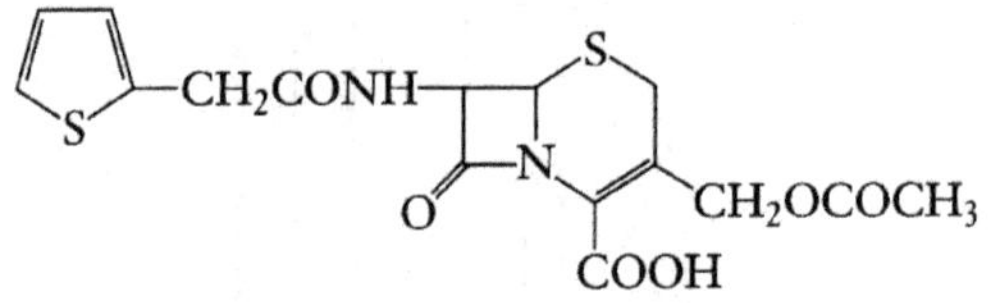

Cephalothin

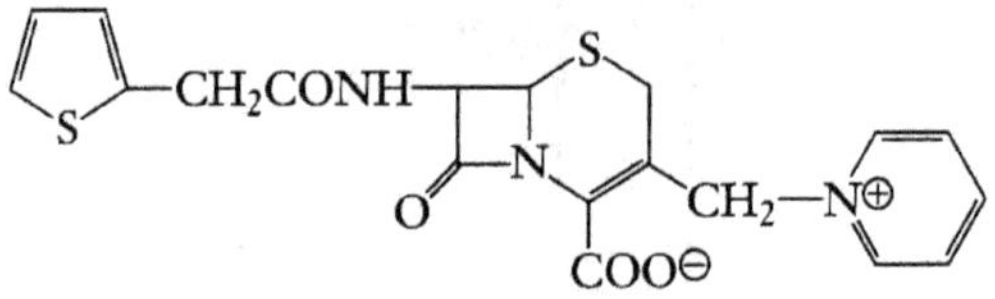

Cephaloridine

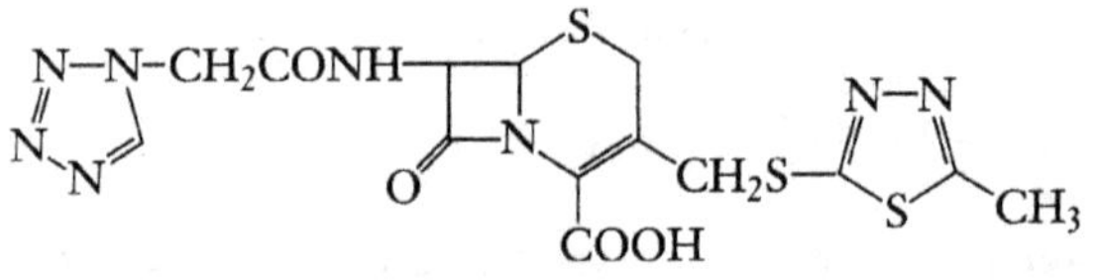

Cefazolin

Fig. 5. First generation Cephalosporins

3.2 Second generation cephalosporins

The second generation cephalosporins have enhanced activity against gram-negative microorganisms (Livermore 1987; Stan *et al.*, 2004). They are more stable to hydrolysis by plasmid-mediated β-lactamases when compared to cefoxitin, to the chromosomal class C cephalosporinase of several *Enterobacteriaceae*. (Medeiros 1997). The second generation cephalosporins include, Cefoxitin, Cefmetazole, Cefuroxime and Cefotetan (Figure 6). Cefuroxime is generally used for respiratory tract and community acquired infections. Cefoxitin has an extra methoxy-group that imparts protection against β-lactamase , but with an added disadvantage that it causes induction of the chromosomal β-lactamases in several bacterial organisms (which can be counterproductive). Cefoxitin (as well as Cefotetan) is well effective against *Bacteroides fragilis*, an enteric anaerobe but not against *Pseudomonas* or *Enterobacter* as it can't enter them.

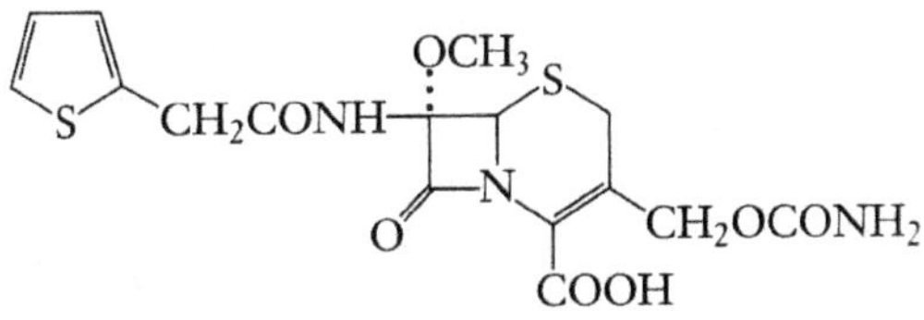

Cefoxitin

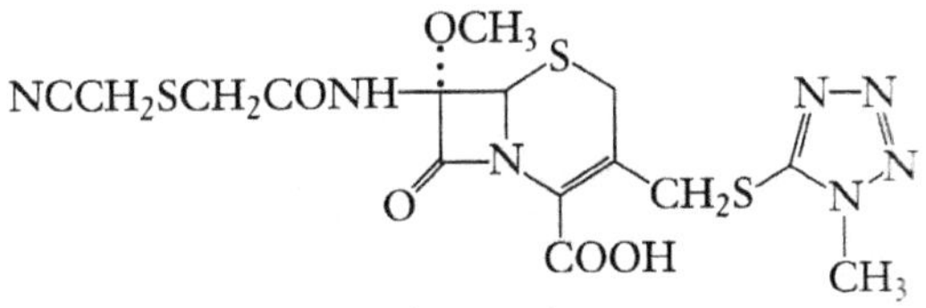

Cefmetazole

Fig. 6. Second generation Cephalosporins

3.3 Third generation cephalosporins

The third generation cephalosporins are less effective than the first generation cephalosporins against gram-positive cocci but are very much potent against *Enterobacteriaceae*, including the β-lactamase-producing strains (Mandell & Sande 1991). The aminothiazolyl and iminomethoxy groups are the substituents in third generation cephalosporins (Neu 1986), which imparted greater stability against the chromosomal class C β-lactamases and with an increased spectrum of activity.These cephalosporins include Cefotaxime, Ceftizoxime and Ceftazidime (Figure 7). The drugs are broad spectrum antibiotics that are effective against both gram-negative and gram-positive microorganisms. The sodium salts of these antibiotics also showed a greater potential.

Cefotaxime has an enhanced affinity to penicillin binding proteins (PBPs) of gram-negative bacteria and thus it could penetrate faster into bacterial cell as compared to older generation cephalosporins.

Also, cefotaxime is the main intermediary in the synthesis of cefpodoxime proxetil, a third generation oral cephalosporin, introduced recently into medical practice (Durckheimer *et al.*, 1985; Reynolds 1989). Third-generation cephalosporins have a broad spectrum of antimicrobial activity including Gram-positive, Gram-negative, and selected anaerobic species. (Neu 1991).

β -lactamase induction or resistant organism selections are an important issue, especially in nosocomial infections (Stratton *et al.*, 1992). Third generation cephalosporins vary in their ability to induce β-lactamases, but none is as effective inducers as the cephamycins, clavams, or carbapenems The discovery of *Klebsiella* isolates resistant to oxyiminocephalosporins imparted more difficulties to β-lactam antibiotics mediated by extended-spectrum β-lactamases (ESBLs). Mutation in the structural genes of plasmid-mediated TEM, SHV, and OXA β-lactamases and to a lesser extent in the PER and CTX enzymes enhanced their affinity for third generation cephalosporins and monobactams, but with varying degrees marking the pavement for newer generations.

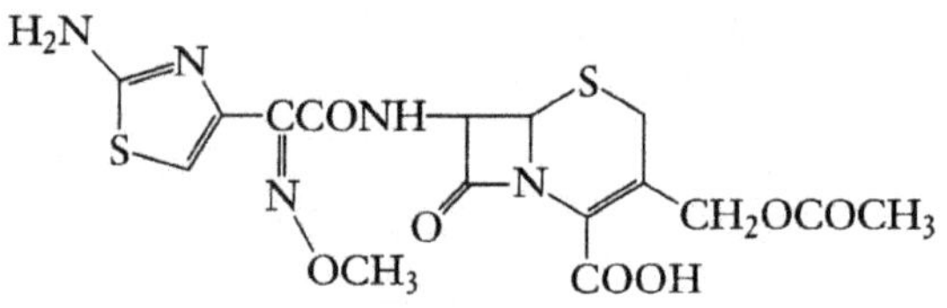

Cefotaxime

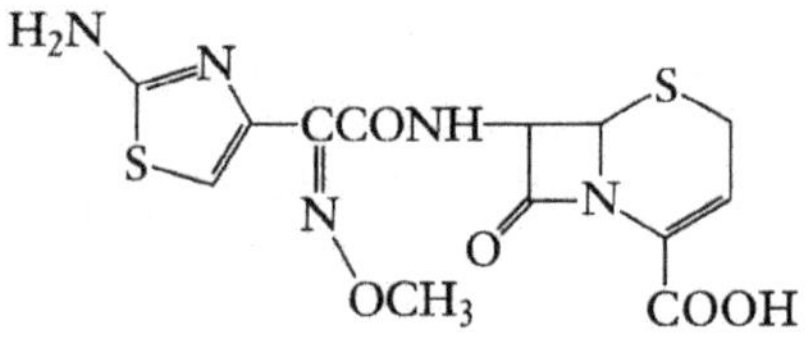

Ceftizoxime

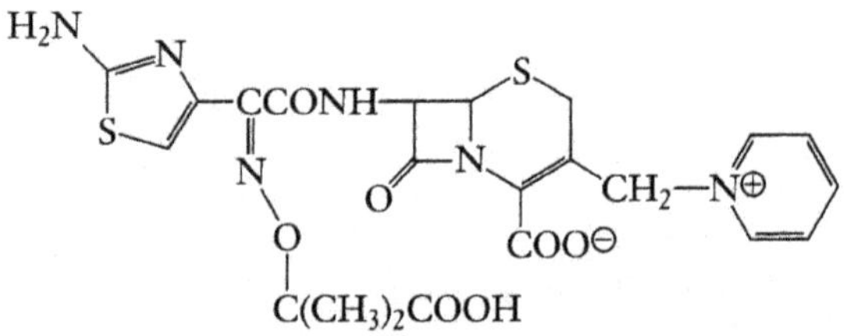

Ceftazidime

Fig. 7. Third generation cephalosporins

3.4 Fourth generation cephalosporins

The fourth generation cephalosporins contains a positively charged quaternary nitrogen atom at C-3, resulting in higher activity (compared to the third-generation cephalosporins) against β-lactamase derepressed mutants of *P. areuginosa* and other enteric bacteria (Georgopapdakau *et al.*, 1989). The fourth generation cephalosporins, Cefepime, Cefpirome and Cefclidin (Figure 8) have the 7-amino-thiazolyl groups [(Livermore & Williams 1996). Cefepime have good potency against gram-negative organisms such as *Pseudomonas aeruginosa*, and gram-positive organism such as *Staphylococcus aureus*, also exhibiting increased stability against β-lactamase-overproducing bacteria. Cefepime is [6 R – [6 α, 7 β (Z)]]-1-[[7-[[[(2-amino-4-thiazolyl) (methoxyimino) acetyl] amino]-2-carboxy-8-oxo-5-thia-1-azabicyclo oct-2-en-3yl] methyl]-1-methylpyrrolidinium inner salt. It is synthesized from 7-aminocephalosporanic acid (7-ACA) with help of trimethylsilyl iodide and N-methylpyrrolidine. It is stable to hydrolysis by the more common chromosomal and plasmid-mediated β-lactamases, and it is quite stable against inducible chromosomally mediated cephalosporinases

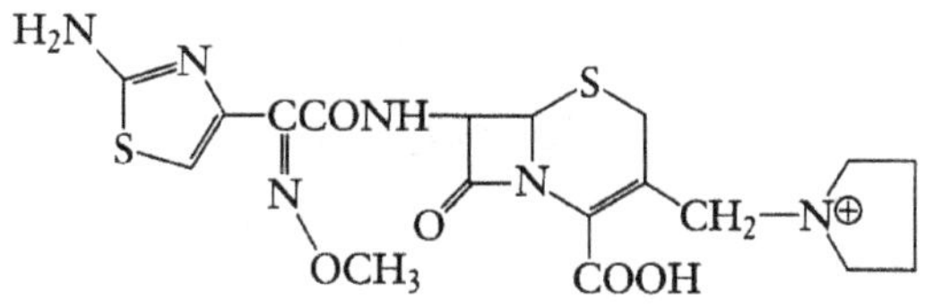

Cefepime

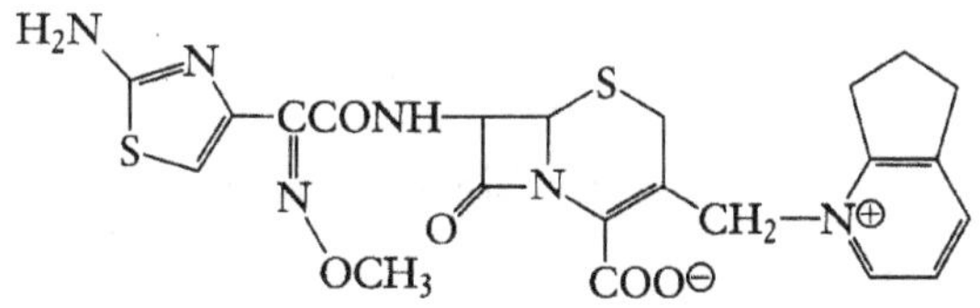

Cefpirome

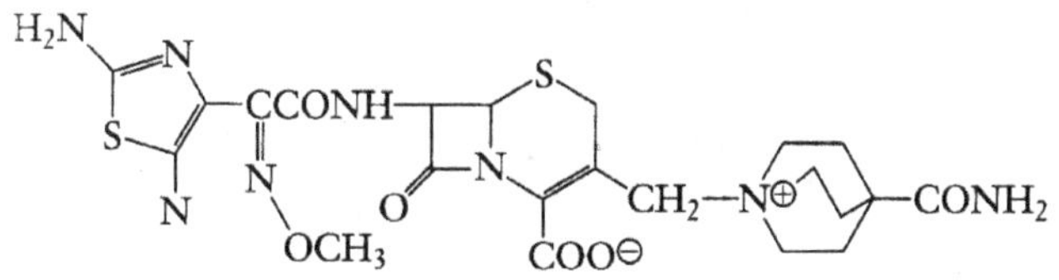

Cefclidin

Fig. 8. Fourth generation Cephalosporins

3.5 Fifth generation cephalosporins

The fifth generation cephalosporin is still an unclear picture with many new modified cephalosporins in the research sector. This generation antibiotic is specifically developed against nosocomial infections of MRSA and Pseudomonas based refractory infection in immuno-compromised patients. Drugs which are in immediate attention of FDA are Ceftobiprole, LB10522 (Kim et al., 1996) and RU-59863 (Figure 9). Ceftobiprole specifically attacks by binding to this penicillin-resistant target. Interactions with cephalosporin side chains occurs in the groove, closed in the free PBP 2a enzyme, binds to the 7-acyl amino side chain, and in another extended groove where it interacts with the 3'-cephem side chain through noncovalent interactions (Lim & Strynadka 2002). It is stable to class A penicillinases produced by S. *aureus* and enteric gram-negative microorganisms and is more stable to few class C beta-lactamases of enteric gram-negative microorganisms (Hebeisen *et al.*, 2001).

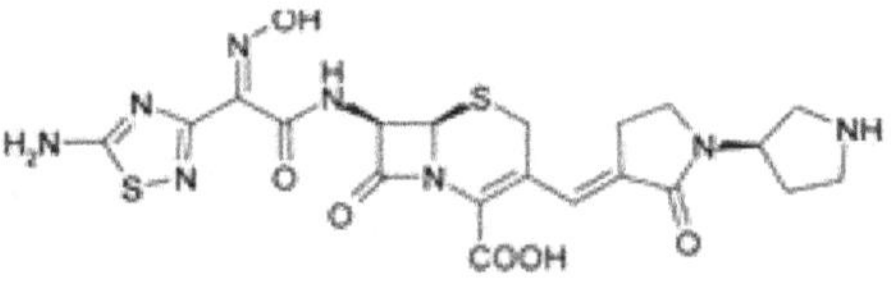

Ceftobiprole

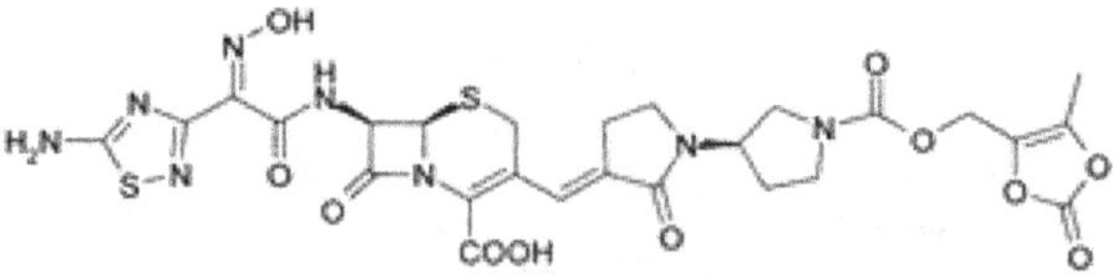

Ceftobiprole medocaril

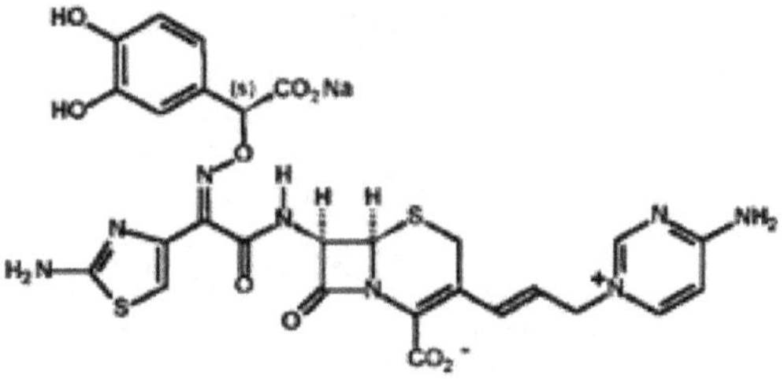

LB10522

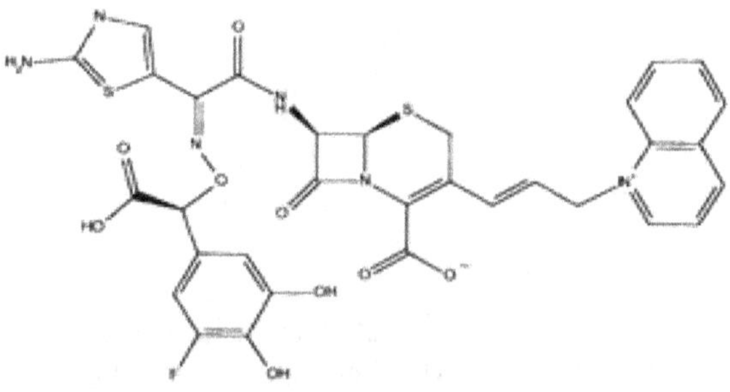

RU-59863

Fig. 9. Fifth generation Cephalosporins

4. Current research in new generation cephalosporins

It is also known that incorporation of a methoxy group in both cephalosporin and penicillin has led to a considerable increase in beta-lactamase stability. These findings prompted us to prepare methoxy and formamido derivatives of Cephalosporin and screen them for their antibacterial activity.

Our research team's current work is to attempt synthesizing some new semi-synthetic cephalosporins and some by modifying already existing semi-synthetic cephalosporins such as cefotaxime (third generation). It is broad spectrum antibiotic with high resistance against beta-lactamases. But the main problem is that it is poorly soluble in water. Hence, the efforts have been made to prepare cephalosporins having better solubility using cefotaxime. All these semi-synthetic cephalosporins are derived from the key intermediate 7- ACA, a product derived from cephalosporin C hydrolysis. They differ in the nature of the substitute attached at the 3 and/ or 7- position of the cephem ring and express various biological and pharmacological effects.

In the present work, enzymatic method has been employed to produce 7-ACA, the key intermediate and this 7-ACA is then utilized for the synthesis of new semi-synthetic cephalosporins. Nicotinic acid, benzimidazole, imidazole or substituted benzimidazole system has been shown to have different pharmacological effects including antifungal, antibacterial and antiviral effects. 2-substituted benzimidazoles, with various types of biological activity, have a close relationship to nucleic acid metabolism. Hence, semi-synthetic cephalosporins containing these nucleuses were prepared and the assessment of these molecules has been checked to interfere with various cellular and metabolic processes. (Figure 10)

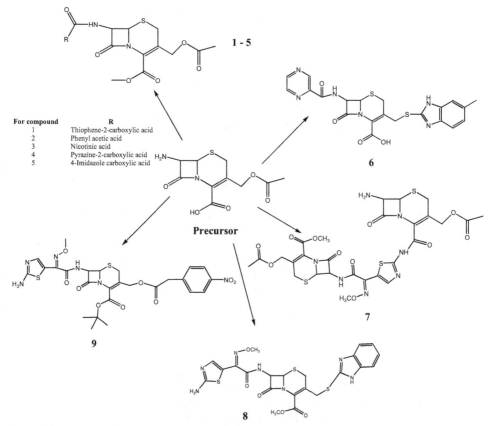

For compound	R
1	Thiophene-2-carboxylic acid
2	Phenyl acetic acid
3	Nicotinic acid
4	Pyrazine-2-carboxylic acid
5	4-Imidazole carboxylic acid

Fig. 10. Formation of new generation Cephalosporins.

In a search for unique and potent cephalosporin antibiotics, we have prepared new semi-synthetic cephalosporins. The motivation for synthesizing these semi-synthetic cephalosporins was to increase the availability of drug at the target site and their oral absorptivity and increased stability. Thus, recurring need for an easily cleaved blocking group for the carboxylic acid in the cephalosporin synthetic chemistry forms the basis of the research. All the synthesised cephalosporins were having easily hydrolysable esters for oral absorption studies; they were also having such suitable blocking groups for the carboxyl, which might be removed later without disruption of the beta-lactam ring. Although simple esters, like the methyl ester, are known to possess diminished antibiotic activity compared to the free acids, the possibility exists that more easily hydrolysable esters (by enzymatic or chemical means) might exhibit significant in vivo activity. A therapeutic advantage might be anticipated from derived compounds if the structural environment of the carboxyl group is a bar to absorption through the gastric or intestinal walls. Activity could be inherent in the derivative or be produced a result of enzymatic cleavage to the parent compound after absorption has occurred. Gastric acidity, often a negative influence in oral absorptibility of penicillins, would send to be an unlikely factor in cephalosporin absorption because of the relatively good acid stability of this class of antibiotics. For the synthesis of these analogues, the methods that are of general applicability are used. To form peptides from a cephalosporin required that the carboxyl at C-4 be appropriately activated for acylation of a protected amino acid. In synthetic organic chemistry, compound containing the carbodiimide functionality are dehydrating agents and are often used to activate carboxylic acids towards amide or ester formation. Additives, such as N-hydroxybenzotriazole are often added to increase yields and decrease side reactions. EDC (acronym for 1-ethyl-3-(3-dimethylaminopropyl) carbodiimide hydrochloride) is a water soluble carbodiimide which is used as a carboxyl activating agent for the coupling of primary amines to yield amide bonds. The possibility that amides derived from a cephalosporanic acid and an amino acid might cross the intestinal wall and be cleaved in the body.

5. Conclusion

In general, attempts to modify the β- lactam thiazolidine ring system of penicillin without loss of antibacterial activity had been unsuccessful. The discovery, structure elucidation and modification of cephalosporin C, which led to important new generations of Cephalosporin group of antibiotics and its large scale production and marketing. In the past decade, even though cephalosporin antibiotics have made remarkable progress and contribution in the treatment of acute disease, many efforts still exist to achieve the well-balanced broad-spectrum and to improve beta-lactamases stability. This work, lead to highly active, acid stable, penicillin resistant, nontoxic antibiotic with increased potency against a wide range of bacteria. Although the progress is in preliminary stage but significance of the work is enormous.

6. References

Babini, G.S. and D.M. Livermore , 2000. Antimicrobial resistance amongst Klebsiella spp. collected from intensive care units in southern and western europe in 1997–1998. *J Antimicrob Chemother.*, Vol. 45, pp. 183–189

Durckheimer, W., Blumbach, J., Lattrell, R. and Scheunemann, K.H. (1985). Recent developments in the field of b-Lactam antibiotics Angew. *Chem. Int. Ed. Engl.*, Vol. 24, pp. 180-182.

Essack, S.Y. (2001). The development of b-Lactam antibiotics in response to the Evolution of b-lactamases. *Pharmaceutical Res.*, Vol.18, pp. 1391-1399.

Gaurav, K., Kundu, K. and Kundu, S. (2007). Microbial Production of 7-aminocepahlosporanic acid and new generation cephalosporins (Cephalothin) by different processing strategies. *Artificial Cells, Blood SubstBiotechnol.* , Vol.35, pp. 345-358.

Gaurav, K., Kundu, K. , Karmakar, S. and Kundu, S. (2011). Development of New Generation Cephalosporins. In Recent advances in life sciences. A.K. Rai (ed.), pp. 173-186, I. K. Publishers, India

Georgopapdakau, N.H. and Bertasso, A. (1993). Mechanisms of action of cephalosporin 3'-quinolone esters,carbamates, and tertiary amines in *Escherichia coli. Antimicrob Agents Chemother.* , Vol.37, pp. 559-565.

Hebeisen, P., Heinze-Krauss, I., Angehrn, P., Hohl, P., Page, M.G.P. and Then, R.L. (2001). *In vitro* and *in vivo* Properties of Ro 63-9141, a novel broad-spectrum cephalosporin with activity against methicillin-resistant Staphylococci. *Antimicrob. Agents Chemother.* , Vol.45, pp. 825-836.

Jacoby, B. K. (2000). Amino acid sequences for TEM, SHV and OXA extended-spectrum and inhibitor resistant β-lactamases. Available from http://lahey.org/studies/webt.htm

Jones, R.N. (1994). Summation the injectable cephalosporins in the treatment of serious infections. *Infection*, Vol. 22, pp. S182-S183.

Kim, M.Y., Oh, J.I., Paek, K.S., Kim, Y.Z., Kim, I.C. and Kwak, J.H. (1996). *In vitro* and *in vivo* activities of LB10522, a new catecholic cephalosporin. *Antimicrob. Agents Chemother.* , Vol. 40, pp. 1825-1831.

Kundu, S., Gupta, S., Bihari, V. and Agrawal, S.C. (2000). Studies on free and immobilized cells of *C. acremonium* on the production of cephalosporins. *Indian J. Microbiol.* , Vol. 40, pp. 141-143.

Kundu, S. and A.C. Mahapatra (1993). Microbial Production of cephalosporin C using co cultures of *Cephalosporium acremonium* and *Chlorella pyrenoidosa* in a packed bed reactor. In: *Recent trends in Biotechnology*. C. Ayanna (ed.), pp. 31-35, Tata McGraw Hill, India,

Kundu, S., Mahapatra, A.C., Nigam, V.K. and Kundu, K. (2003). Continuous production of cephalosporin-C by immobilized microbial cells using symbiotic mode in a packed bed bioreactor. *Artificial Cells, Blood Substitutes and Biotechnology*, Vol. 31, pp. 313-327.

Kundu, S., Singh, S.K. and Nigam, V.K. (1993). Comparative studies of cephalosporin-C production in batch and continuous stirred tank bioreactor. *J. Microb. Biotech.*, Vol.8, pp. 76-84.

Lim, D. and Strynadka, N.C. (2002). Structural basis for the beta lactam resistance of PBP2a from methicillin resistant *Staphylococcus aureus. Nat. Struct. Biol.* , Vol.9, pp. 870-876.

Livermore, D.M. (1987). Mechanisms of resistance to cephalosporin antibiotics. *Drugs* , Vol.34, pp. 64.

Livermore, D.M. (1998). Beta-lactamase-mediated resistance and opportunities for its control. *J. Antimicrob. Chemother.*, Vol. 41, pp. 25-41.

Livermore, D.M. and Williams, J.D. (1996). Lactams: mode of action and mechanisms of bacterial resistance, In: *Antibiotics in laboratory medicine*, Lorian V (Ed.), 4th edn, pp. 502-578, Williams & Wilkins, Baltimore, Md..

Mahapatra, A.C., Kundu, K., Nigam, V.K., Mandava, M.V.P. and Kundu, S. (2002). Comparative studies of CPC production by free and immobilized cells of

Cephalosporium acremonium in different modes of bioreactors. *Indian J. Microbiol.*, Vol. 42, pp. 319-322.

Mandell, G.L. and Sande, M.A. (1991). *Goodman and Gilman's, The Pharmacological Basis of Therapeutics*, 8th Edition. pp. 1065, Pergamon Press, New York..

Medeiros, A. (1997). Evolution and dissemination of b-lactamases. *Clin. Infect. Dis.*, Vol. 24, pp. S19-S45.

Mishra, P., Srivastava, P. and Kundu, S., (2005). A Comparative evaluation of oxygen mass transfer and broth viscosity using cephalosporin C production as a case strategy. *World Journal of Microbiology & Biotechnology*, Vol. 21, pp. 525-530

Neu, H.C. (1986). beta-Lactam antibiotics: structural relationships affecting in vitro activity and pharmacologic properties. *Rev. Infect. Dis.*, Vol. 8, pp. S237–S259.

Neu, H.C. (1991). Cephalosporins-cefotaxime 10 years later, a major drug with continued use. *Infection*, Vol. 19: pp. 309-315.

Nigam,V.K., S. Kundu and P. Ghosh, (2005). Single step conversion of Cephalosporin- C acylase to 7- ACA by free and Immobilized cells of Pseudomonas diminuta. *Appl. Biochem. & Biotechnol*, Vol. 126,pp. 13-21

Nigam, V.K. and Kundu, S (1999). Batch Production of 7-ACA by Different Microorganisms – A Comparative Study. *Ind. Chemical Engg.*, Vol. 41, no. 1, pp. 5-9

Reynolds, J.E.F. (1989). *Martindale-The Extra Pharmacopoeia*, 29th edn, p. 151., Pharmaceutical Press, London.

Srivastava, P. and Kundu, S. (1990). A simple kinetic analysis of ephalosporin-C production using various carbon substrates. *J. Microb. Biotechnol.*, Vol. 5, pp. 34-41.

Srivastava, P. and Kundu, S. (1995). A laboratory air lift reactor for cephalosporin-C. *J. Ind. Chem Engg.* , Vol. 37, pp. 138-139.

Srivastava, P. and Kundu, S. (1999). Studies on cephalosporin-C production in an air lift reactor using different growth modes of *Cephalosporium acremonium*. *Process Biochem.* , Vol. 34, pp. 329-333.

Srivastava, P., Nigam, V.K. and Kundu, S. (1996). A comparative evaluation of Cephalosporin-C production in stirred-tank reactor and air lift reactor. *Ind. J. Chem Tech.*, Vol. 3, pp. 371-372.

Srivastava, P., Mishra, P. and Kundu, S., (2006). Process strategies for Cephalosporin-C Fermentation. *J. of Scientific and Industrial Research*, Vol. 65, pp. 599-602.

Stan, C., Dumitrache, M. and Diaconu, D.E. (2004). Means of purification of cephalexin with a view to therapeutic use. *Rev. Med. Chir. Soc. Med. Nat. Iasi*, Vol. 108, pp. 718-720.

Stratton, C.W., Ratner, H., Johnston, P.E. and Schaffner, W. (1992). Focused microbiologic surveillance by specific hospital unit as a sensitive means of defining antimicrobial resistance problems. *Diagn Microbiol Infect Dis.*, Vol. 15, pp. 11S-18S.

Tzouvelekis, L.S., Tzelepi, E., Prinarakis, E., Gazouli, M., Katrahoura, A., Giakkoupi, P., Paniara, O. and Legakis, (1998). Sporadic Emergence of Klebsiella pneumoniae Strains Resistant to Cefepime and Cefpirome in Greek Hospitals. *J. Clin. Microbiol*, Vol. 36, pp. 266-268

Wilson, W.R., 1998. The role of fourth-generation cephalosporins in the treatment of serious infectious diseases in hospitalized patients. *Diagn Microbiol Infect Dis.*, Vol. 31, pp. 473–477

Zhang, Q.J. and Xu, W.X. (1993). Morphological physiological and enzymatic characteristics of cephalosporin acylase producing *Arthrobacter* strain 45-A. *Arch. Microbiol.*, Vol. 159, pp. 392-395.

13

Antimicrobial Resistance and Potential Probiotic Application of *Enterococcus* spp. in Sea Bass and Sea Bream Aquaculture

Ouissal Chahad Bourouni[1], Monia El Bour[1],
Pilar Calo-Mata[2] and Jorge Barros-Velàzquez[2]
[1]*Institut National des Sciences et Technologies de la Mer (INSTM), Tunis,*
[2]*Department of Analytical Chemistry, Nutrition and Food Science, LHICA,*
School of Veterinary Sciences, University of Santiago de Compostela,
[1]*Tunisia*
[2]*Spain*

1. Introduction

Microbial resistance to antibiotics is a world-wide problem in human and veterinary medicine. It is generally accepted that the main risk factor for the increase in the antibiotic resistance is an extensive use of antibiotics. In fact, for the last 50 years, high levels of antibiotics are commonly used for treatment and prevention of infectious diseases in humans and animals. This led to emergence and dissemination of resistant bacteria and resistance genes in wild populations (Bogaard & Stobberingh 2000). The antimicrobial agents used in animal care are also significant, both in increasing resistance in animal pathogens, and in transmission of resistant bacteria from animals to humans. In part, this is due to the transfer of antimicrobial-resistant normal or commensal microflora of animals, *via* the food chain to humans. Several recent papers reported link between antibiotic use in food producing animals, emergence of antibiotic resistance in *Salmonella, Escherichia coli,* enterococci or *Campylobacter* in treated animals and transfer of these resistances to humans (or their resistance genes to human pathogens) *via* the food chain (Barton 2000; Angulo et al. 2004). However, less attention was paid to potential for antibiotic use in aquaculture industries to compromise human health. In addition to transfer of resistant bacteria through consumption of contaminated fish and shellfish, there is substantial risk of environmental contamination due to practice of using medicated feeds to treat whole pens or cages.

2. Antibiotic resistance in aquaculture

Aquaculture around the Mediterranean basin has increased significantly to satisfy the demand for seafood, which cannot be met by wild fisheries harvesting as this is currently in a state of decline because of over-fishing, pollution and marine habitat destruction. Recent reports of the United Nations Food and Agriculture Organization (FAO), noted approximately more than 290.10^3 tons for the mainly species of marine fish farmed (sea bass and sea bream) and had previously estimated that half of the world's seafood demand will be met by aquaculture in 2020 (FAO, 2008). In Mediterranean aquaculture, the culture practices for most farmed fish species are mostly semi-intensive or intensive and a significant challenge to fish farming however is disease caused by bacteria such as *Aeromonas* sp., *Vibrio* sp., *Pseudomonas* sp. and *Flavobacterium* sp. Both prophylactic and therapeutic treatments utilize drug supplemented feeds to keep farmed fish free of diseases.

Antibiotics such as oxytetracycline (OTC) and quinolone such as oxolinic acid (OA) are the most widely used in Mediterranean aquaculture in feed (Rigos & Troisi, 2005) and treatments discharge drugs directly into the marine environment, where they are relatively resistant to biodegradation. Rigos et al., 2004 found that 60-73% of the OTC and 8-12% of the OA administered to farmed sea bream were excreted with the faeces. Also, the results of ARMed (Antibiotic Resistance in the south-eastern Mediterranean) suggest existence of high resistances of bacteria particularly in the eastern region where the resistance in *E. coli* appears to be more important than in other Mediterranean countries.

Previous reports noted that resistance emergence result directly from infections treatment with antibacterial drugs (Sorum 1998, 1999) and therefore limited their value in control of bacterial diseases of fish (Smith et al., 1994), apart from any public health concerns.

Further, antibacterial drugs were shown to persist in animal tissues and in the sea, including the aquatic food chain (CIESM, 2004) and development of antibiotic resistance is direct consequence of drug pollution. Chelossi et al., 2003 found that antibiotics discharged through faeces or undigested feed, contributed to high incidences of quinolone, tetracyclin and penicillin-resistant benthic bacteria and caused a shift in structure of the benthic microbial assemblage next to fish farms. Moreover, a considerable increase in resistance to several antimicrobial drugs has been discovered in some species of *Vibrio* and *Pseudomonas* recovered from diseased farmed sea bream of south-western Spain (Zorilla et al., 2003).

In Turkey, bacteria isolated from sea bass (*Dicentrarchus labrax*) showed a multidrug resistance to trimethoprim-sulfamethoxazole, cephalothin, tetracyclin and streptomycin suggesting that fish farms act as a reservoir of multidrug-resistant pathogenic bacteria such as *Pseudomonas* and *Vibrio* (Matyar, 2007). Considering the frequent usage of anti-bacterial drugs in Mediterranean fish farming, and serious problems of their rapid increase in resistance and transfer to non-target microflora including human and animal pathogens, there is an urgent need for monitoring drug contamination in aquatic environment and thus, the need for alternative techniques replacing drugs with effective and inexpensive probiotics which became increasingly evident and necessary to avoid resistance in fish farming sites and antibiotic residues in fish flesh destined for human consumption.

In Tunisia, aquaculture fish industry was developed since 1989 and has highly increased during these last ten years and national production passed from 1566 tons in 2000 to 4468 tons in 2009 with an increase in number of aquatic farms multiplied by about five. The production statistics in 2009 noted more than 2800 tons for marine fish farming. Regarded as a strategic activity that can support the fishing sector, aquaculture benefits in Tunisia of a particular interest mainly for the most two marine species farmed sea bass (*Dicentrarchus labrax*) and sea bream (*Sparus aurata*), which were undertaken in almost private farms.

The evolution of antibiotic resistance of the main bacterial species of medical interest is subject to increased surveillance in Tunisia. Since 1999, the research laboratory on antibiotic resistance (LAB MDT-03) established a system for monitoring bacterial resistance to antibiotics (L'Antibio - Résistance en Tunisie or LART). It includes four hospitals regularly monitoring the epidemiology of major bacterial species of medical importance and antibiotic resistance data collected are used in development of recommendations to antibiotic therapy (Boutiba et al., 2007). However, the problem of antibiotic resistance is underestimated in animal production including aquaculture and studies related are scarced. A study of pathogens vibrios isolated from sea bass showed a multi-resistance of *Vibrio alginolyticus* and *Vibrio parahaemolyticus* for almost antibiotics used and sensitivity was only demonstrated for furazolidone and chloramphenicol (Bakhrouf et al., 1995). Bouamama et al., 2001 isolated several multiresistant bacteria from mussel *Mytilus galloprovincialis* with resistance profiles to 12 different antibiotics in *Aeromonas hydrophila* and *Propioni acnes. Vibrio alginolyticus* was isolated from internal organs of sea bream and sea bass reared in two fish farms located in Tunisian coast. Multi-drug resistance to antimicrobial agents was detected, all the 34 strains tested were resistant to ampicillin, 31 strains were resistant to nitrofurantoïne and 12 were resistant to tetracycline (Ben Kahla-Nakbi et al., 2006). The most recent study of Rezgui et al., (2010) showed abundance of antibiotic resistant bacteria isolated mainly from gills and intestinal tract of sea bream and sea bass which belong to several species of the genus *Pseudomonas, Aeromonas, Vibrio* and *Enterobacteriaceae* and were resistant essentially to tetracyclin and penicillin (antibiotics commonly used respectively in veterinary and human clinical).

3. Probiotics as alternative to antibiotics in aquaculture

The increasing problems associated with infectious diseases in fish, the frequent usage of drugs for treatment and prevention of these diseases and the rapid increase in resistance to these antibiotics represent major challenges for this source of food production worldwide. Thus, replacing drugs with effective and inexpensive probiotics was became increasingly evident and necessary to avoid resistance in fish farming sites and antibiotic residues in fish flesh destined for human consumption (Vershuere et al., 2000; Balcazar et al., 2006; Rengpipat et al., 2008).

3.1 Probiotics: definition and principles

The term, probiotic, simply means "for life", originating from the Greek words "pro" and "bios" (Gismondo et al., 1999). The most widely quoted definition was made by Fuller (1989). He defined a probiotic as "a live microbial feed supplement which beneficially affects the host animal by improving its intestinal balance". This definition is still widely referred to, despite continual contention with regard to the correct definition of the term. Current probiotic applications and scientific data on mechanisms of action indicate that non-viable microbial components act in a beneficial manner and this benefit is not limited just to the intestinal region (Salminen et al., 1999). Besides, based on the intricate relationship an aquatic organism has with the external environment when compared with that of terrestrial animals, the definition of a probiotic for aquatic environments needs to be modified. Verschuere et al. (2000a) suggested the definition "a live microbial adjunct which has a beneficial effect on the host by modifying the host-associated or ambient microbial community, by ensuring improved use of the feed or enhancing its nutritional value, by enhancing the host response towards disease, or by improving the quality of its ambient environment".

3.2 Different modes of action

Several studies have demonstrated certain modes of probiotic action in effect in the aquatic environment. Bairagi et al. (2002) assessed aerobic bacteria associated with the gastrointestinal tract (GIT) of nine freshwater fish. They determined that selected strains produced digestive enzymes, thus facilitating feed utilization and digestion. Ramirez & Dixon (2003) reported on the enzymatic properties of anaerobic intestinal bacteria isolated from three fish species, showing the potential role a probiotic could play. In the paper of Bairagi et al. (2004) the benefit of adding *B. subtilis* and *B. circulans* to the diet of rohu, *Labeo rohita*, was shown. In the search to replace fish meal with leaf meal in fish feed, they found that addition of the two fish intestinal *Bacillus spp.* increased performance as judged by several factors (growth, feed conversion ratio, and protein efficiency ratio). They attributed this to the extracellular cellulolytic and amylolytic enzyme production by the bacteria. Although competition for adhesion sites has been widely suggested as a mode of action, there is little evidence in the literature to demonstrate this. Although for not direct attachment competition, Yan et al. (2002) demonstrated that production of antibiotic substances by two seaweed-associated *Bacillus* sp. was dependent on biofilm formation by the bacteria. This study highlighted a factor which might be important for some bacteria to be effective probiotics, i.e. surface attachment. Such observation concurred with Fuller's (1989) definition of a probiotic, i.e. the requirement for GIT colonization. It has been proposed that the mechanism of competitive exclusion for attachment sites could be given a distinct advantage via addition of probiotic bacteria during the initial egg fertilization steps of larviculture, thereby "getting in there first" (Irianto and Austin, 2002a).

Several studies have attributed a probiotic effect to competition for energy sources (Rico Mora et al., 1998; Verschuere et al., 1999; Verschuere et al., 2000b). Beneficial growth and survival was found in Artemia sp. pre-exposed to nine strains of bacteria before challenge with *V. proteolyticus* (Verschuere et al., 1999). It was concluded that the effect was not caused by extracellular products, but required the live bacterial cell. Although it was not specifically tested, they hypothesized that the protective effect probably resulted from competition for energy sources and for adhesion sites.

Itami et al. (1998) found that addition of *Bifidobacterium thermophilum* derived peptidoglycan to kuruma shrimp increased significantly their survival when they were challenged with *V. penaeicida*. They attributed this to an immunostimulatory effect, as the phagocytic activity of shrimp granulocytes was significantly higher in the treated shrimp compared with those of the control animals. Gullian et al. (2004) tested immunostimulation by a live *Vibrio sp.* (P62) and *Bacillus sp.* (P64), using *V. alginolyticus* as a positive control. They concluded that P64 and *V. alginolyticus* were immunostimulants. A review by Smith et al. (2003) provided important information on the potential problems associated with immunostimulants in crustacean aquaculture. They argued that the prolonged use of immunostimulants was in fact detrimental to the host and that much more research was needed before their use during critical periods could be considered safe.

Competition for iron has been reported as an important factor in marine bacteria (Verschuere et al., 2000a). Iron is needed by most bacteria for growth, but is generally limited in the tissues and body fluids of animals and in the insoluble ferric Fe^{3+} form (Verschuere et al., 2000a). Iron-binding agents, siderophores, allow acquisition of iron suitable for microbial growth. Siderophore production is a mechanism of virulence in some pathogens (Gram et al., 1999). Equally, a siderophore producing probiotic could deprive potential pathogens of iron under iron limiting conditions. This was shown by Gram et al. (1999), who found that a culture supernatant of *Pseudomonas fluorescens*, grown in iron-limited conditions, inhibited growth of *V. anguillarum*, whereas the supernatant from iron-available cultures did not.

Possibly the most studied mode of probiotic action in aquatic animals is the production of inhibitory substances. Currently, there are four methods commonly employed to screen for inhibitory substances *in vitro*; the double layer method, the well diffusion method, the cross-streak method, and the disc diffusion method. All methods are based on the principle that a bacterium produces extracellular substance inhibitor to itself or another bacterial strain (the indicator). The inhibitory activity is displayed by growth increase of the producer culture in agar medium.

This *in vitro* screening method has identified very good probiotics in aquaculture (Irianto & Austin, 2002b; Lategan and Gibson, 2003; Vaseeharan et al., 2004; Lategan et al., 2004a,b), with two major limitations for this approach. The first is that other modes of probiotic activity (e.g. immunostimulation, digestive enzymes production, competition for attachment site, or nutrients) will not be expressed in the laboratory on agar plate and, hence, a major source of potential beneficial action will be overlooked. The second drawback is that positive results *in vitro* fail to determine the real *in vivo* effect.

3.3 Developing probiotics for aquaculture

It has been widely published that a probiotic must possess certain properties (Verschuere et al., 2000a). These properties were proposed in order to aid in correct establishment of new, effective and safe products and included:

1.   The probiotic should not be harmful to the host it is desired for,
2.   It should be accepted by the host, e.g. through ingestion and potential colonization and replication within the host,
3.   It should reach the location where the effect is required to take place,
4.   It should actually work *in vivo* as opposed to *in vitro* findings,
5.   It should preferably not contain virulence resistance genes or antibiotic resistance genes.

The future application for probiotics in aquaculture looks bright. There is an ever-increasing demand for aquaculture products and a similar increase in the search for alternatives to antibiotics. The field of probiotics intended for aquacultured animals is now attracting considerable attention and a number of commercial products are available.

3.4 Probiotic strains studied in aquaculture

Most probiotics proposed as biological control agents in aquaculture belong to the lactic acid bacteria (*Lactobacillus* and *Carnobacterium*), although other genera or species have also been studied, belonging to the genus *Vibrio*, to the genus *Bacillus*, or to the genus *Pseudomonas*, and also *Aeromonas* and *Flavobacterium* (Table 1).

Within probiotic group, lactic acid bacteria (LAB) have been recognized for their fermentative ability as well as their health and nutritional benefits since they exert strong antimicrobial activities against many pathogenic microorganisms and were considered as harmless bacteriocin-producing strains which may act antagonistic against fish pathogens (Maugin & Novel, 1994; Ringo & Gatesoupe, 1998). Moreover, LAB were signalled as competing for nutrients or space with spoiling microorganisms due to their ability to produce organic acids, hydrogen peroxide, diacetyl and bacteriocins and therefore should be of applied interest for marine fish and shellfish food bio-preservation (Franz C. et al., 2007).

Animals tested	Potential probiotic	Pathogen tested or type of study conducted	Test method
Gilthead sea bream	Cytophaga sp., Roseobacter sp., Ruergeria sp., Paracoccus sp.,A. sp., Shewanella sp.	Natural larval survival study	In vivo
Gilthead sea bream	V. spp., Micrococcus sp.	L. anguillarum	In vitro and in vivo
Atlantic cod	Carnobacterium divergens	V. anguillarum	In vitro and in vivo
Atlantic cod	Carnobacterium divergens	V. anguillarum	In vitro and in vivo
Atlantic salmon	Lactobacillus plantarum	A. salmonicida	In vitro and in vivo
Atlantic salmon	Carnobacterium sp. (K1)	V. anguillarum, A. salmonicida	In vitro and in vivo
Atlantic salmon	Ps. fluorescens	A. salmonicida	In vitro and in vivo
Atlantic salmon, rainbow trout	Carnobacterium sp.	V. anguillarum, V. ordalii, Y. ruckeri, A. salmonicida	In vitro and in vivo
Eel	Commercial product: Cernivet® LBC (Ent. Faecium SF68), Toyocerin® (B. toyoi)	Ed. tarda	In vivo
Eel.	A. media	Saprolegnia sp	In vitro and in vivo
Eel	A. media	Saprolegnia parasitica	In vivo
Goldfish	Dead cells of A. hydrophila	A. salmonicida	In vivo
Indian major carp	B. subtilis	A. hydrophila	In vivo
Nile tilapia	Str. faecium, Lactobacillus acidophilus, Sacc. cerevisiae	Growth study	In vivo
Pollack	Commercial product: Bactocell (Pediococcus acidilactici), Levucell (Sacc. cerevisiae)	Pollack growth study using enriched Artemia	In vivo
Rainbow trout	Ps.fluorescens	V. anguillarum	In vitro and in vivo
Rainbow trout	Lactobacillus rhamnosus	A. salmonicida ssp. salmonicida	-
Rainbow trout	Ps. spp.	(furunculosis)	
Rainbow trout	A. hydrophila, V. fluvialis, Carnobacterium sp.	V. anguillarum	In vitro and in vivo
Rainbow trout	Dead cells of A. hydrophila, V. fluvialis, Carnobacterium sp.	A. salmonicida	In vitro and in vivo
Rainbow trout	Lactobacillus rhamnosus	A. salmonicida	In vivo
Rainbow trout	Commercial product: BioPlus2B (B. subtilis, B. licheniformis)	Immune enhancement paper	In vivo
Rainbow trout	Lactobacillus rhamnosus	Y. ruckeri Natural immunostimulation measured	In vivo
Rainbow trout	Pediococcus acidilactici, Sacc. boulardii	Prevention of vertebral column compression syndrome	In vivo
Rainbow trout	A. sobria	L. garvieae, Str. iniae	In vivo
Rainbow trout	Lactobacillus rhamnosus	Natural immunostimulation measured	In vivo
Rohu	B. circulans, B. subtilis	Digestive enzyme study	In vivo
Sea bass	Debaryomyces hansenii, Sacc. cerevisiae	Digestive enzyme study	In vivo
Senegalese sole	V. spp., Ps. spp., Micrococcus sp.	V. harveyi	In vitro and in vivo
Silver perch	A. media	Saprolegnia sp.	In vivo
Tilapia	Commercial product: Alchem Poseidon, Korea	Ed. tarda	In vivo
Turbot	2 unidentified marine bacteria	GIT colonization study	In vivo
Turbot	Marine bacteria	Natural survival study	In vivo
Turbot	Roseobacter spp., V. spp.	V. anguillarum, V. splendidus, Psalt. sp.	In vitro and in vivo

Table 1. Summary of research towards probiotics for finfish

The LAB bacteriocin producer widespread in nature, and were isolated from several sources: dairy products, fermented sausages, vegetables, sillage, and mammalian gastro-intestinal tract (Laukova et al., 1993; Kato et al., 1994; Giraffa, 1995; Ennahar et al.,1998). Recently, bacteriocin producing LAB were efficiently tested in attempt to improve aquatic environment for both shrimp and fish aquaculture (Calo-Mata P et al., 2007; Chae-Woo et al., 2009). Among them, bacteria belonging to the genus *Enterococcus* are primarily associated with the indigenous human and animal gastrointestinal flora and are widely distributed, being found in air, water, sewage, soil and vegetation (J. Lukasova & A. sustackova, 2003). Although certain *Enterococcus* spp. have recently been associated with human nosocomial infections (Murray, 1998), a wide variety of enterococcal strains are increasingly being used as probiotics owing to their contribution to the healthy microflora of human mucosal surfaces. They have also been introduced into animal foods owing to their contribution to the health of farmed animals and as biological control agents in aquaculture (Calo-Mata P. et al., 2007).

4. Probiotic development in aquaculture farming in Tunisia

In Tunisia, fish farming of the two species sea bass (*Dicentrarchus labrax*) and gilthead sea bream (*Sparus aurata*) has significantly increased since a great benefit for such aquaculture which was threatened by microbial infections causing high mortalities at larval stages, and therefore decrease in farmed fish production. In addition, widespread use of antibiotics created an ecological problem for coastal ecosystems due to emergence of antibiotic resistant pathogen bacteria (Bouamama, 2001; Dellali, 2001; El Bour et al., 2001). Therefore, selection and use of probiotic bacteria capable of inhibiting pathogenic bacteria in sustainable way without ecosystem alteration would be a useful for specific farming problems. In this scope, for several years the INSTM team in Tunisia, in collaboration with the Department of Analytical Chemistry, Nutrition and Food Science, from the University of Santiago de Compostela in Spain were focusing in isolation and characterization of probiotic group, lactic acid bacteria (LAB) which were recognized for their fermentative ability as well as their health and nutritional benefits.

The study aimed to investigate the occurrence and antibiotic resistance profiles of *Enterococcus* spp. associated to the skin and the gastrointestinal tract of farmed sea bass and sea bream, the main fish species with high economic value cultured in Mediterranean aquaculture. This was accomplished by phenotypic and genotypic analysis, the latter including 16S rRNA sequencing and RAPD-PCR analysis. Besides, and with a view to perform a preliminary screening of potential probiotic LAB, the strains were investigated in their ability to produce antibacterial compounds against spoilage and pathogenic bacteria.

4.1 Methodology

Gilthead sea bream (*Sparus aurata*) and European sea bass (*Dicentrarchus labrax*) were collected from a fish farm in Hergla (Aquaculture Tunisiènne, Monastir, Tunisia). Skin patches were excised and the intestinal content was removed by dissecting the fish, removing the intestine and squeezing out the contents. Eighty four LAB strains were then isolated and investigated. The phenotypic characterization of bacterial isolates was studied to determine their colony morphology, cell morphology, motility, Gram stain and the production of cytochrome oxidase and catalase. The phenotypic identification of LAB strains was carried out by means of miniaturized API 50 CH biochemical tests (BioMérieux, Marcy L'Etoile, France). The results of the identification tests were interpreted using the APILAB PLUS software (BioMérieux).

Production of antibacterial activities was investigated, against a range of 39 pathogenic and spoilage microorganisms (Table2), to select potential producer strains. Detection of bacteriocin activity in LAB strains was screened by means of a standardized agar disk diffusion method.

Code	Genus	Species	Origin
AmH01	*Aeromonas*	*hydrophila*	ATCC 7966
BaC23	*Bacillus*	*cereus*	ATCC 14893
BaP31	*Bacillus*	*pumilus*	ATCC 7061
BaS05	*Bacillus*	*Subtilis ssp. Spizizenii*	ATCC 6633
BxT01	*Brochotrix*	*thermosphacta*	ATCC 11509
CbD21	*Carnobacterium*	*divergens*	ATCC 35677
CbM01	*Carnobacterium*	*maltaromaticum*	LHICA collection
EbA01	*Enterobacter*	*aerogenes*	ATCC 13048
EbC11	*Enterobacter*	*cloacae*	ATCC 13047
HaA02	*Hafnia*	*alvei*	ATCC 9760
KlOx11	*Klebsiella*	*oxytoca*	ATCC 13182
KlP02	*Klebsiella*	*planticola*	ATCC 33531
KlPn21	*Klebsiella*	*Pneumoniae ssp. pneumoniae*	ATCC 10031
Lb30A	*Lactobacillus*	*saerimneri*	LHICA collection
MoM02	*Morganella*	*morganii ssp. morganii*	ATCC 8076H
PhD11	*Photobacterium*	*damselae*	ATCC 33539
PrM01	*Proteus*	*mirabilis*	ATCC 14153
PrP11	*Proteus*	*penneri*	ATCC 33519
PrV21	*Proteus*	*vulgaris*	ATCC 9484
PsF12	*Pseudomonas*	*fluorescens*	ATCC 13525
PsFr51	*Pseudomonas*	*fragi*	ATCC 4973
PsG21	*Pseudomonas*	*gessardii*	LHICA collection
SrM53	*Serratia*	*marcescens ssp. marcescens*	ATCC 274
SyE21	*Staphylococcus*	*epidermidis*	ATCC 35983
SyX11	*Staphylococcus*	*xylosus*	ATCC 29971
StM03	*Stenotrophomonas*	*maltophilia*	ATCC 13637
59	*Staphylococcus*	*aureus*	ATCC 9144
4521	*Staphylococcus*	*aureus*	ATCC 35845
4032	*Lysteria*	*monocytogenes*	NCTC 11994
1112	*Lysteria*	*monocytogenes* 1112	LHICA collection
CI34.1	*Pseudomonas*	*anguilliseptica*	Seabream*
ACR5.1(AS)	*Aeromonas*	*salmonicida*	Turbot*
CI52.1(VCI)	*Vibrio*	*anguillarum*	Seabream*
ACC30.1	*Photobacterium*	*damselae ssp. piscida*	Sole*
V62	*Vibrio*	*anguillarum*	Seabream**
VF	*Vibrio*	*anguillarum*	Seabass***
AF	*Aeromonas*	*salmonicida*	Seabass***
V90.11.287(V287)	*Vibrio*	*anguillarum*	Seabass****
AH2	*Pseudomonas*	*fluorescens*	*Lates niloticus*****

* Strains provided by Pr. J. L. Romalde (Spain). ** Strain provided by Pr. G. Breuil (France). *** Strains provided by Pr. J. C. Raymond (France). **** Strains provided by Pr. L. Gram (Denmark).

Table 2. Pathogenic and spoilage indicator microorganisms used to test the antibacterial activities of LAB isolates.

Genetic characterization of producer LAB strains was then performed by PCR targeted to the 16S rRNA gene using the universal set of primers: p8FPL (forward: 5'-AGTTTGATCCTGGCTCAG-3') and p806R (reverse: 5'-GGACTACCAGGGTATCTAAT-3'), that yield a 800 bp PCR product of the 16S rRNA gene. The PCR products were purified and sequenced. The sequences were compared with others present in GenBank database.

Further genetic characterization of LAB isolates was performed by RAPD-PCR using primers M13 (5′-GAGGGTGGCGGTTCT-3′) (Andrighetto et al., 2004). To check reproducibility, all PCR assays were performed in triplicate. Each reaction we included a tube without template DNA as a negative control.

The antibacterial sensitivity was determined by the agar diffusion method according to Chabbert (1982), using 16 antibiotics that were selected as representative of different classes of antimicrobial agents relevant in human and animal medicine (Penicillin G, Amoxicillin, Oxacilin, Cefoxitin, Ceftriaxon, Streptomycin, Tobramycin, Neomycin, Chloramphenicol, Tetracyclin, Oleandomycin, Nitrofurantoin, Trimethoprim-Sulphonamid, Rifampicin, Oxolinic acid and also Vancomycin). Based on the zones of inhibition a qualitative report of "susceptible", "intermediate" or "resistant" can be determined for the tested bacteria according to French national guidelines (Comité de l'Antibiogramme de la Société Française de Microbiologie, 1996).

4.2 Results and discussion

Eighty four strains of LAB were isolated from both gastrointestinal content and skin of fish studied. All isolates were Gram-positive, catalase-negative, facultatively anaerobic and nonmotile chain-forming cocci. They were tested for assaying inhibitory production against 39 Gram-positives and Gram-negatives bacteria, including pathogenic bacteria in aquaculture and others spoilage bacteria. 58 strains (69%) exhibited inhibitory activity against a large number of the indicator organisms investigated. Greater inhibition was observed against L. monocytogenes, S. aureus, A. hydrophila, A. salmonicida, V. anguillarum and Carnobacterium strains in comparison with the remaining indicators. The diameters of the inhibition halos were within the 7.5–18 mm range. Thus, we selected 35 highly producing strains that generated inhibitory zones with diameters between 12 and 18 mm.

The results allowed the classification of the strains as belonging to the species E. faecium (29 strains) and E. sanguinicola (6 strains) (paper under process) (Table3). Other studies, previously mentioned, also showed that the skin and gastrointestinal tract of various fish species contains lactic acid bacteria which produce antibacterial compounds able to inhibit the growth of several micoorganisms (Ringo 1999; Spanggaard B. et al., 2001; Rengpipat S. et al., 2008; Vijayabaskar P & Somasundaram S. T., 2008; Ringo, 2008).

According to the results obtained, all the strains tested were resistant to at least three different antibiotics. The frequency of resistance to the various antimicrobials for all bacteria is presented in Fig. 1. Differences of resistance rates were noted for amoxicillin, oxacillin, cephalosporins (cefoxitin, ceftriaxon), aminosids (streptomycin, tobramycin and neomycin), macrolids (oleandomycin) and oxolinic acid. In contrast, phenicol, tetracyclin, rifampicin and trimethoprim-sulphamid were the most active antibiotics against the majority of the bacterial isolates (fig1).

In fact, more than half (64.8%) of all the isolates were found to be resistant to amoxicillin and 71.4% were resistant to oleandomycin, 78.1% to ceftriaxon, 80.1% to streptomycin and 85% to cefoxitin. Oxacillin resistance was found in 92.5% of the isolates and tobramycin and oxolinic acid resistance in 94.2%. Resistance to neomycin was found in 98.3% of the isolates. Resistance to chloramphenicol and trimethoprim-sulphamide was detected in 5.1% and 2.2% of the isolates respectively, 8% of the isolates were found to be resistant to tetracyclin. Resistance to rifampicin was seen in 16.9% of the isolates

Strains	Fish	Organ	Identification	Accession number
UPAA 1	Sea bass	GIT	*Enterococcus sanguinicola*	GU460379
UPAA 4	Sea bass	GIT	*Enterococcus faecium*	GU460381
UPAA 7	Sea bass	Skin	*Enterococcus faecium*	GU460383
UPAA 11	Sea bream	GIT	*Enterococcus faecium*	HQ450696
UPAA 15	Sea bass	Skin	*Enterococcus faecium*	GU460385
UPAA 23	Sea bass	GIT	*Enterococcus faecium*	GU460388
UPAA 24	Sea bass	GIT	*Enterococcus faecium*	GU460389
UPAA 25	Sea bass	GIT	*Enterococcus faecium*	GU460390
UPAA 31	Sea bass	Skin	*Enterococcus faecium*	GU460394
UPAA 32	Sea bass	GIT	*Enterococcus faecium*	GU460395
UPAA 33	Sea bass	GIT	*Enterococcus sanguinicola*	GU460396
UPAA 34	Sea bream	Skin	*Enterococcus faecium*	HQ450701
UPAA 35	Sea bream	GIT	*Enterococcus faecium*	HQ450702
UPAA 37	Sea bass	GIT	*Enterococcus faecium*	GU460398
UPAA 39	Sea bream	GIT	*Enterococcus faecium*	HQ450704
UPAA 40	Sea bream	GIT	*Enterococcus faecium*	HQ450705
UPAA 44	Sea bream	Skin	*Enterococcus faecuim*	HQ450706
UPAA 45	Sea bream	GIT	*Enterococcus faecuim*	HQ450707
UPAA 53	Sea bass	GIT	*Enterococcus faecium*	GU460402
UPAA 54	Sea bass	GIT	*Enterococcus faecium*	GU460403
UPAA 56	Sea bass	Skin	*Enterococcus faecium*	GU460404
UPAA 57	Sea bass	Skin	*Enterococcus sanguinicola*	GU460405
UPAA 58	Sea bass	Skin	*Enterococcus faecium*	GU460406
UPAA 63	Sea bass	GIT	*Enterococcus faecium*	GU460409
UPAA 71	Sea bream	GIT	*Enterococcus sanguinicola*	HQ450716
UPAA 80	Sea bass	GIT	*Enterococcus faecium*	GU460416
UPAA 83	Sea bass	Skin	*Enterococcus faecium*	GU460415
UPAA 85	Sea bream	GIT	*Enterococcus faecium*	HQ450721
UPAA 89	Sea bream	GIT	*Enterococcus faecium*	HQ450724
UPAA 105	Sea bass	GIT	*Enterococcus faecium*	GU460417
UPAA 110	Sea bream	GIT	*Enterococcus faecium*	HQ450730
UPAA 111	Sea bass	Skin	*Enterococcus faecium*	GU460420
UPAA 113	Sea bass	GIT	*Enterococcus sanguinicola*	GU460421
UPAA 114	Sea bass	GIT	*Enterococcus faecium*	GU460422
UPAA 116	Sea bass	Skin	*Enterococcus sanguinicola.*	GU460423

Table 3. Antibacterial producing isolates

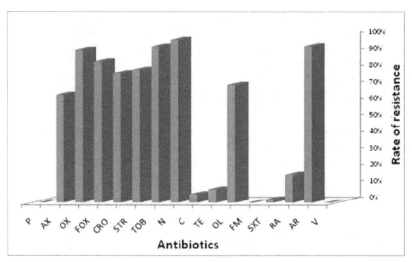

P: penicillin G; Ax: amoxicillin; Ox: oxacillin; Fox: cefoxitin; Cro: ceftriaxon; Str: streptomycin; Tob: tobramycin; N: neomycin; C: chloramphenicol; Te: tetracyclin; Ol: oleandomycin; Fm: furans; Sxt: trimethoprim-sulphamide; Ra: rifampicin; Ar: oxolinic acid; V: vancomycine.

Fig. 1. Profiles of resistance obtained for the different enterococci isolates against the 16 antimicrobial agents tested.

Interestingly, all the strains were sensitive to vancomycin, penicillin and furans and were not haemolytic.

Enterococci have been known to be resistant to most antibiotics used in clinical practice. Multidrug-resistant and vancomycin-resistant enterococci are commonly isolated from humans, animal sources, aquatic habitats, agricultural run-off which indicates their ability to enter the human food chain (Rice et al., 1995). They are naturally resistant to cephalosporins, aminoglycosides and clindamycin and may also be resistant to tetracyclins and erythromycin. They are intermediate sensitive to penicillin and ampicillin and glycopeptides. The strains that produce β-lactamase are rare and Vancomycin-resistant enterococci (VRE) are emerging as a global threat to public health.

Enterococci are known to acquire antibiotic resistance with relative ease and to be able to spread these resistance genes to other species (Kuhn et al., 2000). *Enterococcus faecalis* has been reported to transfer plasmids harbouring antibiotic-resistance traits to other enterococci and to *Listeria monocytogenes* in water treatment plants (Marcinek et al., 1998). *Enterococcus faecium* conjugative transposons can be transferred from animal bacteria to human ones. Such conjugative trasposons can also transfer vancomycin resistance to *Staphylococcus aureus*, streptococci and lactobacilli.

The extremely high level of antibiotic resistance observed in these bacteria has made them feared infectious agents in intensive care wards. Possible pathogenicity factors like hemolysins have been described. The most important species are *E. faecalis* and *E. faecium*, the first being more common in human illnesses, the second one (though less common in human infections) may pose a larger resistance threat (Huycke et al., 1998).

In both species, the evolutionary development of resistance has been attributed to the possession of broad host range and extremely mobile genetic elements like conjugative plasmids and transposons. The molecular details of the structures and functions of these elements are fairly well studied and becoming understood (Clewell et al., 1995; Marra & Scott 1999). It is noteworthy that transcription of the transfer functions of Tn*916* requiring excission of the element is dramatically increased in the presence of tetracyclin (Celli & Trieu-Cuot 1998).

Therefore, antibiotic resistance, notably to vancomycin, and the presence of haemolysins as an indicator of potential pathogenecity, must be evaluated in these microorganisms, before they can be used as probiotics and/or food additives.

The antimicrobial spectra observed for the *Enterococcus* species isolated included several genera indicating a broad spectrum of activity against Gram-positive but also Gram-negative pathogenic and spoilage organisms. A number of earlier studies have also shown that several marine bacteria produce inhibitory substances that inhibit bacterial pathogens in aquaculture systems (Nogami & Maeda, 1992; Austin et al., 1995; Rengpipat et al., 1998; Gram et al., 1999; Chahad et al., 2007). The use of such bacteria to inhibit pathogens by release of antimicrobial substances is now gaining importance in fish farming as a better and more effective alternative than administering antibiotics to manage the health of these organisms (Vijayan et al., 2006). Spanggaard et al. (2001) reported that this antagonism was the most influential factor preventing the establishment of the exogenous bacteria and indicates that the antagonistic part of an indigenous flora may offer a significant contribution to the control of unwanted (pathogenic) bacteria.

LAB isolated from the same environment on which they will be further used as bio-control cultures, ensure that these LAB strains are well ecological adapted. This fact is an important factor for their effectiveness as natural antimicrobial agents. The local results suggest the potential usefulness of the inhibitory-producing strains isolated from fish, as probiotics in aquaculture, in order to prevent bacterial infections caused by *A. salmonicida*, *A. hydrophila* and *V. anguillarum* which are the most common pathogenic bacteria isolated from the marine environment, causing high mortalities of fish and shellfish. Their inhibitory activities show some properties which make it potentially remarkable food preservatives.

5. Conclusion

In comparison with studies on impact of antibio-resistance on terrestrial food producing animals, those related to marine aquaculture enterprises still scarced. The present study supports the view that there is a risk of transfer of resistant bacteria to humans from consumption of aquaculture products. In Tunisian field, although there are no products registered for use in aquaculture, antimicrobial resistance resistance is present in isolates from aquaculture..

The extent of the resistance found and in particular the significant levels of multiple resistance are of concern. Follow-up studies are required to investigate the extent of antibiotic use in Tunisian aquaculture farms and environments and to determine the molecular basis of antimicrobial resistance to the different antibiotics, the potential for transfer of resistance genes from aquaculture isolates to human pathogens, some assessment of the risk of transfer of resistant organisms (or genes) to humans *via* food chain and the threats imposed by environmental contamination with antibiotic resistant bacteria.

The highly antibacterial producing *Enterococcus* strains isolated from both sea bream and sea bass which inhibit growth of pathogenic and spoiling bacteria should have a potential practical interest and offer a natural means for simultaneous application as probiotics and/or for preventing the development of *Listeria* in food stuffs.

6. References

Andrighetto, C.; Knijif E.; Lombardi, A.; Vancanneyt, M.; Kersters, K.; Swings, J. & Dellaglio F (2004). Phenotypic and genetic diversity of enterococci isolated from Italian cheeses. *Journal of Dairy Research*, Vol.68, pp.303-316

Angulo, F. J.; Nargund, V. N. & Chiller, T. C. (2004). Evidence of an Association Between Use of Anti-microbial Agents in Food Animals and Anti-microbial Resistance Among Bacteria Isolated from Humans and the Human Health Consequences of Such Resistance. *Journal of Veterinary Medecine*, Vol. 51, pp.374–379

Austin, B.; Stuckey, L.F.; Robertson, PAW.; Effendi, I. & Griffith, DRW. (1995). A probiotic strain of *Vibrio alginolyticus* effective in reducing diseases caused by *Aeromonas salmonicida,Vibrio anguillarum* and *Vibrio ordalii*. *Journal of Fish Diseases*, Vol.18, pp.93-96

Bairagi, A.; Sakar Ghosh; K., Sen; S.K. & Ray, A.K. (2002). Enzyme producing bacterial flora isolated from fish digestive tracts. *Aquaculture International* , Vol.10, pp.109–121

Bairagi, A.; Sarkar Ghosh, K.; Sen, S.K. & Ray, A.K. (2004). Evaluation of the nutritive value of Leucaena leucocephala leaf meal, inoculated with fish intestinal bacteria *Bacillus subtilis* and Bacillus circulans in formulated diets for rohu, Labeo rohita (Hamilton) fingerlings. *Aquaculture Research*, Vol. 35, pp. 436–446

Bakhrouf, A. ; Ben Ouada, H. & Oueslati, R. (1995). Essai de traitement des vibrioses du loup *Dicentrarchus labrax* dans une zone de pisciculture, à Monastir, Tunisie. *Marine Life*, Vol.5, pp. 47-54

Balcàzar, JL.; de Blas, I.; Ruiz-Zarzuela, I.; Cunningham, D., Vendrell, D. & Muuzquiz, JL. (2006). The role of probiotics in aquaculture. *Veterinary Microbiology*, Vol. 114, pp.173–186

Barton, M.D. (2000). Antibiotic use in animals feed and its impact on human health. *Nuritiont Research Reviews*, Vol.13, pp.79–299

Ben Kahla-Nakbi, A.; K., Chaieb; A., Besbes; T., Zmantar & A., Bakhrouf, (2006). Virulence and enterobacterial repetitive intergenic consensus PCR of *Vibrio alginolyticus* strains isolated from Tunisian cultured gilthead sea bream and sea bass outbreaks. *Veterinary Microbiology*, Vol.117, pp.321-327

Boggard van den, AE. & Stobberingh EE. (2000). Epidemiology of resistance to antibiotics-Links between animals and humans. *International Journal of Antimicrobial Agents*, Vol.*14*, pp.327-335

Bouamama, K. (2001). *Mytilus galloprovincialis* de la lagune de Bizerte : populations bactériennes et Biomarqueurs non spécifiques. Diplôme des études approfondies (DEA). Faculté des Sciences de Tunis, Institut des Sciences et Technologies de la Mer. Tunis, Tunisia

Boutiba, I.; Ghozzi, R.; Jouaihia, W.; Mahjoubi, F.; Thabet, L.. Smaoui, H.; Ben Hassen, A. Hàmmamí, A.; Kechrid, A. & Ben Redjeb, S. (2007). Résistance bactérienne aux antibiotiques en Tunisie : Données de 1999 A 2003, *Revue Tunisienne d'Infectiologie,* Vol. 1, pp. 5-11

Calo-Mata, P.; Arlindo, S.; Boehm. K. ; De Miguel, T. Pascoal A. & Barros-Velazquez, J. (2007). Current application and future trends of lactic acid bacteria and their bacteriocins for biopreservation of aquatic food products. *Food Bioprocess Technology,* Vol.1(1), pp.43-63

Celli, J. & Trieu-Cuot, P. (1998). Circularization of Tn916 is required for expression of the transposon-encoded transfer functions: characterization of long tetracycline-inducible transcripts reading through the attachment site. *Molecular Microbiology,* Vol. 28, pp.103–117

Chabbert Y.A (1982). L'antibiogramme. In : Bactériologie médicaleL. Le Miror, M. véron, (eds): Flammarion. Medecine Science. Paris, 205-212.

Chae-Woo, M.; Yun-Seok, C. & Kye-Heon, O. (2009). Removal of pathogenic bacteria and nitrogens by *Lactobacillus spp.* JK-8 and JK-11. *Aquaculture,* Vol.287, pp.266-270

Chahad Ouissal, B.; El Bour, M.; Mraouna, R.; Abdennaceur, H. & Boudabous, A. (2007). Preliminary selection study of potential probiotic bacteria from aquacultural areas in Tunisia. *Annals of Microbiology,* Vol.57 (2), pp.185-190

Chelossi, E. ; Vezzulli, L. ; Milano, A. ; Branzoni, M. ; Fabiano, M. ; Riccardi, G. & Banat, I.M., (2003). Antibiotic resistance of benthic bacteria in fish-farm and control sediments of the Western Mediterranean. *Aquaculture,* Vol. 219, pp.83–97

CIESM 2004. Novel contaminants and pathogens in coastal waters. CIESM Workshop Monograph N°26, Monaco "www.ciesm.org/online/monographs/Neuchatel.pdf"

Clewell, DB., Flannagan, SE. & Jaworsky. DD. (1995). Unconstrained bacterial promiscuity: the Tn916-Tn1545 family of conjugative transposons. *Trends in Microbiology,* Vol.3, pp.229–236

Comité de l'Antibiogramme de la Société Française de Microbiologie, (1996). Statement 1996 CA-SFM. Zone sizes and MIC breakpoints for non-fastidious organisms. *Clinical Microbiology and Infecion,* Vol.2, Suppl. 1, pp.46-49

Dellali, M., (2001). Utilisation d'indicateurs microbiologiques et biochimiques chez *Ruditapes decussatus* et *Mytilus galloprovincialis* dans la biosurveillance de la lagune de Bizerte : Validation de certains biomarqueurs. Thèse de doctorat, Faculté des Sciences de Bizerte. Tunisia

El Bour, M.; Attia El Hilli, H.; Mraouna, R. & Ayari, W. (2001). Bacterial study of mesophilic Aeromonads distribution in shellfish. Proceeding of the fifth international conference on the Mediterranean coastal environment, *MEDCOAST*, pp.557- 565

Ennahar, S.; Aoude-Werner. D.; Assobhei, O. & Hasselmann, D. (1998). Antilisterial activity of enterocin 81, a bacteriocin produced by *Enterococcus faecium* WHE 81 isolated from cheese, *Journal of Applied Microbiology, Vol.*85, pp.521–526

Franz, CMAP; van Belkum, MJ.; Holzapfel, WH; Abriouel, H. & Galvez, A. (2007). Diversity of Enterococcal bacteriocins and their grouping in a new classification scheme. *FEMS Microbiology Review,* Vol.31, pp.293–310

Fuller, R. (1989). Probiotics in man and animals. *Journal of Applied Bacteriology,* Vol. 66, pp.365–378

Giraffa, G. (1995). Enterococcal bacteriocins: their potential as anti-*Listeria* factors in dairy technology. *Food Microbe,* Vol.12, pp.291–299

Gismondo, M.R.; Drago, L.; Lombardi, A. (1999). Review of probiotics available to modify gastrointestinal flora. *International Journal of Antimicrobial Agents,* Vol. 12, pp.287–292

Gram, L.; Melchiorsen, J.; Spanggaard, B.; Huber, I. & Nielsen, T.F. (1999). Inhibition of Vibrio anguillarum by Pseudomonas fluorescens AH2, a possible probiotic treatment of fish. *Applied and Environmental Microbiology, Vol.*65 (3), pp.969–973

Gullian, M.; Thompson, F. & Rodriguez, J. (2004). Selection of probiotic bacteria and study of their immunostimulatory effect in Penaeus vannamei. *Aquaculture,* Vol.233, pp.1–14

Huycke, MM.; Sahm, DF. & Gilmore, MS. (1998). Multiple-drug resistant enterococci: the nature of the problem and an agenda for the future. *Emerging Infectious Diseases,* Vol.4(2), pp.239-249

Irianto, A. & Austin, B. (2002a). Probiotics in aquaculture. *Journal of Fish Diseases,* Vol.25, pp.633–642

Irianto, A. & Austin, B. (2002b). Use of probiotics to control furunculosis in rainbow trout, Oncorhynchus mykiss (Walbaum). *Journal of Fish Diseases,* Vol.25, pp.333–342

Itami, T.; Asano, M.; Tokushige, K.; Kubono, K.; Nakagawa, A.; Noboru, T.; Nishimura, H.; Maeda, M.; Kondo, M. & Takahashi, Y. (1998). Enhancement of disease resistance of kuruma shrimp, *Penaeus japonicus,* after oral administration of peptidoglycan derived from Bifidobacterium thermophilum. *Aquaculture,* Vol.164, pp.277–288

Murray, BE. (1998). Diversity among multidrug-resistant enterococci. *Emerging Infectious Diseases, Vol.* 4, pp.37–47

Kato, T.; Matsuda, T.; Ogawa, E.; Ogawa, H.; Kato, H.; Doi, U. & Nakamura, R. (1994). Plantaricin-149, a bacteriocin produced by *Lactobacillus pluntarum* NRIC 149. *Journal of Fermentution and Bioengineering,* Vol.77, pp.277-282

Kuhn, I.; Iversen, A.; Burman, L.G.; Olsson-Liljequist, B.; Franklin, A.; Finn, M.; Aarestrup, F.; Seyfarth, A.M.; Blanch, A.R., Taylor, H.; Caplin, J.; Moreno, M.A.; Dominguez, L. & Mollby, R. (2000). Epidemiology and ecology of enterococci, with special reference to antibiotic resistant strains, in animals, humans and the environment. Example of an ongoing project within the European research programme. *International Journal of Antimicrobial Agents.* Vol.14, pp.337–342

Lategan, M.J. & Gibson, L.F. (2003). Antagonistic activity of *Aeromonas media* strain A199 against Saprolegnia sp., an opportunistic pathogen of the eel, *Anguilla australis* Richardson. *Journal of Fish Diseases,* Vol.26, pp.147–153

Lategan, M.J.; Torpy, F.R. & Gibson, L.F. (2004a). Biocontrol of saprolegniosis in silver perch Bidyanus bidyanus (Mitchell) by Aeromonas media strain A199. *Aquaculture,* Vol.235, pp.77–88

Lategan, M.J.; Torpy, F.R. & Gibson, L.F. (2004b). Control of saprolegniosis in the eel *Anguilla australis* Richardson, by *Aeromonas media* strain A199. *Aquaculture,* Vol.240, pp.19–27

Laukova, A.; M., Marekova & P. Javorsky. (1993). Detection and antimicrobial spectrum of a bacteriocin like substances produced by Enterococcus faecium CCM4231. *J. Letters in Applied Microbiology, Vol.*16, pp.257-260

Lukàsova, J. & Sustàckovà, A. (2003). Enterococci and Antibiotic Resistance: Review Article. *Acta. Veterinaria Brno.*, Vol.72, pp.315-323

Marcinek, H.; Wirth, R.; Muscholl-Silberhorn, A. & Gauer, M. (1998). Enterococcus faecalis gene transfer under natural conditions in municipal sewage water treatment plants. *Applied and Environmental Microbiology*, Vol.64, pp.626-632

Mauguin, S. & Novel, G. (1994). Characterization of lactic acid bacteria isolated from seafood. *Journal of Applied Bacteriology*, Vol.76, pp.616–625

Marra, D. & Scott. JR. (1999). Regulation of excision of the conjugative transposon Tn916. *Molecular Microbio*logy, Vol.31, pp.609–621

Matyar, F. (2007). Distribution and antimicrobial multiresistance in Gram-negative bacteria isolated from Turkish sea bass (*Dicentrarchus labrax* L., 1781) farm. *Annals of Microbiology*, Vol.**57**, pp.35–38

Nogami, K. & Maeda, M. (1992). Bacteria as biocontrol agents for rearing larvae of the Crab *Portunus trituberculatus*. *Canadian Journal of Fish. and Aquatic Sciences*, pp.2373-2376

Ramirez, R.F. & Dixon, B.A. (2003). Enzyme production by obligate intestinal anaerobic bacteria isolated from Oscars (*Astronotus ocellatus*), angelfish (*Pterophyllum scalare*) and southern flounder (*Paralichthys lethostigma*). *Aquaculture* , Vol.227, pp.417–426

Rengpipat, S.; Phianphak, W.; Piyatiratitivorakul, S. & Menasveta, P. (1998). Effects of a probiotic bacterium on black tiger shrimp *Penaeus monodon* survival and growth. *Aquaculture* Vol.167, pp.301-313

Rengpipat, S., Rueangruklikhit, T. & Piyatiratitivorakul, S. (2008). Evaluations of lactic acid bacteria as probiotics for juvenile sea bass *Lates calcarifer*. *Aquaculture Research*, Vol.39, pp.134-143

Rezgui, I. (2010). Etude de l'antibioresistance chez deux espèces de poisons aquacoles en Tunisie: le loup (*Dicentrarchus labrax*) et la daurade (*Sparus aurata*). Master of Biology. University of Sciences of Tunis. Institut des Sciences et Technologies de la Mer. Tunis, Tunisia

Rice, E.W.; Messer, J.W.; Johnson, C.H. & Reasoner, D.J. (1995). Occurrence of high-level aminoglycoside resistance in environmental isolates of enterococci. *Applied and Environmental Microbiology*. Vol.61, pp.374–376

Rico-Mora, R.; Voltolina, D. & Villaescusa-Celaya, J.A. (1998). Biological control of Vibrio alginolyticus in Skeletonema costatum (Bacillariophyceae) cultures. *Aquacultural Engineering* Vol.19, pp.1–6

Rigos, G.; Nengas, I.; Alexis, M. & Troisi, G. (2004). Potential drug (oxytetracycline & oxolinic acid) pollution from Mediterranean sparid fish farms. *Aquatic Toxicology*, Vol.69, pp.281-288

Rigos, G. & Troisi, G. (2005). Antibacterial agents in Mediterranean finfish farming: a synopsis of drug pharmacokinetics in important euryhaline fish species and possible environmental implications. *Reviews in Fish Biology and Fisheries*, Vol.15, pp.53-73

Ringo, E. (1999). Lactic acid bacteria in fish: antibacterial effect against fish pathogens.In effects of Anti nutrients on the Nutritional Value of Legume Diets, Vol.8, ed.

Krogdahl, Mathiesen, SD. And Pryme, I. COST 98. 70-75, Luxembourg: EEC Publication.

Ringø, E. & Gatesoupe, F.-J. (1998). Lactic acid bacteria in fish: a review. *Aquaculture,* Vol.160, pp.177-203

Ringo, E. (2008). The ability of *Carnobacteria* isolated from fish intestine to inhibit growth of fish pathogenic bacteria: a screening study. *Aquaculture Research,* Vol.39, pp.171-180

Salminen, S.; Ouwehand, A.; Benno, Y. & Lee, Y.K. (1999). Probiotics: how should they be defined. *Trends in Food Science and Technology,* Vol.10, pp.107-110

Smith, P.; Hiney, M. & Samuelson, O. (1994). Bacterialresistance to antimicrobial agents used in fish farming: a critical evaluation of method and meaning. *Annual Review of Fish Diseases,* Vol.4, pp.273-313

Smith, V.J.; Brown, J.H. & Hauton, C. (2003). Immunostimulation in crustaceans: does it really protect against infection?. *Fish and Shellfish Immunology,* Vol.15, pp.71-90

Sorum, H. (1998). Mobile drug resistance genes among fish bacteria. *APMIS Suppl.,* Vol.106, pp.74-76

Sorum, H. (1999). Antibiotic resistance in aquaculture. *Acta Veterinaria Scandinavica Suppl.,* Vol.92, pp.29-36

Spanggaard, B.; Huber, I., Nielsen, J.; Sick. E.B.; Pipper, C.B.; Martinussen, T.; Slierendrecht, W.J. & Gram, L. (2001). The probiotic potential against vibriosis of the indigenous microflora of rainbow trout. *Environmental Microbiology,* Vol.3(12), pp.755-765

Vaseeharan, B.; Lin, J. & Ramasamy, P. (2004). Effect of probiotics, antibiotic sensitivity, pathogenicity, and plasmid profiles of *Listonella anguillarum* like bacteria isolated from Penaeus monodon culture systems. *Aquaculture,* Vol.241, pp.77-91

Verschuere, L. ; Rombaut, G. ; Huys, G. ; Dhont, J. ; Sorgeloos, P. & Verstraete, W. (1999). Microbial control of the culture of Artemia juveniles through preemptive colonization by selected bacterial strains. *Applied and Environmental Microbiology,* Vol.65, pp.2527-2533

Verschuere, L.; Rombaut, G.; Sorgeloos, P. & Verstraete, W. (2000a). Probiotic bacteria as biological control agents in aquaculture. *Microbiology and Molecular Biology Review,* Vol.64, pp.655-671

Verschuere, L.; Heang, H.; Criel, G.; Sorgeloos, P. & Verstraete,W. (2000b). Selected bacterial strains protect Artemia spp. from the pathogenic effects of Vibrio proteolyticus CW8T2. *Applied and Environmental Microbiology,* Vol.66(3), pp.1139-1146

Vijayabaskar, P. & Somasundaram, S. T. (2008). Isolation of bacteriocin producing lactic acid bacteria from fish gut and probiotic activity against common fresh water fish pathogen *Aeromonas hydrophila. Biotechnology,* Vol.7, pp.124-128

Vijayan, K.K.; Bright Singh, I.S.; Jayaprakash, N.S.; Alavandi, S.V.; Somnath Pai, S., Preetha, R.; Rajan, J.J.S. & Santiago, T.C. (2006). A brackish water isolate of *Pseudomonas* PS-102, a potential antagonistic bacterium against pathogenic vibrios in penaeid and non-penaeid rearing systems. *Aquaculture,* Vol.251, pp.192-200

Yan, L.; Boyd, K.G. & Burgess, J.G. (2002). Surface attachment induced production of antimicrobial compounds by marine epiphytic bacteria using modified roller bottle cultivation. *Marine Biotechnology,* Vol.4, pp.356-366

Zorrilla, I.; M., Chabrillón; S., Arijo; P., Díaz Rosales; E., Martínez-Manzanares; M.C., Balebona & M.A., Moriñigo, (2003). Bacteria recovered from diseased cultured gilthead sea bream (*Sparus aurata* L.) in southwestern Spain. *Aquaculture*, Vol.218, pp.11-20

14

Antibiotic-Free Selection for Bio-Production: Moving Towards a New "Gold Standard"

Régis Sodoyer, Virginie Courtois, Isabelle Peubez and Charlotte Mignon
Sanofi Pasteur,
France

1. Introduction

Antibiotics have shown a proven efficiency profile in therapy against some infectious agents for several decades. Nevertheless, a large-scale spreading of antibiotics in the environment, and emergence of resistant or even multi-resistant pathogenic bacterial strains has become a general concern promise to even further increase. Besides therapeutic applications, antibiotics are often used as a selection pressure to avoid bio-contamination in production processes such as fermentation. In this particular context the problem can show two distinct facets: the antibiotic molecule itself, seen as a contaminant product in a given biological and the antibiotic resistance gene used as a selection marker.

The increasing regulatory requirements to which biological agents are subjected will hopefully have a great impact in the field of industrial protein expression and production. There is an expectation that in a near future, there may be "zero tolerance" towards antibiotic-based selection and production systems. Besides the antibiotic itself, the antibiotic resistance gene is a major subject of consideration. The complete absence of antibiotic-resistance gene being the only way to ensure that propagation in the environment or transfer of resistance to pathogenic strains will not happen.

In order to address these issues, different and complementary approaches can be applied. The first would be to design more stable host/vector couples allowing to set-up and conduct fermentation processes in complete absence of antibiotics. A more achieved strategy would be to substitute the antibiotic-based selection by an alternative mean such as the complementation of an essential gene product, not expressed by the host or sophisticated post-segregational killing mechanism.

For specific therapeutic agents or fields of application such as DNA vaccination or gene therapy the presence of an antibiotic resistance gene in the vector backbone is seen as undesirable to health authorities. In that case the problem is the possibility of horizontal transfer of antibiotic resistance to circulating microbial population.

2. Current selection methods

2.1 Different antibiotic-based systems

Most commercialized vectors use antibiotic-based selection markers. Ampicillin and kanamycin resistance genes are two widely used selection markers.

Ampicillin resistance gene, Amp^R also known as bla$_{TEM1}$, is derived from *Salmonella paratyphi*. It allows the synthesis of the beta-lactamase enzyme, which neutralizes antibiotics of the penicillin group, such as ampicillin. Surprisingly, ampicillin that is the most popular selection marker used in research laboratories is in fact a very inefficient selection mean in liquid cultures. The antibiotic-resistance gene product, β-lactamase, efficiently secreted into the culture supernatant rapidly eliminates the antibiotic, even if used at high concentration.

Chloramphenicol is more rarely used, or for some specific applications, for instance, large plasmid or cosmid DNA amplification. The spectra of activity of this antibiotic being variable between true bactericidal and bacteriostatic effect according to the gram character or nature of the bacterial strain considered (Rahal and Simberkoff 1979).

Kanamycin resistance gene, Kan^R also know as *ntpII* (neomycin phosphotransferase II) was initially isolated from the transposon Tn5 that was present in the bacterium strain *Escherichia coli* K12. The gene encodes the aminoglycoside 3'-phosphotransferase enzyme, which inactivates by phosphorylation a range of aminoglycoside antibiotics such as neomycin and kanamycin.

2.2 Advantages and drawbacks

Even if antibiotic resistance gene are widely use for DNA production and recombinant protein expression in bacteria, regulatory agencies tend to restrict their use because of potential horizontal transfer to environmental bacteria. Indeed, due to several mechanisms of gene transfer between bacteria, a potential risk of antibiotic resistance spread exists.

3. Potential concern

3.1 Safety issue

Antibiotic resistance genes are the most commonly used selectable markers for plasmid production (i.e. for vaccine or therapeutic DNA or for production of recombinant proteins as biotherapeutics).To date, kanamycin resistance gene is the most commonly used as selectable antibiotic marker. Ampicillin resistance gene is not acceptable due to concerns for patients which have reactivity to β-lactam antibiotics. Tetracyclin resistance gene is toxic for *E.coli* (Williams et al., 2009)

The major issue is the horizontal genetic transfer of antibiotic resistance gene to prokaryotic organisms present in the environment for biotherapeutic production or in commensal flora.

3.2 Horizontal transfer

Horizontal genetic transfer (HGT) is the passage of genetic elements between organisms (Tuller et al., 2011). This HGT is a major driving force in bacterial evolution by facilitating the diversity of bacteria. An essential element in HGT is to determine which factors influence the fixation of transferred genes. Some of these factors have already been identified (Tuller et al., 2011) and correspond to the advantage conferred by the transferred gene, the toxicity of its product, the ability of the transferred gene to be integrated into the host genome and to be stabilized, the number of interactions of the transferred gene product and the compatibility of codon usage between the transferred gene and the host. Tuller et al., 2011, have shown a correlation between the number of horizontally transferred gene with different organisms and the similarity between their tRNA pools. Moreover, organisms present in a same ecological environment have similar tRNA pools. These two points increase the probability of integration and fixation of a HTG into a new host genome.

Acquisition of antibiotic resistance is one element of this evolution by HTG. For example, Datta and Kontomichalou in 1965 have shown the importance of the penicillin resistance transfer across the *Enterobacteriaceae*. More recently, acquisition of the virulence factors that distinguish *Salmonella* from *Escherichia coli* has been shown as the result of HTG (Wiedenbeck & Cohan, 2011).

Moreover, one element favoring HTG is the length of DNA and this is the case with plasmid harboring antibiotic resistance gene used in recombinant protein (biotherapeutic) expression.

These elements are potential concerns that have to be taken into account in production of therapeutics or vaccine plasmid products and of biotherapeutics to restrict safety issues.

4. Regulatory point of view

A large number of guidance for industry, have been released by the FDA. Among these some are directly applied to the use of antibiotic resistance marker genes in different contexts such as transgenic plants at large or crops for animal feed. Here we have deliberately decided to restrict our focus on vaccines and biological therapeutics.

The market of "biotherapeutics", derived from recombinant DNA technologies, is entering an exponential growing phase. As much as 34 monoclonal antibodies have been, to date, approved by the FDA for various therapeutic applications. Besides antibodies, other products such as next generation recombinant vaccines and gene therapy constructs are progressively invading new therapeutic areas. As a result of growth in existing markets and the opening of new opportunities, the global demand is largely projected to further increase. A direct consequence is a progressive adaptation and strengthening of the existing regulation. A reasonable expectation is a move towards a "zero tolerance" for antibiotic based selection in production systems.

4.1 North American & European regulation

As soon as in July 1993, the FDA drafted some points to consider in the characterization of cell lines used to produce biological products.

> *'Penicillin or other beta lactam antibiotics should not be present in production cell cultures. Minimal concentrations of other antibiotics or inducing agents may be acceptable [21 CFR 610.15(c)]. However, the presence of any antibiotic or inducing agent in the product is discouraged.'*

The WHO technical report series N° 878: "Requirements for the use of animal cells as *in vitro* substrates for the production of biologicals", published in 1998 goes exactly in the same direction.

> *'Penicillin or other β-lactam antibiotics shall not be present in production cell cultures.*

Minimal concentration of other antibiotics may be acceptable. However the presence of any antibiotic in a biological process or product is discouraged.'

Over the years the recommendation became more precise or specific to some categories of biological products such as DNA vaccines. The potential issue of allergic responses to some classes of antibiotics is evoked, the necessity to document the trace amount of antibiotics in the final product clearly seen as mandatory. And finally appears an interesting allusion to novel strategies to replace antibiotic-based selection.

In December 1996 FDA issued a draft guidance entitled - Points to Consider on Plasmid DNA Vaccines for Preventive Infectious Disease Indications

'Antibiotic resistance is commonly employed as a selection marker. In considering the use of an antibiotic resistance marker, CBER is advising manufacturers against the use of penicillin or other beta-lactam antibiotics as these antibiotics can, in certain individuals, result in allergic reactions ranging in severity from skin rashes to immediate anaphylaxis. When an antibiotic resistance marker is required in a plasmid DNA vaccine construct, CBER advises the use of an antibiotic such as kanamycin or neomycin. These aminoglycoside antibiotics are not extensively used in the treatment of clinical infections due to their low activity spectrum, prevalence of kanamycin-resistant bacteria, and their problematic therapeutic index with toxicities including irreversible ototoxicity and nephrotoxicity. Specifications for the level of antibiotic present in the final container should be established and should consider the minimum level of antibiotic that will give an unintentional clinical effect. The use of alternative antibiotic resistance markers or the use of suppressor tRNA genes in a plasmid construct intended as plasmid DNA vaccine should be discussed with CBER prior to full scale development of a new vaccine product.'

Several updates (2006 and 2009) of this guidance are accessible on the web.

The EMEA is perfectly in line with its North American counterpart, as a matter of example, a 2001 guidance indicates:

'lack of expression in mammalian cells should be verified due to regulatory concerns'

This comment is an illustration of the concern applied to the antibiotic-resistance gene itself.

In a draft review, released from the FDA in November 2004, it is clearly specified that the use of beta-lactams should be avoided or at least very clearly documented in terms of safety for the patient. This recommendation, even if not prohibitive, appears as extremely dissuasive.

Content and Review of Chemistry, Manufacturing and Control (CMC) Information for Human Gene Therapy Investigational New Drug Application (INDs)

'Because some patients may be sensitive to penicillin, we recommend that you, a sponsor, do not use beta-lactam antibiotics during the manufacturing of a therapeutic product for humans. If beta-lactam antibiotics are used, we recommend that you take and describe precautions to prevent hypersensitivity reactions.'

In a recent release from the FDA (October 23, 2009) dedicated to Vaccines, Blood & Biologics, entitled: Common Ingredients in U.S. Licensed Vaccines: Why are antibiotics in some vaccines?

'Certain antibiotics may be used in some vaccine production to help prevent bacterial contamination during manufacturing. As a result, small amounts of antibiotics may be present in some vaccines. Because some antibiotics can cause severe allergic reactions in those children

allergic to them (like hives, swelling at the back of the throat, and low blood pressure), some parents are concerned that antibiotics contained in vaccines might be harmful. However, antibiotics most likely to cause severe allergic reactions (e.g., penicillins, cephalosporins and sulfa drugs) are not used in vaccine production, and therefore are not contained in vaccines.'

In the issue of july 7th 2011 of: Common Ingredients in U.S. Licensed Vaccines, some comments on antibiotics used in vaccine manufacturing processes are somewhat moderated.

'Examples of antibiotics used during vaccine manufacture include neomycin, polymyxin B, streptomycin and gentamicin. Some antibiotics used in vaccine production are present in the vaccine, either in very small amounts or they are undetectable. For example, antibiotics are used in some production methods for making inactivated influenza virus vaccines. They are used to reduce bacterial growth in eggs during processing steps, because eggs are not sterile products. The antibiotics that are used are reduced to very small or undetectable amounts during subsequent purification steps. The very small amounts of antibiotics contained in vaccines have not been clearly associated with severe allergic reactions.'

4.2 Conclusion and future rules

According to the above mentioned information:

- It is not yet prohibited but strongly advised to avoid or minimize the use of any kind of antibiotics in cell or bacterial culture,
- If antibiotics are used, it is mandatory to minimize their amount and to control for the presence of traces in the final product,
- The rationale for the use of antibiotics must be clearly documented in the CTD
- Penicillin, more generally β-lactams and streptomycin must not be used in reason of potential concerns with hyper reactivity of some patients to antibiotics of the β-lactam family
- Kanamycin and neomycin are the preferred choice and still tolerated.

The use of antibiotic resistance markers is generally discouraged, and if used the *in vivo* effect needs to be evaluated.

There are specific mentions for the nature of the gene encoding resistance to kanamycin, as reviewed by Williams et al., (2009). The gene neomycin phosphotransferase III [npt-III, *aph* (3')-III] should be avoided, since it also confers resistance to amikacin, a reserve antibiotic (EMEA, 2008).

As a final comment it is easy to anticipate, what might be the future requirements from health authorities: constructs have to be completely devoid of antibiotic resistance genes in their final structure, even if in use at early stages of construction. Alternative solutions would be available and validated soon.

5. Alternatives to antibiotics in bio-production

5.1 Vector stabilization

One aspect to be considered during recombinant biopharmaceutical expression is the stability of the plasmid used. More than 20 years ago, several studies on natural plasmids have highlighted that some plasmids naturally display regions necessary for their stability.

Ogura & Higara,, 1983a, have shown that plasmid F, that exists only as one to two copies per chromosome and is stably inherited to daughter cells during cell growth, contains stabilization sequences. They did show that these sequences were independent from plasmid replication function. They first identify 3 regions essential for plasmid maintenance: *SopA* and *SopB* that acts in trans and *SopC* that acts in *cis* to stabilize the plasmid by probably interacting with cellular components. These authors also put in evidence that *SopA*, *SopB* and *SopC* were not sufficient for full stability of mini-F plasmid, and identified the *ccd* (control of cell death) region that seemed to control cell division when copy number carrying *ccd* segment decreases (Ogura & Higara, 1983b). The so-called *ccd* region is divided into two functional regions: *ccdB*, which product inhibits the host cell division and *ccdA*, which product is able to inhibit the *ccdB* function. Two years after, Jaffé et al., 1985, demonstrated that cell division is not immediately inhibited and that residual division could take place in the plasmid free-cells before finally being inhibited. Authors concluded that *ccd* region guarantees that plasmid carrying cells could grow preferentially in a population by killing plasmid free daughter cells, introducing the concept of post-segregational killing.

Plasmid R1 has also been shown to contain a stabilization system (Gerdes et al., 1985). As for plamid F, the stabilization system is based on post segregational killing du to the *parAB+* locus. This locus is composed of two genes *Hok* (Host killing) and *Sok* (suppression of killing). The translation of the Hok messenger, encoding a toxin lethal to the bacteria, is completely blocked by the anti-messenger Sok. In the absence of plasmid, Sok, which is less stable than Hok, is lost first, allowing the translation of the Hok mRNA and expression of the toxin lethal to the cell.

Concerning plasmid maintenance, it has been shown that factors reducing mutlimerization of plasmid could increase plasmid stability (Summers & Sherratt, 1984). ColE1 plasmid contains a region, *cer* that seems to be necessary for a recombination event converting multimers to monomers, allowing the plasmid to be more stable. Multimer resolution is achieved through action of the XerCD site-specific recombinase at the *cer* site (see Figure 1). Cloning of the *cer* locus into various expression vectors has been extensively documented and the proof of principle largely established in high-cell density cultures.

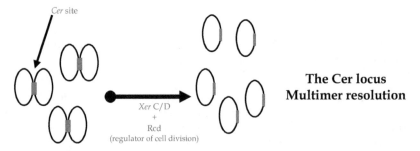

Fig. 1. Multimers resolution of high copy plasmids by XerC/D recombinase at *cer* locus.

5.2 Genomic integration

If mutation and deletion into *E.coli* genome are now widely used, it seems that genomic integration is not the preferred way to express a recombinant protein without antibiotic selection. However, some plasmid-free system have been described (see Figure 2).

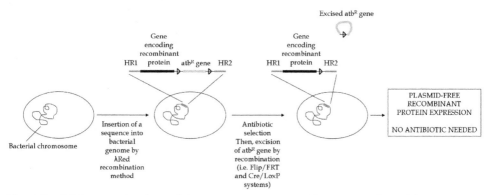

Fig. 2. Establishment of a plasmid-free expression system, illustration adapted from Striedner et al., 2010.

In 2009, a "plasmid-free T7-based *E.coli* expression system" has been developed by inserting a region of a pET plasmid into bacterial genome by λ Red recombination and P1 transduction (Datsenko & Wanner, 2000, as cited in Striedner et al., 2010). The study compared protein expression between plasmid-based and plasmid-free expression system showing an improved protein production with chromosome-based system. This system also conferred a high stability and simple upstream processing as well as high flexibility in process design.(Striedner et al., 2010).

More recently, Lemuth et al., 2011, reported the construction of the first plasmid-free *E. coli* strain that produces astaxanthin. This engineered *E. coli* strain harbors 5 heterologous biosynthetic genes from *P. ananatis* and one from *N. punctiforme* that are required for the formation of astaxanthin. Furthermore, a plasmid-free *E.coli* strain that accumulated astaxanthin as the exclusive carotenoid was engineered. This system presents many advantages compared to a plasmid-based strategy: a reduced metabolic burden, a better stability and obviously the absence of selection markers such as antibiotic resistance genes.

5.3 Complementation of essential gene product and auxotrophy markers

Essential gene complementation requires the engineering of a bacterial strain lacking an essential gene. The activity of the lacking gene product can be complemented by the culture medium or by transforming the bacteria with a plasmid having this gene as selection marker (see Figure 3).

Several antibiotic-free selection systems are based on gene complementation. One of the first systems was based on *dapD* gene (Degryse, 1991). The *dapD* gene, which has a role in the lysine biosynthetic pathway as well as cell wall assembly, has been selected as a preferred candidate by several authors, knowing that mutations in the DAP pathway are lethal. The limitations, in that case, are the intrinsic difficulty in construction of a *dapD* mutant strain and the dependence towards defined culture media composition.

Based on the same gene, a more elaborated strategy called "operator repressor titration" emerged in 2001. In this system, *dapD* gene is engineered in order to be under the control of lac Operon. When not supplemented with IPTG or DAP, *dapD* gene is not expressed

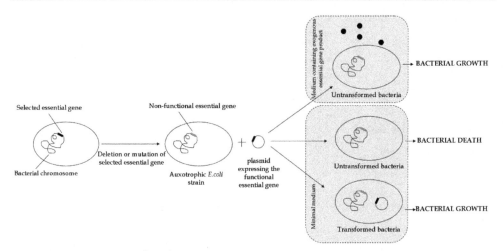

Fig. 3. Antibiotic-free selection system based on essential gene complementation.

inducing bacterial death. When the strain is transformed by a lac operator containing multi copy plasmid, the operator competitively titrates the Lac I repressor and allows the expression of *dapD* from the lac promoter allowing bacterial growth. (Cranenburgh et al., 2001 & 2004)

Other essential genes have been selected for the same purpose, such as *infA*, coding for translation initiation factor 1 (IF1), an essential protein for cell viability. In 2004, Hägg et al. generated a strain in which the *infA* gene has been deleted by a plasmid-based gene replacement method. They used a plasmid encoding a functional IF1 as selection marker and show that the system is tightly regulated and that no cross feeding is observed since initiation factors released into the media from lysed cells are not absorbed by plasmid-free cells.

The *fabI* essential gene has been used in an original way because of its property to reduce the E.coli susceptibility to triclosan when overexpressed. In this system, only plasmid containing cells overexpress *fabI* gene and can grow in presence of triclosan. Even if triclosan is a biocide, it is considered as non-antibiotic and regulatory agencies approve the use of triclosan for clinical use (Goh & Good, 2008).

More recently, Dong et al., 2010, developed a novel antibiotic-free selection system based on complementation of host auxotrophy in the NAD synthesis pathway. NAD can be *de novo* synthesized from tryptophan and aspartate with the quinolinic acid phosphoribosyltransferase (QAPRTase) or synthesized using the salvage pathway according to different substrates such as nicotinamide. Authors constructed a bacterial strain depleted for QAPRTase gene that can only grow if the NAD synthesis pathway is complemented by addition of salvage pathway substrate or QAPRTase gene present on a plasmid. The results obtained with this novel selection system show that the QAPRTase seletion marker does not represent a metabolic burden for bacterial growth and the stability of all plasmid harboring this system were 100% in the ΔQAPRTase strain even after 6 days of continuous growth. In this study, reserchers went further by complementing for the first time in an antibiotic-free selection system a bacterial strain by a mammalian QAPRTase gene with success.

A strain is auxotrophic for one amino-acid if it carries a genetic mutation that renders it unable to synthesize the amino-acid. Such a strain will be able to grow only if the amino-acid is present in the environment or if the functional gene product is expressed from a plasmid. Amino-acid auxotrophy markers had been investigated as novel antibiotic-free selection markers.

In 2001, Fiedler & Skerra developed expression vectors containing the *proAB* gene, in order to complement their proline-auxotrophic K12 strain. Their aim was not to develop an antibiotic-free selection system but to use their strain to obtain a better expression of recombinant antibody Fab fragment. For this reason, the plasmid-mediated complementation is used simultaneously with beta-lactamase selection to completely abolish plasmid loss during high scale fermentation.

In 2008, Vidal et al. described a plasmid selection system, devoid of antibiotic resistance gene and based on glycine auxotrophy. Researchers generated an *E.coli* strain that contains a deletion in the *glyA* gene, which encode for serine hydroxymethyl transferase, an enzyme involved in glycine biosynthesis pathway in *E.coli*. This strain can grow fast on a defined media only if glycine is added to the culture medium or if the bacteria harbor a plasmid expressing a functional *glyA* gene. They show comparable amount of recombinant protein with their system compared to a classical beta-lactamase selection system.

5.4 RNA-based antibiotic-free selection systems

Several antibiotic-free selection strategies are based on RNA, using antisense or anti-messenger properties or using suppressor tRNA.

The principle of down regulating an essential gene upon plasmid loss has been exploited in a very original way for the design of new vectors for gene therapy (Mairhofer et al., 2008). The expression of the essential gene *murA* encoding an enzyme essential for the biosynthesis of cell wall is under control of the Tet repressor, TetR expression is inhibited by an RNA-RNA antisense interaction with RNAI derived from plasmid origin of replication ColE1 (see Figure 4A). The major advantage of this system is that no additional sequence is required on the plasmid. (Pfaffenzeller et al., 2006; see figure 4B)

In a recent paper, RNA based selectable marker, not restricted to ColE1 containing vectors is described (Luke et al., 2009). Briefly, a counter-selectable marker *(sacB)* levansucrase from *Bacillus subtilis*, under control of the RNA-IN promoter is integrated into the bacterial chromosome induces cell death in presence of sucrose. Plasmid maintenance is ensured by the presence of the plasmid-borne regulator RNA-OUT anti-messenger acting as a down regulator of the expression of levansucrase (see Figure 4C).

Another vector system so-called pCOR, based on the complementation of an amber mutation using a suppressor tRNA, and conditional origin of replication has also been established (Soubrier et al., 1999). The original feature of the model is that an additional degree of refinement was introduced, since the dependence created between the host and the vector has become bilateral (see Figure 4D).

Nevertheless, the requirement for a minimal medium for culture means these systems are more likely to be used for DNA production rather than recombinant protein over expression.

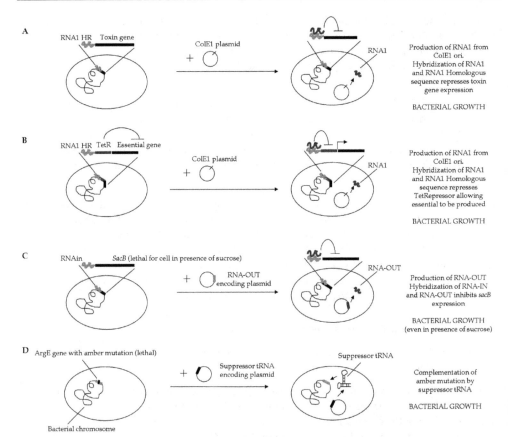

Fig. 4. RNA-based antibiotic-free systems. Illustration adapted from Pfaffenzeller et al., 2006; Luke et al., 2009 & Soubrier et al., 1999.

5.5 Post-segregational killing

Post-segregational killing is a mechanism by which plasmids are stably maintained by expressing a gene product that would be toxic to cells becoming plasmid-free upon division (see Figure 5). This mechanism, discovered on natural plasmid, has been used as selection system devoid of antibiotic.

One of these systems, based on *ccdA/ccdB* genes has been proposed by Szpirer & Milinkovitch, 2005, and is commercialized by the Delphigenetics Company. *ccdB* gene is inserted into the bacterial genome of the *E. coli* strain BL21 (DE3) and encodes a stable protein (100 aa), binding gyrase, essential for cell division. Upon binding gyrase, the *ccdB* gene product impairs DNA replication and induces cell death. *ccdA* gene, plasmid-born, encodes an instable protein (90 aa) under control of the mob promoter, acting as a natural inhibitor of *ccdB*. It has been shown that after 20 generations on a non-selective medium 100% of the bacteria still contain the plasmid. Two hours after induction, the plasmid is still present into all bacteria, which is not the case with a standard pET/BL21λDE3 system.

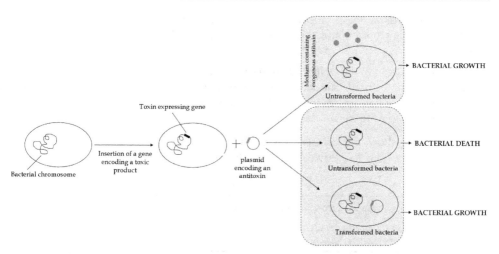

Fig. 5. Antibiotic-free selection system based on Toxin/antitoxin post-segragational killing. Illustration adapted from Szpirer & Milinkovitch, 2005.

To go further, Peubez et al. proposed in 2010 a system combining the *ccdA/ccdB* selection marker to the *cer* fragment to increase plasmid stability among long-term fermentation.

Different toxin/antitoxin (TA) systems have been described and could allow the generation of novel antibiotic-free systems. In order to detect putative TA systems, Milinkovitch's team had developed an algorithm based on predefined similarities and TA-specific structural constraints (Guglielmini et al., 2008).

Interestingly, this TA-based antibiotic-free selection system is starting to be adapted to mammalian cells selection. The toxin Kid (Killing determinant) and its antidote Kis (killing suppressor) have been used to control cell proliferation during expression of a recombinant protein in CHO-K1 cells (Nehlsen et al., 2010). If antibiotics are still used in this study, authors show that the TA strategy can significantly increase the recombinant protein expression level and could be a benefit for "difficult" to produce proteins.

6. Additional benefits

6.1 Recombinant protein production

In many cases, especially for "difficult proteins" the yield of protein production has proven to be higher with antibiotic-free system compared to a conventional one. The presence of an antibiotic resistance gene can indirectly reduce the amount of expressed protein, since even in absence of selection pressure the gene would be transcribed and account for an additional stress for the host during the fermentation process. However, even if the yield of protein is not superior to a conventional system, the antibiotic-free systems remain interesting due to their biosafety.

6.1.1 Plasmid stabilisation cer locus

Most commonly used multicopy plasmids are unstable and are lost during culture. Plasmid stabilization and increased maintenance during a fermentation process can be considered as a first step towards antibiotic starvation. Genetic elements allowing plasmid maintenance during cell division and limiting the probability of plasmid loss over generations should be considered.

To stabilize the plasmid, the well–studied mechanism of site specific recombination of *E.Coli* plasmid ColE1 can be used. The 380 bp *Cer* fragment was inserted into the plasmid carrying the gene of interest and the multimers are resolved to monomers by the Xer recombinase. (Described in 5.1, see Figure 1)

Tables 1 and 2 show the contribution of the cer fragment in increasing the plasmid maintenance over time is clearly established. The plasmid loss is dependant on the antigen expressed.

Culture time	Plasmid without *cer*	With *cer*
2h(IPTG added)	97%	100%
4h	25%	100%
6h	20%	75%
23h	3%	79%

Table 1. Example of *Helicobacter pylori* AlpA protein produced in erlen flask in absence of Kanamycin.

Culture time	Plasmid without *cer*	With *cer*
1h	87%	100%
2h	IPTG addition	
3h	67%	100%
5h	1%	50%
25h	0%	9%

Table 2. Example of *Helicobacter pylori* Urease produced in erlen flask in absence of kanamycin.

6.1.2 ccdA/ccdB

The combination of different genetic elements can allow an increased stability and antibiotic-free selection. In this case, the kanamycin resistant gene present on the vector backbone was eliminated by a restriction enzyme digestion and self–relegation.

The selection system based on the couple poison (gene *ccdB*)/antidote:(gene *ccdA*), proposed by Szpirer & Milinkovitch, 2005, combined with the stabilizing element, the *cer* locus, was tested to express different recombinant proteins.

-   the poison gene (*ccdB*), inserted into the bacterial genome, encodes a stable protein (100 aa), which is an inhibitor of the DNA replication capable to bind to the gyrase (an essential protein for cell division). This interaction induces the cell death.

- the antidote gene (*ccdA*), localized on the plasmid under the control of a constitutive promoter, encodes for a small unstable protein (90aa) which neutralizes the effect of ccdB protein action.

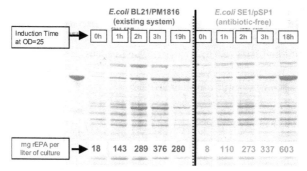

Fig. 6. Protein production evaluation in 1 liter fermenter.

Figure 6 shows a comparison of expression of the same protein with the kanamycin resistant gene (E. coli BL21/pM1816) and the antibiotic-free system (E. coli SE1/pSP1) without the kanamycin resistant gene and with the *ccdA* gene. Both have the *cer* element. Upon induction, the behavior of both systems is comparable but a clear increase in protein production is observed with the antibiotic-free system at the end of fermentation.

6.1.3 Antibiotic resistance gene elimination

Antibiotic-based selection, convenient for cloning steps, must be removed for production.

Even if antibiotic selection pressure is not used during the fermentation process, removal of this antibiotic resistance marker is of major importance to prevent horizontal transfer in the environment. This is particularly true for vectors to be used in gene therapy or DNA vaccination protocols

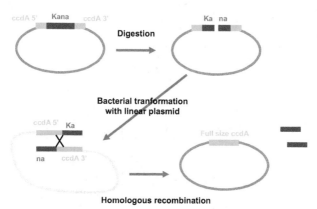

Fig. 7. Homologous recombination process allowing assembly of a functional *ccdA* encoding gene.

In order to overcome the problem of positive pressure of selection, a new apporach has been developed ensuring the elimination of the antibiotic-resistance gene through homologous recombination. In this model the *ccdA* locus is split into 2 parts, containing a common sequence, and cloned at the 5′ and 3′ regions flanking the antibiotic resistance gene (figure 7). After digestion at a unique restriction site located inside the antibiotic selection marker and transformation of ccdB expressing cells with linear DNA, a fully functional *ccdA* would assemble through homologous recombination. Only bacteria containing a recombinant plasmid with a functional *ccdA* can grow upon transformation.

6.1.4 Summary of different antibiotic-free systems

System developed	Mode of action	Protein expressed	Comments/ potential drawbacks	Ref article
Plasmid-free system	Chromosome based expression system	GFP Human superoxide dismutase(SOD)	Modified *E coli* strain, required	Striedner et al., 2010
Fabl-triclosan	Endogenous essential gene	None	Chemical Biocid utilisation	Goh & Good, 2008
E. coli strain **ΔQAPRTase gene**	Complementation	EGFP	Modified *E coli* strain, required	Dong et al., 2010
Pro BA	Complementation	Fab fragment	Modified *E coli* strain, required Presence of antibiotic	Fiedler & Skerra, 2001
E coli strain **ΔglyA**	Glycine auxotrophy	RhuA	Modified *E coli* strain, required. Comparable to the conventional system	Vidal et al., 2008
RNA/RNA interference	RNA/RNA interaction	EGFP	Modified *E coli* strain, required	Pfaffenzeller et al., 2006
RNA out	RNA/RNA interaction	EGFP HA vaccine candidate		Luke et al., 2009
pCOr	Complementation of amber mutation tRNA suppressor	Luciferase	Modified *E coli* strain, and minimum medium required	Soubrier et al., 1999
ccdA/ccdB	Toxin/antitoxin	AlpA/rEPA vaccine candidates	Modified *E coli* strain required	Peubez et al., 2010
Kid/Kis	Toxin/antitoxin	EGFP	Presence of antibiotic	Nehlsen et al., 2010

6.2 DNA immunization and gene therapy

Requirement can also be variable according to the nature of the therapeutic product, the presence of an antibiotic resistance gene, tolerated on a vector expressing a recombinant biopharmaceutical, will be totally undesirable on a gene therapy plasmid.

Among systems described in paragraph 5, some have been developed especially for DNA vaccine production such as pCOR (Soubrier et al., 1989), RNA/RNA interference (Pfaffenzeller et al., 2006) and RNA out (Luke et al., 2009).

To go further, Carnes et al., 2009, have proposed a combination of antibiotic-free selection system and an autolytic *E.coli* strain to improve both upstream and downstream processes. The antibiotic-free selection is based on RNA selectable marker described by Luke et al., 2009 and the autolytic plasmid DNA extraction method uses integrated bacteriophage endolysin gene (λR), encoding a peptidoglycan hydrolase (lysozyme) enzyme to permeabilize the bacterial cell wall, and to selectively extract the plasmid DNA from the cells in an acetate buffer. Authors found that their autolytic strain allowed efficient plasmid DNA recovery, similar to alkaline lysis plasmid DNA purification.

7. Conclusion and perspectives

Antibiotic-free selection is a general and ultimate goal that can be reached by the implementation of various and combined approaches. An increasing knowledge of bacterial physiology will give access to comprehensive information on essential genes or pathways that would be an unlimited source of inspiration for the design of novel selection means.

The major driver for the definition of antibiotic-free systems is an anticipation of fulfilling future recommendations from health authorities to overcome safety concerns. It is easy to imagine that, upon availability and functional validation, these alternative selection means will progressively gain the status of "preferred", "strongly recommended" and finally "mandatory".

In addition to their safety profile, some antibiotic-free systems can give access to unexpected properties such as a marked increase in recombinant protein production or plasmid recovery.

The complete elimination of any antibiotic resistance gene is, for different reasons, of critical importance for recombinant protein production, DNA immunization and gene therapy vectors.

It is likely to think that upon validation at industrial scale, antibiotic-free selection might be an added value for biotherapeutics in terms of safety profile of the product and become an important element of the marketing strategy as well. A direct consequence would be the emergence of a new "gold standard".

8. References

Carnes, A.E.; Hodgson, C.P.; Luke, J.M.; Vincent, J.M. & Williams, J.A. (2009). Plasmid DNA production combining antibiotic-free selection, inducible high yield fermentation, and novel autolytic purification. *Biotechnol Bioeng.*, Vol.104, No.3, (Oct 2009), pp.505-515

Cranenburgh, R.M.; Hanak, J.A.; Williams, S.G. & Sherratt, D.J. (2001). Escherichia coli strains that allow antibiotic-free plasmid selection and maintenance by repressor titration. *Nucleic Acids Res.*, Vol. 29, No.5, (Mar 2001), E26

Cranenburgh, R.M.; Lewis, K.S. & Hanak, J.A. (2004). Effect of plasmid copy number and lac operator sequence on antibiotic-free plasmid selection by operator-repressor titration in Escherichia coli. *J Mol Microbiol Biotechnol.*, Vol.7, No.4, (2004), pp.197-203

Datsenko, K.A. & Wanner, B.L. (2000). One-step inactivation of chromosomal genes in Escherichia coli K-12 using PCR products. *Proc Natl Acad Sci U S A.*, Vol.97, No.12, (Jun 2000), pp.6640-6645

Datta, N. & Kontomichalou, P.(1965). Penicillinase synthesis controlled by infectious R factors in Enterobacteriaceae. *Nature. Vol.208, No.5007,* (Oct 1965), pp.239-241

Degryse, E. (1985). Stability of a host-vector system based on complementation of an essential gene in Escherichia coli. *J Biotechnol.*, Vol.18, No.1-2, (Apr 1991), pp.29-39

Dong, W.R.; Xiang, L.X. & Shao, J.Z. (2010). Novel antibiotic-free plasmid selection system based on complementation of host auxotrophy in the NAD de novo synthesis pathway. *Appl Environ Microbiol.*, Vol.76, No.7, (Apr 2010), pp.2295-2303. Epub 2010 Jan 29

Durany, O.; Bassett, P.; Weiss, A.M.; Cranenburgh, R.M.; Ferrer, P.; López-Santín, J.; de Mas, C. & Hanak, J.A. (2005). Production of fuculose-1-phosphate aldolase using operator-repressor titration for plasmid maintenance in high cell density Escherichia coli fermentations. *Biotechnol Bioeng.*, Vol. 91, No.4, (Aug 2005), pp.460-467

Fiedler, M. & Skerra, A. (2001). proBA complementation of an auxotrophic E. coli strain improves plasmid stability and expression yield during fermenter production of a recombinant antibody fragment. *Gene*, Vol.274, No.1-2, (Aug 2001), pp.111-118

Gerdes, K.; Larsen, J.E. & Molin, S. (1985). Stable inheritance of plasmid R1 requires two different loci. *J Bacteriol.* Vol.161, No.1, (Jan 1985), pp.292-298

Goh, S. & Good, L. (2008). Plasmid selection in Escherichia coli using an endogenous essential gene marker. *BMC Biotechnol.*, Vol.11, No. 8, (Aug 2008), pp.61

Guglielmini, J.; Szpirer, C.Y. & Milinkovitch, M.C. (2008). Automated discovery and phylogenetic analysis of new toxin-antitoxin systems. *BMC Microbiol.* Vol.25; No.8, (Jun 2008), pp.104

Hägg, P.; de Pohl, J.W.; Abdulkarim, F. & Isaksson, L.A. (2004). A host/plasmid system that is not dependent on antibiotics and antibiotic resistance genes for stable plasmid maintenance in Escherichia coli. *J Biotechnol.*, Vol.111, No.1, (Jul 2004), pp.17-30

Jaffé, A.; Ogura, T. & Hiraga, S. (1985). Effects of the ccd function of the F plasmid on bacterial growth. *J Bacteriol.*, Vol.163, No.3, (Sep 1985), pp.841-849

Lemuth, K.; Steuer, K. & Albermann, C. (2011). Engineering of a plasmid-free Escherichia coli strain for improved in vivo biosynthesis of astaxanthin. *Microb Cell Fact.*, Vol.26, No.10, (Apr 2011), pp.29

Luke, J.; Carnes, A.E.; Hodgson, C.P. & Williams, J.A. (2009). Improved antibiotic-free DNA vaccine vectors utilizing a novel RNA based plasmid selection system. *Vaccine.*, Vol.27, No.46, (Oct 2009), pp.6454-6459. Epub 2009 Jun 24

Mairhofer, J.; Pfaffenzeller, I.; Merz, D. & Grabherr, R. (2008). A novel antibiotic free plasmid selection system: advances in safe and efficient DNA therapy. *Biotechnol J.*, Vol.3, No.1, (Jan 2008), pp.83-89

Nehlsen, K.; Herrmann, S.; Zauers, J.; Hauser, H. & Wirth, D. (2010). Toxin-antitoxin based transgene expression in mammalian cells. *Nucleic Acids Res.*, Vol.38, No.5, (Mar 2010), e32.

Ogura, T. & Hiraga, S. (1983). Partition mechanism of F plasmid: two plasmid gene-encoded products and a cis-acting region are involved in partition. *Cell*. Vol.32, No.2, (Feb 1983), pp.351-360

Ogura, T. & Hiraga, S. (1983). Mini-F plasmid genes that couple host cell division to plasmid proliferation. *Proc Natl Acad Sci U S A*, Vol.80, No.15, (Aug 1983), pp.4784-4788

Peubez, I.; Chaudet, N.; Mignon, C.; Hild, G.; Husson, S.; Courtois, V.; De Luca, K.; Speck, D. & Sodoyer, R. (2010). Antibiotic-free selection in E. coli: new considerations for optimal design and improved production. *Microb Cell Fact.*, Vol.7, No.9, (Sep 2010), pp.65.

Pfaffenzeller, I.; Mairhofer, J.; Striedner, G.; Bayer, K. & Grabherr, R. (2006). Using ColE1-derived RNA I for suppression of a bacterially encoded gene: implication for a novel plasmid addiction system. *Biotechnol J.*, Vol. 1, No.6, (Jun 2006), pp.675-681.

Rahal, J.J. Jr.& Simberkoff, M.S. (1979). Bactericidal and bacteriostatic action of chloramphenicol against memingeal pathogens. *Antimicrob Agents Chemother*. Vol.16, No.1, (Jul 1979), pp.13-18

Soubrier, F.; Cameron, B.; Manse, B.; Somarriba, S.; Dubertret, C.; Jaslin, G.; Jung, G.; Caer, C.L.; Dang, D.; Mouvault, J.M.; Scherman, D.; Mayaux, J.F. & Crouzet, J. (1999). pCOR: a new design of plasmid vectors for nonviral gene therapy. *Gene Ther.*, Vol.6, No.8, (Aug 1999), pp.1482-1488

Summers, D.K. & Sherratt, D.J. (1984). Multimerization of high copy number plasmids causes instability: CoIE1 encodes a determinant essential for plasmid monomerization and stability., *Cell*, Vol. 36, No.4, (Apr 1984), pp.1097-1103

Striedner, G.; Pfaffenzeller, I.; Markus, L.; Nemecek, S.; Grabherr, R. & Bayer, K. (2010). Plasmid-free T7-based Escherichia coli expression systems. *Biotechnol Bioeng.*, Vol. 105, No.4, (Mar 2010), pp.786-794

Szpirer, C.Y. & Milinkovitch, M.C. (2005). Separate-component-stabilization system for protein and DNA production without the use of antibiotics. *Biotechniques.*, Vol.38, No.5, (May 2005), pp.775-781

Tuller, T.; Girshovich, Y.; Sella, Y.; Kreimer, A.; Freilich, S.; Kupiec, M.; Gophna, U. & Ruppin, E. (2011). Association between translation efficiency and horizontal gene transfer within microbial communities. *Nucleic Acids Res*. Vol.39, No.11, (Jun 2011), pp.4743-4755

Vidal, L.; Pinsach, J.; Striedner, G.; Caminal, G. & Ferrer, P. (2008). Development of an antibiotic-free plasmid selection system based on glycine auxotrophy for recombinant protein overproduction in Escherichia coli. *J Biotechnol*, Vol.134, No.1-2, (Mar 2008), pp.127-136

Wiedenbeck, J. & Cohan, F.M. (2011), Origins of bacterial diversity through horizontal genetic transfer and adaptation to new ecological niches. *FEMS Microbiol Rev*. doi: 10.1111/j.1574-6976.2011.00292.x. (Jun 2011), [Ahead of print]

Williams, J.A.; Carnes, A.E. & Hodgson, C.P. (2009). Plasmid DNA vaccine vector design: impact on efficacy, safety and upstream production. *Biotechnol Adv.* Vol.27, No.4, (Jul-Aug 2009), pp.353-370

15

Antibiotic Susceptibility of Probiotic Bacteria

Zorica Radulović[1], Tanja Petrović[1] and Snežana Bulajić[2]
[1]University of Belgrade, Faculty of Agriculture
[2]University of Belgrade, Faculty of Veterinary Medicine
Republic of Serbia

1. Introduction

Lactic acid bacteria (LAB) are a heterogeneous group of bacteria widely distributed in nature. These bacteria are found in gastrointestinal (GI) and urogenital tract of humans and animals; they are present on plant material, in milk and meat, and numerous fermented foods. Lactic acid bacteria have been associated with traditional dairy products, cereals, vegetable and meat fermented foods, due to their natural presence leading to spontaneous fermentation. They are also used as starter cultures in industrial food production, as well as in the production of probiotic products due to their potential health benefits to consumer. Milk and dairy products are the most examined food system for the delivery of probiotic bacteria to the human gut. The probiotic concept has progressed and is now in the focus of different research. Significant improvements have been made in selection and characterization of new cultures and their application in food production.

The food products, which are produced by traditional methods, exhibit a rich biodiversity with the respect to bacterial contents. From these products, new probiotic strains with the potential functional properties can been isolated and selected. The selected strains have to be further characterized in order to be used in the food industry. Before the probiotics can benefit human health, they must fulfill several criteria including: a) scientifically validated health properties; b) good technological properties meaning that they can be manufactured and incorporated into food products without loosing viability, functionality and technological performance; c) high survival through the upper gastrointestinal tract and high viability at its site of action; d) antagonistic activity to pathogens; e) antibiotic susceptibility; and f) to be able to function in the gut environment. Bearing in mind importance of antibiotic resistance of LAB in food chain, antibiotic susceptibility of potential probiotic strains is a very important criteria for their selection.

In the recent decade, releasing of antibiotics in biosphere seriously increased, leading to a strong selective pressure for the emergence and persistence of resistant LAB strains. Since LAB are naturally present in traditionally made fermented food and GI tract and are also added as starter culture or probiotic bacteria in industrial food production, concerns have been raised about the antibiotic resistance of these beneficial bacteria strains. Probiotic bacteria can help maintaining balance in gastrointestinal tract in cases of diarrhea caused by antibiotic treatment. However, there is high risk associated with the ability of these resistant strains to transmit the resistance gene to pathogenic bacteria in gut microbiota. This can complicate the treatment of a patient with an antibiotic resistant bacterial infection or disease. The circulation of genes coding for antibiotic resistance from beneficial LAB in the food chain via animals to humans is a complex problem. Therefore, there is a need to evaluate the safety of potential probitic strains regarding their ability to acquire and disseminate antibiotic resistance determinants in selection of LAB.

In this study, importance of LAB in the food chain will be reviewed. Morphological and biochemical characteristics of lactobacilli, bifidobactera and enterococci, as well as criteria for probiotic selection and role of probiotics in health benefit will be discussed. Antibiotic susceptibility as criteria for potential probiotic bacteria selection and mechanisms of gene transfers will be considered.

2. Lactic acid bacteria in the GI tract

The human GI tract represents a complex ecosystem in which interactions between food, microbes and the host cells occur. The bacterial population of normal gut of an adult comprise of more than 500 different species. The quantity of microbes present in the intestine (about 10^{14}) exceeds 10-fold the total number of all human cells (Backhed et al., 2005). The most important function of this intestinal microbiota is to act as a microbial barrier against pathogens, by so-called competitive exclusion mechanisms, but also influence the humoral and cellular mucosal immune responses during the neonatal phase of life, and thereafter to maintain a physiologically-normal steady-state condition throughout life (Tancrede, 1992). The gut microflora profoundly influences nutritional, physiologic and protective processes. Both direct and indirect defensive functions are provided by the normal microbiota. Specifically, gut bacteria directly prevent colonization by pathogenic organisms by competing for essential nutrients or for epithelial attachment sites. By producing antimicrobial compounds, volatile fatty acids, and chemically modified bile acids, indigenous gut bacteria also create a local environment that is generally unfavourable for the growth of enteric pathogens. This phenomenon is called Colonization Resistance, which can be defined as the ability of microorganisms belonging to the normal gut microflora to impede the implantation of pathogens (van der Waaij, 1988). This function of the microflora is also known as the barrier effect. While probiotic bacteria improve colonization resistance, consensus thinking is that the importance of LAB as probiotic agents lies more in the indirect mechanisms such as immunomodulation. When the genetic repertoire of these bacteria is considered, the GI tract translates into a reservoir of genes encoding numerous physiological functions from which the human GI tract can benefit. Bacteria represent the most extensively investigated group of microorganisms. Which species of bacteria will be long-term colonized in GI tract depends on the biochemical capability of the microorganisms, the microenvironment determined by the host cells and the available foodstuffs. Lactobacilli are probably the most well known representative of favourable microorganisms in GI tract. There is a number of species of lactobacilli reside in the human intestine in a symbiotic relationship with each other and with other microorganisms (Claesson et al., 2007). They are generally considered essential for maintaining gut microfloral health; however, it is the overall balance of the various microorganisms which is ultimately of most importance.

2.1 The composition of the GI tract

The composition of the GI microflora undergoes considerable changes from the day of birth until adulthood. The GI tract of a normal fetus is sterile, but colonization begins immediately after birth and is influenced by the mode of delivery, the infant diet, hygiene levels and medication (Benett et al., 1986; Gronlund et al., 1999). During the first months of life diet has a significant influence on the development of the intestinal flora (Heavey & Rowland, 1999; Stark & Lee, 1982). Within one to two days facultative anaerobes predominate and create a reduced environment that allows the growth of strict anaerobes. Within three to four days, bifidobacteria appear and become predominant. The average number of bifidobacteria in breast-fed infants is 10^{10}–10^{11} cfu/g. In formula fed infants, bifidobacteria have also been demonstrated to be a numerically important species, but they generally occur in lower numbers than in breastfed infants of the same age (Mountzouris et al., 2002). The predominance of beneficial bacteria in the gut microbiota of breast-fed infants is thought to result from the fermentation of oligosaccharides-non-digestible carbohydrates consisting of several linked monosaccharides (typically 3-10 simple sugars) in breastmilk (Agostoni et al., 2004). Oligosaccharides pass unabsorbed through the small intestine into the colon, where they are fermented by resident bifidobacteria to short-chain fatty acids and lactic acid, reducing the gut pH to approximately 5.7, thus providing the protection against enteric infections (Newburg, 2000, Coppa et al., 2004). In contrast, the gut microflora of formula-fed infants produces a different profile of short-chain fatty acids and a pH in the local microenvironment of approximately 7.0 (Ogawa et al., 1992). Infant faecal flora appears to be stabilized at 4 weeks of age and until weaning when introduction of solid foods takes place (Mountzouris et al., 2002). During weaning, bifidobacteria decrease by 1 log, the microbiota alters from infant-type to adult-type, and a remarkable proliferation of bacteroides, eubacteria, peptostreptococcaceae, and clostridia occur. The faecal flora of children closely resembles that of adults, where the numbers of bacteroidaceae, eubacteria, peptococcaceae, and usually clostridia outnumbered bifidobacteria, which constitute 5-10% of the total flora.

An adult individual's GI tract is extremely stable and it is very difficult to introduce new species. There are several factors that can alter the composition of the GI flora such as medications (especially antibiotics), diet, climate, aging, illness, stress, pH, infections, geographic location, and even race (Murphy et al., 2009). Thus it is not surprising to find out that the composition of the GI flora not only differs among individuals, but also differs during the life within the same individual. Furthermore, indigenous bacteria are not distributed randomly throughout the gastrointestinal tract but instead are found at population levels and in species distributions that are characteristic of specific regions of the tract.

As shown in Figure 1, there are three main regions that offer very different conditions for the survival of various microorganisms in the GI environment. In the stomach, microbial growth is greatly reduced by the high acidity and presence of oxygen provided by the swallowing. As a result, in the stomach acidotolerant microorganisms and facultative anaerobes such as lactobacilli, streptococci, yeasts, etc. are present. In the second region (small intestine), the microflora consists mainly of facultative anaerobic bacteria such as lactobacilli, streptococci and enterobacteria, and anaerobes such as bifidobacteria, bacteroides and clostridia. In the last region (colon), the number of bacteria is considerably high, due to the low redox potential and relatively high concentration of short-chain fatty acid, and counts 10^9–10^{12} cfu/ml (Cummings et al. 1989). The colon has an important role in food digestion, and microflora in this region participates in the transformation of many carbohydrates, proteins and amino acids. The microflora of the colon is very complex and dominated by anaerobic bacteria (*Bacteroides* spp., *Clostridium* spp, *Bifidobacterium* spp., etc), while the facultative anaerobic bacteria are less numerous and represented by lactobacilli, enterococci, streptococci and *Enterobacteriaceae*. Yeasts (eg., *Candida albicans*) are relatively poorly represented.

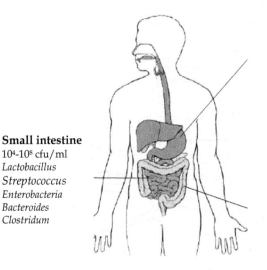

Stomach
10^1-10^4 cfu/ml
Helicibacter pylori,
Lactobacillus
Streptococcus
Candida albicans

Small intestine
10^4-10^8 cfu/ml
Lactobacillus
Streptococcus
Enterobacteria
Bacteroides
Clostridum

Colon
10^9-10^{12} cfu/ml
Bacteroides
Bacillus
Eubacterium
Bifidobacterium
Clostridium
Peptococcus
Peptostreptococcus
Ruminococcus
Actinomyces
Lactobacillus
Enterobacteriacae
Enterococcus

Fig. 1. The average concentration of microorganisms in the GI tract (adapted from Ouwehand & Vesterlund, 2003)

As part of gut microbiota, it is estimated that lactobacilli are present in following concentrations: 10^3–10^6 cfu/ml in the oral cavity; 10^3 cfu/ml in the stomach; 10^4 cfu /ml in the duodenum and jejunum; 10^8 cfu /ml in the ileum and 10^9 cfu /ml in the colon (Reuter, 2001; Koll et al., 2008; Ryan et al., 2008). An overview of lactobacilli commonly found in the GI tract microbiota is shown in Table 1.

Considering that lactobacilli and bifidobacteria constitute a significant population in the GI tract, this environment represents a good source for the isolation of new strains of LAB.

3. Lactic acid bacteria as probiotic bacteria

By definition probiotics are described as „living microorganisms, which upon ingestion in certain numbers, exert health benefits beyond inherent basic nutrition" (Guarner & Schaafsma, 1998). Regarding the probiotics, the majority of research is focused on bacterial genera *Lactobacillus* and *Bifidobacterium* (Table 2).

Oral cavity	Stomach	Small intestine	Faeces	Colon epithelial biopsies
L. paracasei	L. gasseri	L. gasseri	L. gasseri	L. plantarum
L. rhamnosus	L. reuteri	L. reuteri	L. paracasei	L. rhamnosus
L. fermentum	L. ruminis	L. rhamnosus	L. ruminis	L. paracasei
L. plantarum			L. reuteri	
L. gasseri			L. plantarum	
			L. salivarius	
			L. sakei	

Table 1. *Lactobacillus* species distribution in different parts of the GI tract (Lönnermark, 2010)

Lactobacillus sp.	Bifidobacteriim sp.	Enterococcus sp.	Others
L. acidophilus	B. bifidum	E. faecium	Lactococcus lactis ssp. lactis
L.plantarum	B. infantis	E. faecalis	Lactococcus lactis ssp. cremoris
L. casei	B. adolescentis		Leuconostoc mesenteroides
L. rhamnosus	B. longum		Pediococcus acidilactici
L. delbrueckii ssp. bulgaricus	B. breve		Propionibacterium freudenreichii
L. fermentum	B. lactis		Streptococcus thermophilus
L. johnsonii			
L. gasseri			
L. salivarius			
L. reuteri			

Table 2. Lactic acid bacteria used as probiotics (adapted from Gardnier et al., 2002)

They have a reputation of health promoters and they have a significant role as probiotic bacteria in the production of different foods, particularly in the production of fermented dairy products. Central position of lactobacilli and bifidobacteria in probiotic formulation is argumented due to (a) the association of these bacteria with human health, (b) the fact that they possess the Generally Regarded As Safe (GRAS) status. Enterococci, although not GRAS organisms, have been used as probiotics too. Some other LAB such as lactococci, pediococci, *Leuconostoc*, propionibacteria have also received attention as potential probiotic cultures (Table 2).

3.1 *Lactobacillus*

The genus *Lactobacillus* is large heterogeneous group of microorganisms, which lacks catalase and cytochromes and is usually microaerophilic, with growth improved under anaerobic conditions (Kandler & Weiss, 1989). They are Gram-positive nonmotile rods, often in pairs or chains, coccobacilli to long rods. They have a strictly fermentative metabolism and convert glucose solely or partly to lactic acid. They are classified as homofermentative (producing mainly lactic acid) or heterofermentative (producing carbon dioxide, ethanol, acetic acid and lactic acid). The optimum growth temperature is in the mesophilic range (30-40°C), but some strains can grow below 15°C and some at temperatures up to 55°C. Differentiation of *Lactobacillus* species depends on physiological criteria, carbohydrate fermentation, biochemical and molecular characterization (Petrovic et al., 2006). Lactobacilli play crucial role in the production of fermented foods: vegetables, meats and dairy products. Non starter lactic acid bacteria (NSLAB) are lactobacilli which form significant proportion of the microflora of most cheese varieties during ripening. Many species of mesophilic *Lactobacillus* have been isolated from cheese; the ones most frequently encountered are *L. casei, L. paracasei, L. pantarum, L. rhamnosus* and *L. curvatus* (Beresford et al., 2001). For example, *L. plantarum, L. casei* ssp. *casei* and *L. brevis* have been isolated from Armada cheese, a Spanish goat milk cheese (Herreros et al., 2003), *L. plantarum, L. paraplantarum, L. paracasei* ssp. *tolerans, L. sake, L. curvaus* and *L. pentosus* from Batzos, a traditional Greek cheese made from raw goat's milk (Psoni et al., 2003) and *L. para.paracasei, L. plantarum, L. curvatus* and *L. brevis* from Sjenica cheese, traditional Serbian white brined cheese (Radulović, 2010). Traditional homemade dairy products have great potential for isolation of new strains, which could be used as starter cultures in food industry, as adjunct cultures for improving flavour of cheeses, or as probiotic in production of functional foods.

3.2 *Bifidobacterium*

Species from the genus *Bifidobacterium* are generally characterized as Gram-positive, non-spore forming, nonmotile and catalase negative. They are strict anaerobes, although some species and strains may tolerate oxygen in the presence of carbon dioxide. Within the genus *Bifidobacterium* pleomorphism exists and it is described as short regular, thin cells with pointed ends, long cells with slight bends with a large variety of branching; single or in chains of many elements; in star-like clusters or disposed in "V" or palisade arrangements (Scardovi, 1986). In bifidobacteria, glucose catabolism occurs through the fructose 6-phosphate phodphoketolase pathway, which can be used as distinguishing feature of bifidobacteria. During fermentation, acetic and lactic acids are produced in molar ratios 3:2. The optimum temperature for growth is 31-41°C within the range 25-45°C. Bifidobacteria are less acid tolerant than lactobacilli and no growth occurs at pH values less than 4.5 (Scardovi, 1986). Nutritional requirements for growth of bifidobacteria are less complex than those of lactobacilli, but in some cases bifidobacteria do require specific factors for optimal growth (Modler et al., 1990). Bifidobacteria are natural habitants of GI tract and strains with probiotic properties are mainly of human origin. *Bifidobacterium* species constitute a significant portion of probiotic cultures used in functional food production.

3.3 *Enterococcus*

Although lactobacilli and bifidobacteria are most commonly used as probiotics, some enterococci can also be used as health-promoting bacteria. Species *E. faecium* and *E. faecalis* have been used as probiotic bacteria, although they are not recognized as GRAS organisms. All species of genus *Enterococcus* are Gram-positive, non-spore forming, catalasa negative, facultative anaerobes. They are spherical or ovoid cocci in pairs or short chains. Their properties, such as the ability to grow at 10°C and 45°C in 6.5%NaCl and at pH 9.6 and their survival heating to 60°C for 30 min, are used to differentiate enterococci from other Gram-positive catalase-negative cocci (Franz et al., 1999). Enterococci are homofermentative with respect to glucose metabolism, although some amounts of formic and lactic acid may be produced in some media. As the other LAB, enterococci do require B vitamins, amino acids, purine and pyramidine bases for optimal growth (Garg & Mital, 1991).

3.4 LAB associated with therapeutic properties

In recent years an increasing number of probiotic pharmaceutical preparations as well as food supplements are being promoted with health claims. The application of LAB has been more developed for the production of functional foods, where probiotic bacteria have an important role. The commercial probiotic strains, used in functional food production, must be well-substantiated with scientific evidence.

The health benefits of probiotic bacteria can be considered as nutritional or therapeutic/prophylactic. Nutritional benefits are mainly connected with their role in enhancing the bioavailability of vitamins and minerals, and an increase of the digestibility of protein (Tamime et al., 2003). Many researchers (Begley et al., 2006; Ouwehand et al., 2003; Rodrigeuz et al., 2010) investigated the therapeutic/prophylactic benefits of probiotics and confirmed their effects:

- Prevention of diarrhoea caused by certain pathogenic bacteria and viruses;
- Regulation of intestinal microflora after an antibiotic therapy;
- Treating the infection with *Helicobacter pylori*, responsible for the development of gastritis, ulcers and gastric cancer;
- Improvement of digestion in "lactose-intolerant" individuals, who have reduced capability for lactose digestion;
- Anticancer effect, as a result of the production of certain compounds during its growth;
- Reducing cholesterol levels;
- Stimulation of γ-interferon production, which contributes to increased resistance to some infections;
- Increasing antibody titar (IgG immunoglobulins), which enhances the immune response of an organism;

Health effects are related to microflora modification and strengthening of the gut mucosal barrier. Some scientific data indicated that probiotic strains have potential in the prevention and treatment of intestinal and urogenital infections and these cultures may be useful as an alternatives to antibiotic therapy. The World Health Organization (WHO) has recommended the reconsideration of microbial interference therapy for infection control (Bengmark, 1998). Certain probiotic strains have been shown multiple effects including prevention of pathogen attachment and invasion in cell culture, inhibiting of the growth of enteropatogens *in vitro* and enhancement the immune response. Considering thee effects, the usage of probiotics may decrease antibiotics dependence. Fooks et al., (1999) have suggested that probiotic bacteria can control the infection in several ways such as the competition for nutrients, secretion of antimicrobial substances, reduction of pH, blocking of adhesion sites, reduction of virulence, blocking of toxin receptor sites, immune stimulation and suppression of toxin production.

Infections by bacterial or viral agents most frequently result in diarrhea. One of the most investigated probiotic, *L.rhamnosus* GG, has been very effective in the treatment of viral diarrhea in children, most cases of which were caused by rotavirus. Other probiotic strains such as *Lactocacillus casei Shirota, B. bifidum* and *S. thermophillus* have also been shown to be effective in the treatment and prevention of rotavirus diarrhea in children (Korhonen, et al., 2007; Saavedra et al., 1994).

Antibiotic-associated diarrhea (AAD) is a major clinical problem that occurs following antibiotic use. The most serious form of this kind is pseudomembranous colitis. Diarrhea is caused by pathogen overgrowth and in 20% cases the etiological agent is *Clostridium difficile*, a pathogen that is especially persistent and difficult to treat (Lewis & Freedman, 1998). Antibiotics are often used to treat for pseudomembranous colitis or other AAD, although the relapse may occurs when the probiotic therapy may be especially useful. Oral therapy with *L. rhamnosus* GG was effective in the prevention of AAD, in treatment of colitis, as well as in traveller's diarrhea (Shah, 2007). A combination of *B. bifidum, S. thermophilus, L. delbrueckii spp. bulgaricus* and *L. acidophilus* have been also effective in the prevention of traveller's diarrhea (Black et al., 1989).

On the other hand, many studies have shown no effect of probiotic treatment (Lewis & Freedman, 1998). There is still some doubts regaring the quality and efficacy of probiotic products. Nevertheless, the probiotic food industry is flourishing. In many European counties the market is expanding resulting in sell of probiotic yogurts that account for over 10% of all yogurts sold in Europe (Stanton et al., 2001).

4. Criteria associated with probiotic bacteria

Consortium of LAB constitute a major part of the natural microflora of human intestine and when present in sufficient numbers create a healthy equilibrium between beneficial and potentially harmful microflora in the gut (Dune et al., 2001). For some positive effects on human health, a probiotic strain has to reach the large intestine at a concentration of about 10^7 viable cells/g (Stanton et al., 2001). Microorganisms ingested with food begin their journey to the lower intestinal tract via the mouth and are exposed during their transit through the GI tract to successive stress factors that influence their survival. The time from entrance to release from the stomach is about 90 min, but further digestive processes have longer residence times (Berrada et al., 1991). Probiotic bacteria must overcome physical and chemical barriers in the GI tract, especially acidic environment of the stomach, and then the activity of hydrolytic enzymes and bile salts in the small intestine. In a typical acid tolerance tests, the viability of potential probiotic organisms is determined by exposing them to low pH in a buffer solution or medium for a certain period of time, during which the number of surviving probiotic bacteria is determined. The generally requirements for probiotics are shown in Table 3.

Acid and bile stability
Adherence to human intestinal cells
Ability to reduce the adhesion of pathogens to surfaces
Colonization of human GI tract
Antagonism against carcinogenic and pathogenic bacteria
Production of anti-microbial substances
Survive the various technological processes of production
Safety evaluation: nonpathogenic, nontoxic, nonallergic, nonmutagenic
Desirable metabolic activity and antibiotic resistance/sensitivity
Clinically validated and documented health effects

Table 3. The desired properties of probiotic strains (adapted from Mattila & Sarraela, 2000)

Bile plays an essential role in lipid digestion; it emulsifies and solubilizes lipids and functions as biological detergent. Prior to secretion into the duodenum, bile acids, which are synthesized from cholesterol, are conjugated to either glycine or taurine in liver (Begley et al., 2006). In the colon conjugated bile undergoes to the various chemical changes including deconjugation, dehydroxylation, dehydrogenation, and deglucuronidation, almost solely by microbial activity (Begley et al., 2006). Bile reduces the survival of bacteria by destroying their cell membranes, whose major components are lipids and fatty acids and these modifications may affect not only the cell permeability and viability, but also the interactions between the membranes and the environment. Bile salt hydrolases (BSHs) are generally intracellular, oxygeninsensitive enzymes that catalyze the hydrolysis of bile salts (Liong & Shah, 2005). A number of BSHs have been identified and characterized in probiotic bacteria (Franz et al., 2001a).

The adhesion ability as well as interaction with pathohens is regarded as important selection criteria for potential probiotic strains (Salminen et al. 2010). Adhesive properties of LAB depend on a variety of factors, including non-specifc adhesion determined by electrostatic or hydrophobic forces and specific binding dependent on particular molecules. To examine the adhesive property of LAB, several models have been developed. These include binding to tissue culture cells (Tuomola & Salminen, 1998), radiolabelling (Bernet et al., 1993), intestinal mucus (Ouwehand et al., 2001), extracellular matrix proteins (de Leeuw et al., 2006) and resected colonic tissue (Vesterlund et al., 2005). Although none of these models reflect the complex interactions occurring in the mucosal layer of the digestive tract, they represent a rapid method for the screening of potential probiotic strains.

Other functional property used to characterize probiotics is the production of antimicrobial compounds. Several antimicrobial substances that have considerable advantages in competition with pathogens and other harmful bacteria are produced by LAB (Klare et al., 2007; Radulović et al., 2010a). These substances include fatty acids, organic acids, hydrogen peroxide, and diacetyl, acetoin and the most studied inhibitory peptides called 'bacteriocins' (Todorov et al., 2011). The ability of probiotics to establish in the GI tract is enhanced by their ability to eliminate competitors. Some examples of antimicrobial substances produced by probiotic bacteria are presented in Table 4.

Probiotic	Compaund
Lactobacillus GG	Wide spread antibiotic
L. acidophilus	Acidolin,Acidophilin, Lactocidin
L. delbrueckii ssp. bulgaricus	Bulgarican
L. plantarum	Lactolin
L. brevis	Lactobacillin,Lactobrevin
L. reuteri	Reuterin

Table 4. Antimicrobial substances (Fuller, 1992)

Antibiotic susceptibility of potential probiotic strains is also considered as an important selection criterion for potential probiotic status (Hummel et al., 2007). Some LAB may carry potentially transmissible plasmid-encoded antibiotic resistance genes. The transmission of antibiotic resistance genes to unrelated pathogenic or potentially pathogenic bacteria in the gut is a major health concern related with the probiotic application (see detailed information in paragraph 6).

Along with above mentioned criteria, selected probiotic strains have to be able to survive well in the food and to have the appropriate technological properties (e.g. acidification during fermentation if required). In addition, it is important that the added probiotic does not adversely affect the taste, smell, and texture of the food or beverage.

In vitro tests based on these selection criteria, although not a definite means of strain selection, may provide an useful initial information. A validation model system, such as a Simulator of the Human Intestinal Microbial Ecosystem (SHIME), which aims to mimic complex physiological and physiochemical in vivo reactions, may also be of value in strain selection. However, the ultimate proof of probiotic effects requires validation in well designed statistically sound clinical trails. Generally, tools that may be employed in such an assessment include *in vitro* studies, studies of strain properties, pharmacokinetic studies, animal studies, use of intestinal models, human studies and epidemiological surveillance. Each strain needs to be tested separately.

It is evident that the selection of new potential probiotic bacteria is an enormous and time-consuming task with uncertain results.

5. Antibiotic resistance of LAB in the food chain

During the recent years, there has been great concern about the possibility of spreading the antibiotic resistance in the environment. According to the European Commission (2005), it has been estimated that one to ten million tons of antibiotics has been released into the biosphere over the last 60 years. This has lead to very strong selective pressure for the emergence of resistant bacterial strains. Since LAB are present in the GI tract in large amounts, LAB resistant to certain antibiotics could benefit the host organism. Nevertheless, there is a risk associated with the ability of these resistant strains to transmit the resistance gene to pathogenic bacteria. Literature data pointed out that some LAB, the predominant microbiota in fermented dairy and meat products, may serve as reservoirs of antibiotic resistance genes potentially transferable to human pathogens (Mathur & Singh, 2005).

The food chain could be regarded as one of the main pathways for the transmission of antibiotic resistant bacteria from animals to humans (Singer et al., 2003). Molecular analysis of resistance genes localized on transferable genetic elements showed they are identical in humans and animals, which confirm that food of animal origin, particularly sausages and cheeses made from raw milk, serve as a vehicle for the transmission of resistant bacteria and antibiotic resistance determinants. The antibiotics application in sub-therapeutic levels in animal's drinking water and feed increases the selective pressure and amplify the transfer of antibiotic resistance between bacterial species. Thus there is a direct correlation between the indigenous microflora of the GI tract of animals with the GI tract of humans. Although many species of LAB used as starter and probiotic cultures possess GRAS status, potential risk to human health caused by the genes transfer of antibiotic resistance has not yet been fully defined. To address this aspect, the safety of LAB should be verified with the respect of their ability to acquire and disseminate resistance determinants (Kastner et al., 2006). Particular concern is due to the evidence of a widespread occurrence in this bacterial group of conjugative plasmids and transposons. The presence of transmissible antibiotic resistance markers in the safety evaluation of LAB strains is a very important task since genes conferring resistance to several antimicrobials (e.g. chloramphenicol, erythromycin, streptomycin, tetracycline, and vancomycin) located on transferable genetic elements (plasmids or transposons) have already been characterized in lactococci (Perreten et al., 1997), lactobacilli (Axelsson et al., 1988; Danielsen, 2002) and enterococci (Eaton & Gasson, 2001; Huys et al., 2002) isolated from food. However, the transfer of antibiotic resistance genes from LAB reservoir strains to bacteria in the resident microflora of human GI tract and hence to pathogenic bacteria, has not been fully addressed.

Irrespective of the antibiotic resistance mechanisms and the bacterial taxon involved, the possibility of spreading an antibiotic resistance determinant through horizontal transfer relies on its genetic basis. Therefore, a distinction between intrinsic and acquired resistance has to be made. Antibiotic resistance may be intrinsic for bacterial species or a genus, and it is characterized by the ability of an organism to survive in the presence of certain antimicrobial agents, due to its inherent characteristics of resistance. Intrinsic or "natural" resistance mechanisms involve the absence of the target, low cell permeability, antibiotic inactivation and the presence of efflux mechanisms. Enterococci are intrinsically resistant to cephalosporins and low levels of aminoglycoside and clindamycin (Teuber et al., 1999). Lactobacilli, pediococci and *Leuconostoc* spp. have been reported to have a high natural resistance to vancomycin, a property that is useful to separate them from other Gram-positive bacteria (Hamilton- Miller & Shah, 1998; Simpson et al., 1988). Some lactobacilli have a high natural resistance to bacitracin, cefoxitin, ciprofloxacin, fusidic acid, kanamycin, gentamicin, metronidazole, nitrofurantoin, norfloxacin, streptomycin, sulphadiazine, teicoplanin, trimethoprim/sulphamethoxazole, and vancomycin (Danielsen & Wind, 2003). For a number of lactobacilli a very high frequency of spontaneous mutation to nitrofurazone (10^{-5}), kanamycin and streptomycin was found (Curragh & Collins, 1992). From these data it is clear that inter-genus and inter-species differences exist, and consequently identification at species level is required in order to interpret phenotypic susceptibility data. Acquired resistance is a characteristic of some strains within a species usually susceptible to certain antibiotics and can be horizontally spread among the bacteria. The acquisition of antibiotic resistance occurs via the mutation of pre-existing genes or by horizontal transmission of resistance determinants. With some exception, intrinsic resistance and resistance by mutation are unlikely to be disseminated, although any gene responsible for intrinsic resistance may spread provided that it is flanked by insertion sequences (European Commissions); horizontally transferred genes, particularly those carried on mobile genetic elements, are those most likely to be transmitted (Normark & Normark, 2002). Among the three well-known mechanisms for horizontal gene exchange between bacteria, namely free DNA mediated transformation, bacteriophage induced transduction, and conjugation, the last is acknowledged to be the most relevant for antibiotic resistance gene transfer (Salyers, 1995). Resistance genes are frequently carried by the mobile genetic elements involved in these mechanisms, such as plasmids and conjugative transposons, which can be freely exchanged irrespective of genus or species barriers, resulting in resistance transfer or co-transfer (Levy, 1986). Recently it has been discovered that the so-called "mobilome" also involves other genetic elements: the transposon can carry integrons, which are not self-transmissible but carry a gene encoding an integrase, which in turn mobilises resistance genes borne on the integron as cassettes (Clementi & Aquilanti, 2011). This mechanism seems to be active only in the context of resistance gene exchange and it surely determines a substantial increase in the horizontal mobility of these genes.

5.1 Procedure for antimicrobial susceptibility/resistance patterns of LAB

As mentioned above, an intrinsic resistance and resistance by mutation are unlikely to be disseminated, so the risk is mainly characterized by horizontally transferred genes. Therefore, distinction between natural and acquired antibiotic resistance among the population of LAB is of a great importance. Analysis of Minimal Inhibitory Concentration (MIC) and their distributions in defined species/antibiotic combinations helps to differentiate between these two resistance mechanisms. When a bacterial strain demonstrates higher resistance to a specific antibiotic than the other strains of the same taxonomical unit, the presence of acquired resistance is indicated and there is a need for further analysis to confirm the genetic basis of resistance.

According to Murray et al., (2003) the MIC distribution of a given antibiotic for a single bacterial species in the absence of resistance mechanisms should approach statistical normality while bimodal distribution of MIC values suggest acquired resistance. For the purpose of identifying bacterial strains with acquired and potentially transferable antibiotic resistance, microbiological breakpoints have been defined. Microbiological breakpoints are set by studying the MIC distribution in the bacterial population and the part of population that clearly deviates from a susceptible majority is considered resistant (Olsson-Liljequist et al., 1997).

The data used for the definition of microbiological breakpoints, as reported in Table 5, were derived from the published body of research and from national and European monitoring procedures. The antibiotics listed: ampicillin, vancomycin, gentamicin, kanamycin, streptomycin, erythromycin, clindamycin, quinupristin+dalfopristin, tetracycline and chloramphenicol were chosen to maximise the identification of resistance genotypes by assessing the resistance phenotypes.

In Gram-positive, bacteria acquired trimethoprim resistance, although occasionally detected is relatively rare. The data available (Korhonen et al., 2007) indicate that within species of lactobacilli the range of apparent trimethoprim resistances can be wide with no clear breakpoint values. Therefore, the MIC testing of trimethoprim for LAB was not considered relevant. Furthermore, testing for linezolid and neomycin is no longer considered necessary. The extremely rare non-mutational resistance to linezolid is due to the acquisition of the *cfr* gene, which also confers resistance to chloramphenicol (Arias et al., 2008; Toh et al., 2007). Testing for chloramphenicol resistance will efficiently cover for the hazard of acquiring resistance to linezolid. Neomycin is removed from the list since testing for the remaining three aminoglycosides efficiently covers the hazard of acquiring resistance to aminoglycosides.

Antibiotic susceptibility testing may be performed using different phenotypic test methods. In Clinical and Laboratory Standards Institute (CLSI), formerly National Committee on Clinical Laboratory Standards (NCCLS), the approved standards state that the methods of choice are agar dilution and broth microdilution (Anonym, 2007). Other widely used methods include the agar gradient method and commercial methods, such as Etest, which consists of a predefined gradient of antibiotic concentrations on a plastic strip (AbBiomerieux, Sweden). In addition to phenotypic antibiotic resistance determinations, also genotypic detection of particular genes causing resistance may be performed. These genotypic methods include different PCR –based methods, southern hybridization, plasmid profiling and microarray (Ammor et al., 2008; Aquilanti et al., 2007). The situation is clearest

Lactic acid bacteria	ampicillin	vancomycin	gentamicin**	Kanamycin**	streptomycin**	erythromycin	clindamycin	quinupristin+ dalphopristin	tetracycline	chloramphenicol
Lactobacillus obligate homofermentative	1	2	16	16	16	1	1	4	4	4
Lactobacillus helveticus	1	2	16	16	16	1	1	4	4	4
Lactobacillus acidophilus group	1	2	16	16	16	1	1	4	4	4
Lactobacillus delbrueckii	1	2	16	16	16	1	1	4	4	4
Lactobacillus obligate heterofermentative	2	n.r.	16	16	64	1	1	4	8	4
Lactobacillus reuteri	2	n.r.	8	16	64	1	1	4	16	4
Lactobacillus fermentum	1	n.r.	16	32	64	1	1	4	8	4
*Lactobacillus facultative heterofermentative**	4	n.r.	16	64	64	1	1	4	8	4
Lactobacillus plantarum	2	n.r.	16	64	n.r.	1	1	4	32	8
Lactobacillus rhamnosus	4	n.r.	16	64	32	1	1	4	8	4
Lactobacillus paracasei	2	n.r.	32	64	n.r.	1	1	4	4	4
Bifidobacterium	2	2	64	n.r.	128	0.5	0.25	1	8	4
Enterococcus	4	4	32	512	128	4	4	4	2	8
Pediococcus	4	n.r.	16	64	64	1	1	4	8	4
Leuconostoc	2	n.r.	16	16	64	1	1	4	8	4
Lactococcus lactis	2	4	32	64	64	2	4	4	4	8
Streptococcus thermophilus	2	4	32	64	64	2	2	4	4	4
Bacillus spp.	n.r.	4	4	8	8	4	4	4	8	8
Propionibacterium	2	4	64	64	64	0.5	0.25	0.5	2	2
Other Gram (-)	1	2	4	16	8	0.5	0.25	0.5	2	2

n.r. not required;
*including *Lactobacillus salivarius*;
**possible interference of the growth medium

Table 5. Microbiological breakpoints categorizing bacteria as resistant (mg L^{-1}). Strains with MIC higher than the breakpoints below are considered as resistant.

when the phenotypic and genotypic resistance patterns are in agreement. However, a phenotypically resistant strain may be genotypically "susceptible". This is usually due to the fact that appropriate genes are not included in the test patterns, or there might be unknown resistance genes. Tetracycline, for example, has more than 40 different genes conferring antibiotic resistance discovered at the moment, and the number of tetracycline resistance genes continues to increase (Roberts, 2005). In contrast, a susceptible phenotype may also carry silent genes, which are observed with genotyping.

However, there is still a lack of agreement on the resistance-susceptibility breakpoints for most antibiotics in LAB (Charteris et al., 1998; Danielsen & Wind, 2003; Katla et al., 2001). Generally, the choice of medium has been shown to have a profound impact on the MICs of

LAB. The recommended growth media by the National Committee for Clinical Laboratory Standards (Mueller-Hinton agar) (NCCLS, 2002) and by the British Society for Antimicrobial Chemotherapy (Iso-Sensitest agar) (Andrews, 2001) do not support growth of all LAB. MRS medium, that generally supports the growth of LAB much better, is not always compatible to the Iso-Sensitest medium for the use in susceptibility testing, as was reported for various classes of antibiotics (Huys et al., 2002). Furthermore, there are still no guidelines available for the interpretation of susceptibility test results of commensal or food-associated bacteria. Additionally, MIC breakpoints values have been shown to be species specific and thus vary between species of the same genera (Danielsen & Wind, 2003). Also, distinguishing between intrinsic, non-specific and acquired resistance is difficult and requires, besides the evaluation of genetic base of resistance, that the antimicrobial-resistance patterns of many LAB species from different sources may be compared (Teuber et al., 1999).

5.2 Mobile genetic elements in LAB

A prerequisite for LAB to acquire antibiotic resistance genes from other bacteria is their ability to communicate actively and passively with these bacteria with the aid of conjugative plasmids and transposons. Conjugative plasmids and transposons are common in LAB, and due to their wide environmental distribution, it is possible that these commensal bacteria act as vectors for the dissemination of antibiotic resistance determinants to the consumer via the food chain. Plasmids are found in many genera of LAB, characterized by different size, function and distribution (Davidson et al., 1996; Wang & Lee, 1997). The functions related to the plasmids include hydrolysis of proteins, metabolism of carbohydrates, amino acids and citrate, production of bacteriocins and exopolysaccharides, and resistance to antibiotics, heavy metals and phages. At least 25 species of lactobacilli contain native plasmids (Wang & Lee, 1997), and often appear to contain multiple (from 1 to 16) different plasmids in a single strain. R-plasmids encoding tetracycline, erythromycin, chloramphenicol, or macrolide-lincomycin-streptogramin resistance have been reported in *L. reuteri* (Lin et al., 1996; Tannock et al., 1994), *L. fermentum* (Fons et al., 1997; Ishiwa & Iwata, 1980), *L. acidophilus* (Vescovo et al., 1982), and *L. plantarum* (Danielsen, 2002) isolated from raw meat, silage and faeces. The reported prevalence of antibiotic resistance genes such as erythromycin, vancomycin, tetracycline, chloramphenicol, and gentamicin resistance genes, on transferable genetic elements in enterococci is more extensive, both on plasmids (Murray et al., 1988) and transposons (Clewell et al., 1995; Perreten et al., 1997a; Rice & Marshall, 1994;). A multiple antibiotic resistance plasmid was reported in a *L. lactis* strain isolated from cheese (Perreten et al., 1997b), encoding streptomycin, tetracycline and chloramphenicol resistance.

Conjugative transposons are the major vehicle regarding antibiotic resistance transport in LAB. They have been discovered in *E.faecalis* (Tn916, Tn918, Tn920, Tn925, Tn2702), *E. faecium* (Tn5233) and *L. lactis* (Tn5276, Tn5301). In enterococci and streptococci, resistances to tetracycline (tet (M)), erythromycin (ermAM, erm), chloramphenicol (cat) and kanamycin (aphA-3) have been determined. In lactococci, code for nisin (nis) production and sucrose fermentation (sac) has been observed. These transposons vary in size between 16 and 70 kb and may be inserted into plasmids or the chromosome in one or multiple copies. They may mobilize plasmids or chromosomal genes. The most remarkable observation is the extreme host range, which is the property of the Tn916/Tn1545 family.

5.3 Horizontal transferability of antibiotic resistance from LAB in food chain

The possible transfer of antibiotic resistance genes between bacterial species have been studied mostly in harmful or pathogenic species, but also recently in LAB. The vast majority of the experiments have been made *in vitro*, using methods such as filter-mating (Klare et al., 2007, Ouoba et al.,2008), although these *in vitro* methods do not mimic the circumstances in nature, and results obtained cannot be compared with the results achieved or expected using *in vivo* methods. The transferability of antibiotic resistance genes in the GI tract from LAB is not straightforward, since the GI tract is a hostile environment to many allochthonous bacteria. Moreover, studies made *in vivo* usually are based on "worst-case scenario", simulating very high daily intake of food products containing the resistant bacteria (Jacobsen et al., 2007). The potentially transferable genes in LAB have been described in multiple studies and have been reviewed in Ammor et al. (2007). Two of the most commonly observed resistance genes in LAB found so far are *tet*(M) for tetracycline resistance and *erm*(B) for erythromycin, followed with *cat* genes coding for chloramphenicol resistance (Cataloluk & Gogebakan 2004; Danielsen, 2002).

Enterococci are known to be very well receptive for conjugation (Clewell & Weaver, 1989), but are also successful donor organisms for the transfer of antibiotic resistance genes to unrelated enterococci (Rice et al., 1998), lactobacilli (Shrago & Dobrogosz, 1988), other Gram-positives including *Bacillus subtilis* (Christie et al., 1987), *Staphylococcus* (Young et al., 1987) and *Listeria* spp. (Charpentier et al., 1997; Perreten et al., 1997b), and even Gram-negative bacteria (Courvalin, 1994). Moreover, the transfer of conjugative elements, including a plasmid-encoded kanamycin resistance and a transposon-encoded tetracycline and erythromycin resistance (Doucet-Populaire et al., 1991), were shown to be transferable from *E. faecalis* to *Escherichia coli* and *Listeria monocytogenes*, respectively, in the digestive tract of mice. In contrast, reports of conjugative transfer of antibiotic resistance genes in other LAB are rare. Two *in vivo* studies were performed, to examine the possibility of conjugative transfer between native Gram-positive members of the gut. Therefore, the broad host range conjugative plasmid pAMβ1 was transferred in vitro to *L. reuteri* (Morelli et al., 1988) and *L. lactis* (Igimi et al., 1996) and administered orally or using gastric intubation to mice. By analysis of faecal content, plasmid transfer to *E. faecalis* was observed in both studies.

In order to fully understand the extent to which LAB strains transfer resistance genes in the natural environment, it is essential to study genetic exchange in this context. Toomey et al., (2009) reported on the ability of wild-type antibiotic resistance determinants [*erm*(B) and *tet*(M)], present in LAB strains isolated from food sources, to be transferred to recipient strains. In vitro mating, using a traditional filter mating technique, showed that all four LAB mating pairs transferred their resistance determinants at high frequencies. By employing two in vivo models, an alfalfa sprout plant and an animal rumen model Toomey et al., (2009) demonstrated the transfer of resistance determinants between all four LAB mating pairs in these models. Previously, in vivo transfer between LAB has only been shown in the gastrointestinal tracts of gnotobiotic rats (Jacobsen et al., 2007) and mice (McConnell et al., 1991; Morelli et al., 1988). The transfer frequencies have been observed to increase when the animals have received the antibiotic in question at subtherapeutic levels (Igimi et al., 1996; Licht et al., 2003; Salyers & Shoemaker 1996) in their drinking water or feed, suggesting that increasing the antibiotic pressure can amplify the transfer of antibiotic resistance between bacterial species. All of these above studies indicate that antibiotic resistant factors may be transferred from food related bacterium species (LAB) to other, potentially pathogenic species. The risks associated need to be considered, in light of the increasing concerns related to food as a potential reservoir for antibiotic resistance determinants.

6. Antibiotic resistance/susceptibility patterns of specific LAB genera applicable as probiotics

Some features appeared to be shared by the majority of LAB; in particular, it was reported that most LAB species are resistant to metronidazole and that they are all intrinsically resistant to sulphonamides and trimethoprim, while they are usually susceptible to piperacillin and piperacillin plus tazobactam. On the other hand, clear differences were highlighted among different LAB genera, although well-defined species-specific profiles were not always identifiable. A high resistance to cefoxitin was acknowledged for *Lactococcus*, *Leuconostoc*, and *Lactobacillus*, whereas, as regards vancomycin, *Leuconostoc*, *Pediococcus* and most lactobacilli species were recognised as intrinsically resistant and most *Lactococcus* isolates as highly susceptible.

Lactobacilli widely used in starter cultures or as probiotics in dairy products enter human intestines in large numbers and there interact with the intestinal microbiota (Teuber et al., 1999). Therefore they have the potential to serve as hosts for antibiotic-resistance genes, with the risk of transferring the genes to opportunistic or pathogenic bacteria. Routine antibiotic susceptibility testing has been advocated as an essential selection criterion for potentially starter or probiotic *Lactobacillus* cultures (Charteris & Kelly, 1993). The *Lactobacillus* species have been found susceptible to many cell wall synthesis inhibitors, like penicillins and ampicillin (Danielsen & Wind 2003, Coppola et al., 2005), in contrast to glycopeptides such as vancomycin, most *Lactobacillus* species, excluding obligate heterofermentative species, have been found to be resistant to these types of antibiotics. However, the resistance towards vancomycin has been demonstrated being as intrinsic (Tynkkynen et al., 1998) due the presence of D-alanine: D-alanine ligase-related enzymes (Elisha & Courvalin, 1995) and should not be compared with transmissible, plasmid–mediated resistance found in enterococci (Leclercq et al., 1992). As a general rule, lactobacilli have a high natural resistance to bacitracin, cefoxitin, ciprofloxacin, fusidic acid, kanamycin, gentamicin, metronidazole, nitrofurantoin, norfloxacin, streptomycin, sulphadiazine, teicoplanin (Danielsen & Wind, 2003). In addition, resistance against inhibitors of nucleic acid synthesis, such as trimethoprim, seems to be intrinsic, although further characterizations are required on this topic (Ammor et al., 2007). Resistance to tetracycline has been observed more often among *Lactobacillus* species, and it has been shown to have a wide range of MICs (Korhonen et al., 2008), also with a multimodal distribution of MICs, probably due to the extensive variability of tetracycline resistance mechanisms conferring diverse levels of susceptibility (Roberts, 2005). Especially with tetracycline, molecular methods should be applied in order to reveal the nature of resistance, i.e. is it due to intrinsic mechanisms, mutation or added, mobile genes.

Screening of antibiotic-resistance profile among *Lactobacillus* strains used in dairy products such as probiotics or as starters is now tending to become systematic. Coppola et al., (2005) pointed out that all of 63 *L. rhamnosus* strains isolated from Parmigiano Reggiano cheese showed resistance to six antibiotics (cefixime, vancomycin, neomycin, enoxacin, peflxacin, and sulphamethoxazole plus trimetoprim). Investigating the current antibiotic-resistance situation in microbial food additives in Switzerland, Kastner et al., (2006) determined that among 74 *Lactobacillus* isolates applicable as starter or probiotic cultures, two antibiotic resistances were detected in probiotic cultures. The genetic base of those resistances was confirmed; the tetracycline resistance gene tet(W) in *L. reuteri* SD 2112 (residing on a plasmid) and the lincosamide resistance gene lnu(A) in *L. reuteri* SD 2112. The similar trend was noticed in study of Katla et al., (2001). Only one of the 189 *Lactobacillus* strains isolated from Norwegian dairy products such as yoghurt, sour cream, fermented milk and cheese was classified as high level resistant to streptomycin. In contrast, a study conducted on "home-made" spanish cheese (Serena, Gamonedo, Cabrales) revealed the presence of lactobacilli resistant to penicillin G, cloxacillin, streptomycin, gentamycin, tetracycline, erythromycin and chloramphenicol (Herrero et al., 1996).

L. lactis strains were sensitive to amikacin, ampicillin, 1st generation cephalosporin, chloramphenicol, erythromycin, gentamicin, imipenem, oxacillin, penicillin, pipericillin, sulphonamide, tetracycline, trimethoprim/sulfomethoxazole, and vancomycin (de Fabrizio et al., 1994). A slightly lowered susceptibility was observed towards carbenicillin, ciprofloxacin, dicloxacillin and norfloxacin. Intrinsic resistances were recorded towards colistin, fosfomycin, pipemidic acid and rifamycin. Orberg & Sandine (1985) demonstrated that investigated strains of *L. lactis* subsp. *cremoris* and subsp. *lactis* were all resistant to thrimethoprim and almost all to sulphathiazole. Resistance to gentamicin, kanamycin, lincomycin, neomycin, rifampin and streptomycin varied.

The enterococcal strains are naturally tolerant to β-lactams, cephalosporins, lincosamides and polymyxins. A specific cause for concern and a factor contributing to the pathogenesis of enterococci is the resistance they acquire to aminoglycosides, tetracyclines, macrolides, chloramphenicol, penicillin, and ampicillin (Gray et al., 1991) and their capacity to exchange genetic information by conjugation. Enterococcal food isolates (mainly *E. faecalis* and *E. faecium*) were analysed for resistances to a broader range of different antibiotics using phenotypic susceptibility testing, both in raw meat (Knudtson & Hartman, 1993; Quednau et al., 1998) and fermented milk and meat products (Franz et al., 2001; Teuber & Perreten, 2000). Their data suggest a high prevalence of (multiple) antibiotic resistant enterococci in foods, which nevertheless were mostly susceptible to the clinically relevant antibiotics ampicillin and vancomycin. Enterococci from European cheeses, mainly belonging to *E. feacalis* and *E. faecium*, are susceptible to different antibiotics in different proportions (Teuber et al., 1999; Franz et al., 2001). From the study of European cheeses Teuber et al. (1999) ascertained that the incidence for vancomycin resistance among enterococcal isolates was as low as 4%. When Franz et al. (2001) tested 47 *E. faecalis* strains, isolated mostly from cheeses, they were all susceptible to vancomycin. Bulajić & Mijačević (2011) pointed out that among enterococcal strains isolated from autochthonous Sombor cheese, only one strain showed vancomycin resistance. In contrast, Citak et al. (2004) have shown resistance to vancomycin among the population of enterococci isolated from Turkish white cheeses and was found in 96.8% of *E. faecalis* isolates, and 76% of *E. faecium* strains. The susceptibility to vancomycin is of great importance as this glycopeptide antibiotic is one of the last therapeutic options in clinical therapy.

Bifidobacteria are generally considered to be food-grade organisms that do not impose health risks on the consumer or the environment. Nevertheless, it should be noted that rare cases of *Bifidobacterium*-associated gastrointestinal and extra-intestinal infections have been described. In contrast to susceptibility testing of clinically important bacteria, no standard procedures are specifically dedicated to the determination of resistance phenotypes in *Bifidobacterium* strains. To date, a large variety of methods and protocols have been described for antimicrobial susceptibility testing of bifidobacteria, including agar (overlay) disc diffusion, broth dilution and agar dilution. In addition, various growth media have been used primarily on the basis that they meet the complex growth requirements of bifidobacteria. As opposed to conventional susceptibility test media such as Mueller–Hinton and Iso-Sensitest medium none of these *Bifidobacterium*-specific media are well defined in terms of minimal interaction between specific antimicrobial agents and growth medium components. Recently, a newly defined medium formulation referred to as the Lactic acid bacteria Susceptibility test Medium supplemented with cysteine (LSM + cysteine) was proposed for susceptibility testing of bifidobacteria.

Moubareck et al., (2005) were tested the fifty bifidobacterial strains, isolated from humans, animals or probiotic products for susceptibility to 30 antibiotics by disc diffusion test on *Brucella* agar supplemented with 5% laked sheep blood and vitamin K (1mg/L). All strains were sensitive to penicilins: penicillin G, amoxicillin, piperacillin, ticarcillin, imipenem, and usually anti-Gram-positive antibiotics (macrolides, clindamycin, vancomycin and teicoplanin). Most isolates (70%) were resistant to fusidic acid and, as expected, high resistance profile were observed for aminoglycosides. Potentially acquired resistance was only observed against tetracycline and minocycline, in 14% of the tested strains. For the first time, Moubareck et al., (2005) identified *tet*(W) as the gene responsible for tetracycline resistance in *Bifidobacterium pseudocatenulatum* and *B. bifidum*. Interestingly, the tet(W) gene was previously found in human *B. longum* and three genera of rumen obligate anaerobes, suggesting intergenic transfer of this resistance gene between anaerobic bacteria (Scott et al., 2000). In the study of Masco et al., (2006), the LSM + cysteine medium was used to determine the susceptibility profile of 100 bifidobacterial isolates (strains of animal and human origin, isolates from probiotic products and strains from clinical sources) to 15 common antimicrobial agents. All strains tested were susceptible to amoxicillin, chloramphenicol, erythromycin, quinupristin/dalfopristin, rifampicin and vancomycin. The date from this study (Masco et al., 2006) also reinforce earlier observations indicating that bifidobacteria are intrinsically resistant to gentamicin, sulfamethoxazole and polymyxin B. Susceptibility to trimethoprim, trimethoprim/sulfamethoxazole, ciprofloxacin, clindamycin, tetracycline and minocycline was variable. The tet(W) gene was responsible for tetracycline resistance in 15 strains including 7 probiotic isolates belonging to the taxa *Bifidobacterium animalis* subsp. *lactis* and *B. bifidum*. This gene was present in a single copy on the chromosome and did not appear to be associated with the conjugative transposon TnB1230 previously found in tet(W)-containing *Butyrivibrio fibrisolvens*.

7. Conclusion

The selective pressure imposed by the use of antimicrobial agents plays a key role in the emergence of resistant bacteria. Under selective pressure, the numbers of these bacteria increase and some may transmit their resistance genes to other members of the population.. The food chain was considered as the main route of transmission of antibiotic resistant lactic acid bacteria between the animals and human population. Fermented dairy products and fermented meats, which are not heat-treated before consumption, provide a vehicle for antibiotic resistant LAB with a direct link between the animal indigenous microflora and the human gastrointestinal tract. There is the potential health risk, due to the transfer of antibiotic resistance genes from LAB to bacteria in the human gastrointestinal tract, especially to pathogenic bacteria.

Lactic acid bacteria used as starter cultures or probiotic bacteria, enter into human intestines in large number where they interact with the intestinal microflora. Since there has been a significant rise in the consumption of probiotic products, it is important that probiotics are well documented regarding antibiotic resistance profile. The ability to transfer antibiotic resistance genes must be considered as an important parameter for the selection of the probiotic strains. Continuous attention should be paid to the selection of probiotic strains free of transferable antibiotic-resistance determinants. Without doubt, the uncontrolled use of antimicrobial agents in farming practice has assisted the spread of resistant organisms. Therefore a much stricter control over the use of these drugs is essential.

8. Acknowledgment

This work was supported by Ministry of Education and Science of Republic of Serbia (Project No. 46010).

9. References

Agostoni, C., Axelsson, I., Goulet, O., Koletzko, B., Michaelsen, K.F. & Puntis, J. W., (2004). Prebiotic Oligosaccharides in Dietetic Products for Infants: A Commentary by the ESPGHAN Committee on Nutrition. *Journal of Pediatric Gastroenterology Nutrition,* Vol. 39, pp. 465-473.

Ammor, M. S., Florez, A. B. & Mayo, B. (2007). Antibiotic Resistance in Nonenterococcal Lactic Acid Bacteria and Bifidobacteria. *Food Microbiology,* Vol. 24, pp. 559-570.

Ammor, M. S., Florez, A. B., van Hoek, A. H., de Los Reyes-Gavilan, C. G., Aarts, H. J., Margolles, A. & Mayo, B. (2008). Molecular Characterization of Intrinsic and Acquired Antibiotic Resistance in Lactic Acid Bacteria and Bifidobacteria. *Journal of Molecular Microbiology and Biotechnology,* Vol. 14, pp. 6-15.

Andrews, J. M. (2001). BSAC Standardized Disc Susceptibility Testing Method. *Journal of Antimicrobial Chemotherapy,* Vol. 48 Suppl .1, pp. 43-57.

Anonym (2007). Methods for Antimicrobial Susceptibility Testing of Anaerobic Bacteria. Approved Standard. CLSI document M11-A7. *Applied and Environmental Microbiology,* 72, pp. 1729-1738.

Aquilanti, L., Silvestri, G., Zannini, E., Osimani, A., Santarelli, S. & Clementi, F. (2007). Phenotypic, Genotypic and Technological Characterization of Predominant Lactic Acid Bacteria in Pecorino Cheese from Central Italy. *Journal of Applied Microbiology,* Vol. 103, pp. 948-960.

Arias, C. A., Vallejo, M., Reyes, J., Panesso, D., Moreno, J., Castaneda, E., Villegas, M. V., Murray, B. E. & Quinn, J. P. (2008). Clinical and Microbiological Aspects of Linezolid Resistance Mediated by the *cfr* Gene Encoding a 23S rRNA Methyltransferaze. *Journal of Clinical Microbiology,* Vol. 46, pp. 892-896.

Axelsson, L.T., Ahrne, S., Andersson, M.C. & Stahl, S.R. (1988). Identification and Cloning of a Plasmid-Encoded Erythromycin Resistance Determinant from *Lactobacillus reuteri* G4. *Plasmid*, Vol. 20, pp. 171-174.

Backhed, F.; Ley, R.E.; Sonnenburg, J.L.; Peterson, D.A. & Gordon, J.I. (2005). Host-Bacterial Mutualism in the Hhuman Intestine. *Science*, Vol. 307, pp. 1915-1920.

Begley, M, Hill, C., & Gahan, C. G. M., (2006). Bile Salt Hydrolase Activity in Probiotics. *Applied and Environmental Microbiology*, Vol. 72, No. 3, pp. 1729-1738.

Bengmark, S. (1998). Ecological Control of the Gastrointestinal Tract. Rhe Role of Probiotic Flora. *Gut*, Vol. 27, pp. 2-7.

Bennet, R., Eriksson, M., Nord, C.E. & Zetterström, R. (1986). Fecal Bacterial Microflora of Newborn Infants During Intensive Care Management and Treatment with Five Antibiotic Regimens. *Pediatric Infectious Disease*, Vol. 5, pp. 533-539.

Beresford, T. P., Fitzimons, N. A., Brenan, N. L. & Cogan, T. M. (2001). Recent Advances in Cheese Microbiology. *International Dairy Journal*, Vol. 11, pp. 256-274.

Bernet, M. F., Brassart, D., Neeser, J. R. & Servin, A. L. (1994). *Lactobacillus acidophillus* LA 1 Binds to Cultured Human Intestinal Cell Lines and Inhibits Cell Attachment and Cell Invasion by Enterovirulent Bacteria. *Gut*, Vol. 35, pp. 483-489.

Bernet, M. F., Brassart, D., Neeser, J.R. & Servin, A.L. (1993). Adhesion of Human Bifidobacterial Strains to Cultured Human Intestinal Epithelial Cells and Inhibition of Enteropathogen–Cell Interactions. *Applied and Enviromental Microbiology.*, Vol. 59, pp. 4121-4128.

Berrada, N., Lemeland, J.F., Laroche, G., Thovenot P. & Piaia,M. (1991). *Bifidobactrium* from Fermented Milk: Survival During Gastic Transit. *Journal of Dairy Science*, Vol. 74, pp. 409-413.

Black, F. T. Anderson, P.L., Oeskov, J., Gaarskev, K. & Laulund, S. (1989). Prophylactic Efficacy of Lactobacilli on Traveler's Diarrhea. *Travel Medicine*, Vol. 7, pp. 333-335.

Bulajić, S. & Mijačević, Z. (2011). Antimicrobial Susceptibility of Lactic Acid Bacteria Isolated from Sombor Cheese. *Acta Veterinaria*, Vol. 61, No. 2-3, pp. 247-258.

Cataloluk, O. & Gogebakan, B. (2004). Presence of Drug Resistance in Intestinal Lactobacilli of Dairy and Human Origin in Turkey. *FEMS Microbiology Letters*, Vol. 236, pp. 7-12.

Charpentier, E. & Courvalin, P. (1997). Emergence of the Trimethoprim Resistance gene *dfr*D in *Listeria monocytogenes* BM4293. *Antimicrobial Agents and Chemoterapy*, Vol. 41, pp. 1134-1136.

Charteris, W. P., Kelly, P. M., Morelli, L. & Collins, J. K. (1998). Antibiotic Susceptibility of Potentially Probiotic *Lactobacillus* Species. *Journal of Food Protection*, Vol. 61, pp. 1636-1643.

Charteris, W. P. & Kelly, P. M. (1993). In Vitro Antibiotic Susceptibility of Potentially Probiotic Lactobacilli and Bifidobacteria. In *Second Annual Report, EU FLAIR Project No. AGRF-CT91-0053* ed. Morelli, L. Brussels: Commission of the European Communities.

Christie, P. J., Korman, R. Z., Zahler, S. A., Adsit, J. C. & Dunny, G. M. (1987). Two Conjugation Systems Associated with *Streptococcus faecalis* plasmid pCF10: Identification of a Conjugative Transposon that Transfers Between *S. facealis* and *Bacillus subtilis. Journal of Bacteriology*, Vol. 169, pp. 2529-2536.

Citak, S., Yucel, N. & Orhan, S. (2004). Antibiotic Resistance and Incidence of *Enterococcus* Species in Turkish White Cheese. *International Journal of Dairy Technology*, Vol. 57, pp. 27-31.

Claesson, M. J., van Sinderen, D. & O'Toole, P. W. (2007). The genus *Lactobacillus* – A Genomic Basis of Understanding its Diversity. *FEMS Microbiology Letters*, Vol. 269, No.1, pp. 22-28.

Clementi, F. & Aquilanti, F. A. (2011). Recent Investigations and Updated Criteria for the Assessment of Antibiotic Resistance in Food Lactic Acid Bacteria. *Anaerobe* (2011) 1-5, *Article in Press*.

Clewell, D. B. Weaver, K. E. (1989). Sex Pheromones and Plasmid Transfer in *Enterococcus faecalis*. *Plasmid*, Vol. 21, pp. 175-184.

Coppa, G., Bruni, S., Morelli, L., Soldi, S. & Gabrielli, O. (2004). The First Prebiotics in Humans: Human Milk Oligosaccharides. *Journal of Clinical Gastroenterology*, Vol. 38, pp. 80-83.

Coppola, R., Succi, M., Tremonte, P., Reale, A., Salzano, G. & Sorrentino, E. (2005). Antibiotic Susceptibility of *Lactobacillus rhamnosus* Strains Isolated from Parmigiano Reggiano Cheese. *Lait*, Vol. 85, pp. 193-204.

Courvalin, P. (1994). Transfer of Antibiotic Resistance Genes Between Gram-positive and Gram-negative Bacteria. *Antimicrobial Agents and Chemotherapy*, Vol. 38, pp. 1447-1451.

Cummings, J. H., Gibson, G. R. & Macfarlane, G. T. (1989). Qualitative Estimates of Fermentation in the Hind Gut of Man. *Acta Veterinaria Scandinavica* Suppl. Vol. 86, pp. 76-82.

Curragh, H. J. & Collins, M. A. (1992). High-levels of Spontaneous Drug-Resistance in *Lactobacillus*. *Journal of Applied Bacteriology*, Vol. 73, pp. 31-36.

Danielsen, M. & Wind, A. A. (2003). Susceptibility of *Lactobacillus* spp. to Antimicrobial Agents. *International Journal of Food Microbiology*, Vol. 82, pp. 1-11.

Danielsen, M. (2002). Characterization of the Tetracycline Resistance Plasmid pMD5057 from *Lactobacillus plantarum* 5057 Reveals a Composite Structure. *Plasmid*, Vol. 48, pp. 98-103.

Davidson, B. E., Kordias, N., Dobos, M. & Hillier, A. J. (1996). Genomic Organization of Lactic Acid Bacteria. *Antonie Van Leeuwenhoek International Journal of General and Molecular Microbiology*, Vol. 70, pp. 161-183.

de Leeuw, E., Li, X. & Lu, W. (2006). Binding Characteristics of the *Lactobacillus brevis* ATCC 8287 Surface Layer to Extracellular Matrix Proteins. *FEMS Microbiology Letters*, Vol. 260, pp. 210-215.

deFabrizio, S. V., Parada, J. L. & Torriani, S. (1994). Antibiotic Resistance of *Lactococcus lactis* – an Approach of Genetic Determinants Location through the Model System. *Microbiologie-Aliments-Nutritions*, Vol. 12, pp. 307-315.

Doucet-Populaire, F., Trieu-Cuot, P., Dosbaa, I., Andremont, A. & Courvalin, P. (1991). Inducible transfer of conjugative transposon Tn1545 from *Enterococcus faecalis* to *Listeria monocytogenes* in the digestive tracts of gnotobiotic mice. *Antimicrobial Agents and Chemotherapy*, Vol. 35, pp. 185-187.

Dunne, C., O'Mahony, L., Murphy, L., Thornton, G., Morrissey, D., O'Halloran, S., Feeney, M., Flynn, S., Fitzgerald G., Daly, C., Kiely, B., O 'Sullivan, G.C., Shanahan, F. & Collins, J.K. (2001). *In vitro* Selection Criteria for Probiotic Bacteria of Human

Origin: Correlation with *In vivo* Findings. *American Journal of Clinical Nutrition*, Vol. 73, pp. 386-392.

Eaton, T. J. & Gasson, M. J. (2001). Molecular Screening of *Enterococcus* Virulence Determinants and Potential for Genetic Exchange between Food and Medical Isolates. *Applied and Environmental Microbiology*, Vol. 67, pp. 1628-1635.

EFSA. (2008). Technical Guidance Prepared by the Panel on Additives and Products or Substances used in Animal Feed (FEEDAP) on the Update of the Criteria Used in the Assessment of Bacterial Resistance to Antibiotics of Human and Veterinary Importance. *The EFSA Journal*, pp. 1-15.

Elisha, B. G. & Courvalin, P. (1995). Analysis of Genes Encoding Dalanine: d-Alanine Ligase-Related Enzymes in *Leuconostoc mesenteroides* and *Lactobacillus* spp. *Gene*, Vol. 152, pp. 79-83.

European Commissions (2005). Opinion of the Scientific Committee on Animal Nutrition on the Criteria for Assessing the Safety of Micro-organisms Resistant to Antibiotics of Human Clinical and Veterinary Importance. European Commissions, Health and Consmer protection Directorate General, Directorate C, Scientific Opinions, Brussels, Belgium.

Fons, M., Hege, T., Lafire, M., Raibaud, P., Ducluzeau, R. & Maguin, E. (1997). Isolation and Characterization pf a Plasmid from *Lactobacillus fermentum* Connferring Erythromycin Resistance. *Plasmid*, Vol. 37, pp. 199-203.

Fooks, L. J., Fuller, R. & Gibson, G. R. (1999). Prebiotics, Probiotic and Human Gut Microbiology. *International Dairy Journal*, Vol. 9, pp. 53-61.

Franz, C. M. A. P., Holzapfel, W. H. & Stiles, M. E. (1999). Enterococci at the Crossroads of Food Safety. *International Journal of Food Microbiology*, Vol. 47, pp. 193-197.

Franz, C. M., Muscholl-Silberhorn, A. B., Yousif, N.M.K., Vancanneyt, M., Swings, J. & Holzapfel, W. H. (2001). Incidence of Virulence Factors and Antibiotic Resistance among Enterococci Isolated from Food. *Applied and Environmental Microbiology*, Vol. 67, pp. 4385-4389.

Franz, C.M.A.P., Specht I., Haberer P. & Holzapfel W. H. (2001a). Bile Salt Hydrolase Activity of Enterococci Isolated from Food: Screening and Quantitative Determination. *Journal of Food Protection*, Vol. 64, No 5, pp. 725-729.

Fuller, R. (1992). *Probiotics: The scientific basis*, ISBN 0-412-40850-3, Chapman & Hall, London,

Gardnier, E. G., Ross, P. R., Kellz, M. P., Stanton, K., Collins, K. K. & Fitzgerald, G. (2002). Microbiology of Therapeutic Milks, In: *Dairy Microbiology Handbook, Third Edition*, R. K. Robinson (Ed.), Wiley-Interscience, Inc., 431-478, ISBN 0-471-38596-4, New York, USA.

Garg, S. K. & Mital, B. K. (1991). Enterococci i n Milk and Milk Products. *Critical Reviews in Microbiology*, Vol. 18, pp. 15-45.

Gevers, D., Huys, G. & Swings, J. (2003). In Vitro Conjugal Transfer of Tetracycline Resistance from Lactobacillus Isolates to Other Gram-positive Bacteria. *FEMS Microbiology Letters*, Vol. 225, pp. 125-130.

Gray, C. M., Stewart, D. & Pedler, S. J. (1991). Species Identification and Antibiotic Susceptibility Testing of Enterococci Isolated from Hospitalized Patients. *Antimicrobial Agents and Chemotherapy*, Vol 35, pp. 1943-1945.

Gronlund, M. M., Lehtonen, O. P., Erola, E.& Kero, P. (1999). Fecal Microflora in Healthy Infants Born by Different Methods of Delivery: Permenent Changes in Intestinal

Flora after Cesarean Delivery. *Journal of Pediatric Gastroeneterological Nutrition*, Vol. 28, pp. 19-25.

Guarner, F. & Schaafsma, G. J. (1998). Probiotics. *International Journal of Food Microbiology*, Vol. 39, pp. 237-238.

Hamilton-Miller, J. M. T & Shah, S. (1998). Vancomycin Susceptibility as an Aid to the Identification of Lactobacilli. *Letters in Applied Microbiology*, Vol. 26, pp. 153-154.

Herrero, M., Mayo, B. Ganzales, B. & Suarez, J.E. (1996). Evaluation of Technologically Important Traits in Lactic Acid Bacteria Isolated from Spontaneous Fermentations. *Journal of Applied Bacteriology*, Vol. 81, pp. 567-570.

Herreros, M. A., Fresno, J.M., Gonzalez Prieto, M. J. & Tornadijo, M. E. (2003). Technological Characterization of Lactic Acid Bacteria Isolated from Armada Cheese (a Spanish Goat 's milk Cheese). *International Dairy Journal*, Vol.13, pp. 469-479.

Hevey, P. & Rowland, I. (1999). The Gut Microflora of The Developing Infant: Microbiology and Metabolism. *Microbial Ecology in Health and Disease*. Vol. 11, pp. 75-83.

Hummel, A.S.; Hertel, C.; Holzapfel, W.H. & Franz, C. (2007). Antibiotic Resistances of Starter and Probiotic Strains of Lactic Acid Bacteria. *Applied and Enviromental Microbiology*, Vol.73, pp. 730-739.

Huys, G., D'Haene, K. & Swings, J. (2002). Influence of the Culture Medium on Antibiotic Susceptibility Testing of Food-Associated Lactic Acid Bacteria with the Agar Overlay Disc Diffusion Method. *Letters in Applied Microbiology*, Vol. 34, pp. 402-406.

Igimi, S., Ryu, C.H., Park, S.H., Sasaki, Y., Sasaki, T. & Kumagai, S.. (1996). Transfer of Conjugative Plasmid pAM beta 1 from *Lactococcus lactis* to Mouse Intestinal Bacteria. *Letters of Applied Microbiology*, Vol. 23, pp. 31-35.

Ishiwa, H & Iwata, S. (1980). Drug Resistance in *Lactobacillus fermentum*. *Journal of General and Applied Microbiology*, Vol. 26, pp. 71-74.

Jacobsen, I., Wicks, A., Hammer, K., Huys, G., Gevers, D. & Andersen, S.R. (2007). Horizontal Transfer of tet(M) and erm(B) Resistance Plasmids from Food Strains of *Lactobacillus plantarum* to *Enterococcus faecalis* JH2-2 in The Gastrointestinal Tract of Gnotobiotic Rats. *FEMS Microbiology Ecology*, Vol. 59, pp. 158-166.

Kandler, O. & Weiss, N. (1989). Genus *Lactobacillus*, In: *Bergeys Manual of Systematic Bacteriology*, P. H. Snearh, N. S. Mair, M. E. Sharpe, J. G. Holt (Ed.), Vol. 2, 1418-1434, ISBN 0-683-07893-3, Williams & Wilkins Baltimore, USA.

Kastner, S., Parreten, V., Bleuler, H., Hugenschmidt, G., Lacroix, C & Meile, L.. (2006) Antibiotic Susceptibility Patterns and Resistance Genes of Starter Culture and Probiotic bacteria Used in Food. *Systematic and Applied Microbiology*, Vol. 29, pp. 145-55.

Katla, A. K., Kruse, H., Johnsen, G. & Herikstad, H. (2001). Antimicrobial Susceptibility of Starter Culture Bacteria Used in Norwegian Dairy Products. *International Journal of Food Microbiology*, Vol. 67, pp. 147-152.

Klare, I., Konstabel, C., Werner, G., Huys, G., Vankerckhoven, V., Kahlmetrr, G., Hildebrandt, B., Muller Bertling , S., Witte, W & Goossens, H. (2007). Antimicrobial Susceptibilities of *Lactobacillus, Pediococcus* and *Lactococcus* Human Isolates and Culture Intended for Probiotic or Nutritional Use. *Journal of Antimicrobial Chemotherapy*, Vol. 59, pp. 900-912.

Knudtson, L. M. & Hartman, P.A. (1993). Antibiotic Resistance among Enterococcal Isolates from Environmental and Clinical Sources. *Journal of Food Protection*, Vol. 56, pp. 489-492.

Koll, P., Mandar, R.., Marcotte, H., Leibur, E., Mikelsaar, M. & Hammarstrom, L. (2008). Characterization of Oral Lactobacilli as Potential Probiotics for Oral Health. *Oral Microbiol Immunol.*, Vol. 23, No 2, pp. 139-147.

Korhonen, J. M. Sclivagnotis, Y. & von Wright, A. (2007). Characterization of Dominant Cultivable Lactobacilli and their Antibiotic Resistance Profiles from Fecal Samples of Weaning Piglets. *Journal of Applied Microbiology*, Vol. 103, pp. 2496-2503.

Leclercq, R., Dutka-Malen, S., Brisson-Noel, A., Molinas, C., Derlot, E., Arthur, M., Duval, J. & Courvalin, P. (1992). Resistance of Enterococci to Aminoglycosides and Glycopeptides. *Clinical Infectious Diseases*, Vol. 15, pp. 495-501.

Levy, S. B. (1986). Ecology of Antibiotic Resistance Determinants. In:Levy, SB, Novick, RP (eds) *Antibiotic resistance genes: ecology, transfer and expression.* Cold Spring Harbor Press, New York, pp. 17-29.

Lewis, S. J. & Freedman, A. R. (1998). The Use of Biotherapeutic Agents in the Prevention and Treatment of Gastrointestinal Disease. *Alimentary Pharmacology and Therapeutics*, Vol. 12, pp. 807-822.

Licht, T. R., Struve, C., Christensen, B. B., Poulsen, R. L., Molin, S. & Krogfelt, K. A. (2003). Evidence of Increased Spread and Establishment of Plasmid RP4 In The Intestine Under Sub-inhibitory Tetracycline concentrations. *FEMS Microbiology Ecology*, Vol. 44, pp. 217-233.

Lin, C. F., Fung, Z .F, Wu, C. L. & Chung, T. C. (1996). Molecular Characterization of a Plasmidborne (pTC82) Chloramphenicol Resistance Determinant (cat-Tc) from *Lactobacillus reuteri. Plasmid*, Vol. 36, pp. 116-124.

Liong, M.T. & Shah, N.P. (2005). Bile Salt Deconjugation Ability, Bile Salt Hhydrolase Activity and Cholesterol Co-precipitation Ability of Lactobacilli Strains. *International Dairy Jounal*, Vol. 15, No 4, pp. 391-398.

Lönnermark, E. (2010). Lactobacilli in the Normal Microbiota and Probiotic Effects of *Lactobacillus plantarum. PhD Thesis*, Department of Infectious medicine, Sahlgrenska Academy, University of Gothenburg, Sweden.

Masco, I., Van Hoorde, De Brandt, E., Swings, J. & Huys, G. (2006). Antimicrobial Susceptibility of *Bifidobacterium* Strains from Humans, Animals and Probiotic Products. *Journal of Antimicrobial Chemotherapy*, Vol. 58, pp. 85-94

Mathur, S. & Singh, R. (2005). Antibiotic Resistance in Lactic Acid Bacteria-a review. *International Journal of Food Microbiology*, Vol. 105, pp. 281-95.

Mattila, T. & Saarela, M. (2000). Probiotic Functional Foods. In: *Functional foods*, Williams and Gibson R.G. (Ed), 287-313. CRC Press LLC. Boca Raton, Boston, New York, Washington, DC.

McConnell, M. A., Mercer, A. A. & Tannock, G. W. (1991). Transfer of Plasmid pAM-1 between Members of Microflora Inhabiting the Murine Digestive Tract and Modification of the Plasmid in a *Lactobacillus reuteri* Host. *Microbial Ecology in Health and Disease*, Vol. 4, pp. 343-355.

Modler, H. V., McKellar, R. C. & Yaguchi, M. (1990). Bifidobacteria and Bifidogenic Factors. *Canadian Institute of Food Science and Technology Journal*, Vol. 23, pp. 29-41.

Morelli, L., Sarra, P.G. & Bottazzi, V. (1988). In Vivo Transfer of pAM-beta-1 from *Lactobacillus reuteri* to *Enterococcus faecalis*. *Journal of Applied Bacteriology*, Vol. 65, pp. 371-375.

Moubareck, C., Gavini, F., Vaugien, L., Butel, M. J. & Doucet-Populaire, F. (2005). Antimicrobial Susceptibility of Bifidobacteria. *Journal of Antimicrobial Chemotherapy*, Vol. 55, pp. 38-44.

Mountzouris, K.C; McCartney, A.L; & Gibson, G.R. (2002). Intestinal Microflora of Human Infants and Current Trends for its Nutritional Modulation. *British Journal of Nutrition*, Vol. 87, pp. 405–420.

Murphy, E., Murphy, C. & O'Mahony, L. (2009). Influence of the Gut Microbiota with Aging. In: *Microbiology and Aging: Clinical Manifestations*, S.L. Percival, (Ed.), Springer-Verlag, ISBN 1588296407, New York, USA.

Murray, B. E., An, F. Y. & Clewell, D. B. (1988). Plasmid and Pheromone Response of the Betalactamase Producer *Streptococcus* (*Enterococcus*) *faecalis* HH22. *Antimicrobial Agents and Chemotherapy*, Vol. 32, pp. 547-551.

Murray, P. R., Baron, E. J., Jorgensen, J. H., Pfaller, M. A. & Yolken R. H. (2003). *Manual of Clinical Microbiology*, American Society for Microbiology, Washington.

National Committee for Clinical Laboratory Standards (NCCLS). (2002). Performance Standards for Antimicrobial Susceptibility Testing, *Twelfth informational supplement* (M100-S12)

Newburg, D.S. (2000). Oligosaccharides in Human Milk and Bacterial Colonization. *Journal of Pediatric Gastroenterological Nutrition*, Vol. 30, 2, pp. 8-17.

Normark, B. H. & Normark, S. (2002). Evolution and Spread of Antibiotic Resistance. *Journal of International Medicine*, Vol. 252, pp. 91-106

Ogawa, K., Ben, R.A., Pons, S., de Paolo, M. I. & Bustos Fernández, L. (1992). Volatile Fatty Acids, Lactic Acid, and pH in the Stools of Breast-fed and Bottlefed infants. *Journal of Pediatric Gastroenterological Nutrition*, Vol. 15, pp. 248-252.

Olsson-Liljequist, B., Larsson, P., Walder, M. & Miorner, H. (1997). Antimicrobial Susceptibility Testing in Sweden, III. Methodology for Susceptibility Testing in Sweden. *Scandinavian Journal of Infectious Disease*, 105S, pp. 13-23

Orberg, P. K. & Sandine, W.E. (1985). Survey of Antimicrobial Resistance in Lactic Streptococci. *Applied and Environmental Microbiology*, Vol. 49, pp. 538-542

Ouoba, L. I., Lei, V. & Jensen, L. B. (2008). Resistance of Potential Probiotic Lactic Acid Bacteria and Bifidobacteria of African and European Origin to Antimicrobials: Determination and Transferability of the Resistance Genes to Other Bacteria. *International Journal of Food Microbiology*, Vol. 121, pp. 217-224

Ouwehand, A. C. & Vesterlund, S. (2003). Health Aspects of Probiotics. *Drugs*, Vol. 6, pp. 573-580.

Ouwehand, A. C., Bianchi, Salvadori, B., Fonden, R., Mogensen, G., Salminen, S. & Sellara, R. (2003). Health Effects of Probiotics and Culture-Containing Dairy Products in Humans. *Bulliten of the International Dairy Federation*, Vol. 380, pp. 4-19.

Ouwehand, A. C., Tuomola, E. M., Tolkko, S. & Salminen, S. (2001). Assessment of Adhesion Properties of Novel Probiotic Strains to Human Intestinal Mucus. *International Journal of Food Microbiology*, Vol. 64, pp. 119-126.

Perreten, V., Schwarz, F., Cresta, L., Boeglin, M., Dasen, G. & Teuber, M. (1997a). Antibiotic Resistance Spread in Food. *Nature*, Vol. 389, pp. 801-802.

Perreten, V., Kolloffel, B. & Teuber, M. (1997b). Conjugal Transfer of the Tn916-like Transposon TnFO1 from *Enterococcus faecalis* Isolated from Cheese to Other Gram-positive Bacteria. *Systematic and Applied Microbiology*, Vol. 20, pp. 27-38.

Petrovic, T., Niksic, M. & Bringel, F. (2006). Strain Typing with ISLpl1 in Lactobacilli. *FEMS Microbiology Letters*, Vol.255, pp. 1-10.

Psoni, L., Tzanetakis, N. & Litopoulou-Tzanetaki, E. (2005). Microbiological Characteristics of Batzos, a Traditional Greek Cheese from Raw Goat's Milk. *Food Microbiology* Vol. 20, No. 5, pp. 575-582.

Quednau, M., Ahrne, S., Petersson, A.C. & Molin, G. (1998). Antibiotic-Resistant Strains of *Enterococcus* Isolated from Swedish and Danish Retailed Chicken and Pork. *Journal of Applied Microbiology*, Vol. 84, pp. 1163-1170

Radulović, Z. (2010). *Autochthonous Lactic Acid Bacteria as Starter Cultures*. Faculty of Agriculture University of Belgrade, ISBN 978-86-7843-081-9, Belgrade, Serbia.

Radulović, Z., Petrović, T., Nedović, V., Dimitrijević, S., Mirković, N., Petrušić, M. & Paunović, D. (2010a). Characterization of autochthonous *Lactobacillus paracasei* strains on potential probiotic ability. *Mljekarstvo*, Vol. 60, No.2, pp. 86-93.

Reuter, G. (2001). The *Lactobacillus* and *Bifidobacterium* Microflora of The Human Intestine: Composition and Succession. *Current Issues Intestinal Microbiology*, Vol. 2, pp. 43-53.

Rice, L. & Marshall, S. H. (1994). Insertions of IS256-like Element Flanking the Chromosomal Beta-lactamase Gene of *Enterococcus faecalis* CX19. *Antimicrobial Agents and Chemotherapy*, Vol. 38, pp. 693-701

Rice, L.B., Carias, L.L., Donskey, C.L. & Rudin, S.D. (1998). Transferable, Plasmid-Mediated VanB-type Glycopeptide Resistance in *Enterococcus faecium*. *Antimicrobial Agents and Chemotherapy*, Vol. 42, pp. 963-964

Roberts, M.C. (2005). Update on Acquired Tetracycline Resistance Genes. *FEMS Microbiology Letters*, Vol. 245, pp. 195-203

Rodriguez, C., Medici, M., Mozzi, F. & de Valdez, G. F. (2010). Therapeutic Effect of *Streptpcoccus thermophilus* CRL 1190 – Fermented Milk on Chronic Gastritis. *World Journal of Gastroenerology*, Vol. 16, pp. 1622-1630.

Ryan, K.A.; Jayaraman, T.; Daly, P.; Canchaya, C.; Curran, S.; Fang, F.; Quigley, E.M. & O'Toole, P.W. (2008) Isolation of Lactobacilli with Probiotic Properties from the Human Stomach. *Letters of Applied Microbiology*, Vol.47, pp. 269-274.

Saavedra, J. M., Bauman, N., Oung, I., Perman, J. & Yolken, R. (1994). Feeding of *Bifidobacterium bifidum* and *Streptococcus thermophilus* to Infants in Hospital for Prevention of Diarrhoea and Shedding of Rotavirus, *The Lancet*, Vol. 344, pp. 1046-1049.

Salminen, S., Nybom, S., Meriluoto, J., Carmen Collado, M., Vesterlund, S. & El-Nezami, H. 2010. Interaction of Probiotics and Pathogens — Benefits to Human Health? *Current Opinion in Biotehnology*, Vol. 21, pp. 157-167.

Salyers, A. A. & Shoemaker, N.B. (1996). Resistance Gene transfer in Anaerobes: New Insights, New problems. *Clinical Infectious Diseases*, Vol. 23 Suppl. 1, S36-43

Salyers, A. A. (1995). Antibiotic Resistance Transfer in the Mammalian Intestinal Tract: Implications for Human Health, *Food Safety and Biotechnology*, Heidelberg:Springer-Verlag, New York, USA.

Scardovi, V. (1986). Genus *Bifidobacterium*, In: *Bergeys Manual of Systematic Bacteriology*, P. H. Snearh, N. S. Mair, M. E. Sharpe, J. G. Holt (Ed.), Vol. 2, 1418-1434, ISBN 0-683-07893-3, Williams & Wilkins Baltimore, USA.

Scott, K. P., Melville, C.M., Barbosa, T.M. et al. (2000). Occurrence of the New Tetracycline Resistance Gene tet(W) in Bacteria from the Human Gut. *Antimicrobial Agents and Chemotherapy*, Vol. 44, pp. 775-777.

Shah, P. N. (2007). Functional Cultures and Health Benefits. *International Dairy Journal*, Vol. 17, pp. 1262-1277.

Shrago, A.W. & Dobrogosz, W.J. (1988). Conjugal Transfer of Group-B Streptococcal Plasmids and Comobilization of *Escherichia coli-Streptococcus* Shuttle Plasmids to *Lactobacillus plantarum*. *Applied and Environmental Microbiology*, Vol. 54, pp. 824-826.

Simpson, W. J., Hammond, J.R.M. & Miller, R.B. (1988). Avoparcin and Vancomycin-Useful Antibiotics for the Isolation of Brewery Lactic Acid Bacteria. *Journal of Applied Bacteriology*, Vol. 64, pp. 299-309.

Singer, R. S., Finch, R., Wegener, H.C., Bywater, R., Walters, J. & Lipstich, M. (2003). Antibiotic resistance - The Interplay Between antibiotic use in Animals and Human Beings. *Lancet Infectious Diseases*, Vol. 3, pp. 47-51.

Stanton, C., Gardiner, G., Meehan, H., Collins, J. K., Fitzgerald, G., Lynch, P. B. & Ross, R. P. (2001). Market Potential for Probiotics. *The American Journal of Clinical Nutrition*, Vol. 73 (suppl.), pp. 4765-4835.

Stark, P.L., & Lee, A. (1982). The Microbial Ecology of the Large Bowel of Breast-fed and Formula-fed Infants During the First Year of Life. *Journal of Medical Microbiology*, Vol. 15, pp. 189-203.

Tamime, A., Božanić, R., Rogelj, I. (2003). Probiotički fermentirani mliječni proizvodi. *Mljekarstvo*, Vol. 53, pp. 111-134.

Tancrede, C. (1992). Role of Human Microflora in Health and Disease. *European Journal of Clinical Microbiology Infection Disease*, 11, pp. 1012–1015.

Tannock, G.W., Luchansky, J.B., Miller, L., Connell, H., Thodeandersen, S., Mercer, A.A. & Kalenhammer, T.R. (1994). Molecular Characterization of a Plasmid Borne (pGT633) Erythromycin Resistance Determinant (ermGT) from *Lactobacillus reuteri* 100-63. *Plasmid*, Vol. 31, pp. 60-71

Teuber, M & Perreten, V. (2000). Role of Milk and Meat Products as Vehicles for Antibiotic Resistant Bacteria. *Acta Veterinaria Scandinavica*, pp. 75-87.

Teuber, M., Meile, L. & Schwarz, F. (1999). Acquired Antibiotic Resistance in Lactic Acid Bacteria from Food. *Antonie van Leeuvenhoek*, Vol. 76, pp. 115-137.

Todorov, S.D., Furtado, D.N., Saad, S. M. I. & Tome, E. (2011). Potential Beneficial Properties of Bacteriocin-Producing Lactic Acid Bacteria Isolated from Smoked Salmon. *Journal of Applied Microbiology*, 110, No 4, pp. 971-986.

Toh, S. M., Xiong, L., Arias, C. A., Villegas, M. V., Lolans, K., Quinn, J. & Mankin, A. S. (2007). Acquisition of a Natural Resistance Gene Renders a Clinical Strains of Methicilllin Resistant *Staphylococcus aureus* Resistant to the Synthetic Antibiotic Linezolid. *Molecular Microbiology*, Vol. 64, pp. 1506-1514.

Toomey, N., Monaghan, A., Fanning, S. & Bolton, D. (2009). Transfer of Antibiotic Resistance Marker Genes Between Lactic Acid Bacteria in Model Rumen and Plant Environments. *Applied and Environmental Microbiology*, Vol. 75, No. 10, pp. 346-3152.

Tuomola, E.M. & Salminen, S.J. (1998). Adhesion of Some Probiotic and Dairy Lactobacillus Strains to Caco-2 Cell Cultures. *International Journal of Food Microbiology*, Vol.41, pp. 45–51.

Tynkkynen, S., Singh, K. V. & Varmanen, P. (1998). Vancomycin Resistance Factor of *Lactobacillus rhamnosus* GG in Relation to Enterococcal Vancomycin Resistance (van) Genes. *International Journal of Food Microbiology*, Vol. 41, pp.195-204. UK.

van der Waaij, D. (1988). Evidence of Imunoregulation of the Composition of Intestinal Microflora and Its Practical Consequences. *European Journal Clinical Microbiology Infectious Diseases*, Vol. 7, pp. 103-106.

Vescovo, M., Morelli, L. & Botazzi, V. (1982). Drug resistance plasmids in *Lactobacillus acidophilus* and *Lactobacillus reuteri*. *Applied and Environmental Microbiology*, Vol. 43, pp. 50-56.

Vesterlund, S., Paltta, J., Karp, M. & Ouwehand, A. C. (2005). Adhesion of Bacteria to Resected Human Colonic Tissue: Quantitative Analysis of Bacterial Adhesion and Viability. *Research in Microbiology*, Vol. 156, pp. 238–244.

Wang, T.T. & Lee, B.H. (1997). Plasmids in *Lactobacillus*. *Critical Reviews in Biotechnology*, Vol. 17, pp. 227-272.

Young, H.K., Skurray, K.A. & Amyes, S.K. (1987). Plasmid-Mediated Trimethoprim-Resistance in *Staphylococcus aureus*. Characterization of the First Gram-Positive Plasmid Dihydrofolate Reductase (type S1). *Biochemistry Journal,* Vol. 243, No. 1, pp. 309-312.

Permissions

The contributors of this book come from diverse backgrounds, making this book a truly international effort. This book will bring forth new frontiers with its revolutionizing research information and detailed analysis of the nascent developments around the world.

We would like to thank Dr. Marina Pana, for lending her expertise to make the book truly unique. She has played a crucial role in the development of this book. Without her invaluable contribution this book wouldn't have been possible. She has made vital efforts to compile up to date information on the varied aspects of this subject to make this book a valuable addition to the collection of many professionals and students.

This book was conceptualized with the vision of imparting up-to-date information and advanced data in this field. To ensure the same, a matchless editorial board was set up. Every individual on the board went through rigorous rounds of assessment to prove their worth. After which they invested a large part of their time researching and compiling the most relevant data for our readers. Conferences and sessions were held from time to time between the editorial board and the contributing authors to present the data in the most comprehensible form. The editorial team has worked tirelessly to provide valuable and valid information to help people across the globe.

Every chapter published in this book has been scrutinized by our experts. Their significance has been extensively debated. The topics covered herein carry significant findings which will fuel the growth of the discipline. They may even be implemented as practical applications or may be referred to as a beginning point for another development. Chapters in this book were first published by InTech; hereby published with permission under the Creative Commons Attribution License or equivalent.

The editorial board has been involved in producing this book since its inception. They have spent rigorous hours researching and exploring the diverse topics which have resulted in the successful publishing of this book. They have passed on their knowledge of decades through this book. To expedite this challenging task, the publisher supported the team at every step. A small team of assistant editors was also appointed to further simplify the editing procedure and attain best results for the readers.

Our editorial team has been hand-picked from every corner of the world. Their multi-ethnicity adds dynamic inputs to the discussions which result in innovative outcomes. These outcomes are then further discussed with the researchers and contributors who give their valuable feedback and opinion regarding the same. The feedback is then collaborated with the researches and they are edited in a comprehensive manner to aid the understanding of the subject.

Apart from the editorial board, the designing team has also invested a significant amount of their time in understanding the subject and creating the most relevant covers. They scrutinized every image to scout for the most suitable representation of the subject and create an appropriate cover for the book.

The publishing team has been involved in this book since its early stages. They were actively engaged in every process, be it collecting the data, connecting with the contributors or procuring relevant information. The team has been an ardent support to the editorial, designing and production team. Their endless efforts to recruit the best for this project, has resulted in the accomplishment of this book. They are a veteran in the field of academics and their pool of knowledge is as vast as their experience in printing. Their expertise and guidance has proved useful at every step. Their uncompromising quality standards have made this book an exceptional effort. Their encouragement from time to time has been an inspiration for everyone.

The publisher and the editorial board hope that this book will prove to be a valuable piece of knowledge for researchers, students, practitioners and scholars across the globe.

List of Contributors

Guido Werner
Robert Koch-Institute, Wernigerode Branch, Germany

Elizabeth A. Ohneck
Emory University Laney Graduate School, USA

Jonathan A. D'Ambrozio, Anjali N. Kunz and Ann E. Jerse
Uniformed Services University of the Health Sciences, USA

William M. Shafer
Emory University School of Medicine, USA

William M. Shafer
Laboratories of Bacterial Pathogenesis, VA Medical Center (Atlanta, GA), USA

Tomasz Jarzembowski, Agnieszka Jóźwik, Katarzyna Wiśniewska and Jacek Witkowski
Medical University of Gdańsk, Poland

Alina Olender
Department of Medical Microbiology, Medical University of Lublin, Poland

Mohamed O. Ahmed
Department of Microbiology and Parasitology, Faculty of Veterinary Medicine, Tripoli university, Tripoli, Libiya

Nicola J. Williams and Peter D. Clegg
Department of Comparative Molecular Medicine, School of Veterinary Science, University of Liverpool, Leahurst, UK

Mohamed O. Ahmed and Malcolm Bennett
Department of Animal and Population Health, School of Veterinary Science, University of Liverpool, Leahurst, UK

Keith E. Baptiste
Department of Large Animal Sciences, Faculty of Life Sciences, University of Copenhagen, Taastrup, Denmark

Thirumananseri Kumarevel
Biometal Science Laboratory, RIKEN Spring-8 Center, Harima Institute, Japan

Yong Chong
Department of Blood and Marrow Transplantation, Hara-Sanshin Hospital, Fukuoka, Japan

María Consuelo Vanegas Lopez
Universidad de los Andes, Colombia

Lingling Wang and Zhongtang Yu
Department of Animal Sciences, The Ohio State University, USA

Zhongtang Yu
Environmental Science Graduate Program, The Ohio State University, USA Public Health Preparedness (PHP) Program, The Ohio State University, USA

Khalid Oufdou and Nour-Eddine Mezrioui
Laboratory of Biology and Biotechnology of Microorganisms, Faculty of Sciences, Semlalia, Cadi Ayyad University, Morocco

Masanori Fukao and Nobuhiro Yajima
Research Institute, KAGOME Co., Ltd., Japan

Kumar Gaurav, Sourish Karmakar, Kanika Kundu and Subir Kundu
Institute of Technology & MMV, Banaras Hindu University, Varanasi, India

Ouissal Chahad Bourouni and Monia El Bour
Institut National des Sciences et Technologies de la Mer (INSTM), Tunis, Tunisia

Pilar Calo-Mata and Jorge Barros-Velàzquez
Department of Analytical Chemistry, Nutrition and Food Science, LHICA, School of Veterinary Sciences, University of Santiago de Compostela, Spain

Régis Sodoyer, Virginie Courtois, Isabelle Peubez and Charlotte Mignon
Sanofi Pasteur, France

Zorica Radulović and Tanja Petrović
University of Belgrade, Faculty of Agriculture, Republic of Serbia

Snežana Bulajić
University of Belgrade, Faculty of Veterinary Medicine, Republic of Serbia

Printed in the USA
CPSIA information can be obtained
at www.ICGtesting.com
JSHW011453221024
72173JS00005B/1060